Clinical Pathways in Stroke Rehabilitation

Thomas Platz
Editor

Clinical Pathways in Stroke Rehabilitation

Evidence-based Clinical Practice
Recommendations

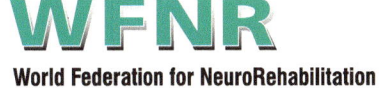

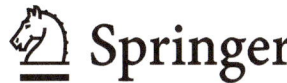

Editor
Thomas Platz
Institute for Neurorehabilitation and Evidence-based Practice
("An-Institute", University of Greifswald), BDH-Klinik Greifswald
Greifswald
Germany

Neurorehabilitation Research Group
University Medical Centre Greifswald (UMG)
Greifswald
Germany

Special Interest Group Clinical Pathways
World Federation Neurorehabilitation (WFNR)
North Shields
UK

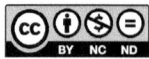

This book is an open access publication.
ISBN 978-3-030-58504-4   ISBN 978-3-030-58505-1   (eBook)
https://doi.org/10.1007/978-3-030-58505-1

This Springer imprint is published by the registered company Springer Nature Switzerland AG
The registered company address is: Gewerbestrasse 11, 6330 Cham, Switzerland

This book is dedicated to all stroke survivors in need of rehabilitation to combat impairments and activity limitations and promote a life after stroke with the least possible stroke-related disability and the greatest possible autonomy and quality of life. In addition, it is there to support all health care professionals involved in stroke rehabilitation by providing guidance for their clinical decision-making in the best interest of those they are taking care of.

Preface

Brain injury caused by stroke is a leading cause of disability with a tendency for an increasing societal burden of stroke-related disability globally. At the same time, our knowledge about effective rehabilitation treatment is rapidly increasing as indicated by the multitude of clinical trials, systematic reviews and meta-analyses being published. For the individual health care professionals involved in stroke rehabilitation, it is hardly possible to keep track with the evolution of clinical evidence and hence there is a risk for an increasing gap between the state of the art in clinical stroke rehabilitation research and clinical practice and decision-making.

Guidelines help to bridge this gap, if systematically evidence-based. Usually written for a specific (national) background they are, however, frequently not readily applicable to other health care situations limiting their usefulness elsewhere.

The authors of this book, mainly coming from the various Special Interest Groups of the World Federation for NeuroRehabilitation (WFNR) with a multidisciplinary and regionally diverse background, had a different goal: the development of international evidence-based stroke practice recommendations that focus on the link between evidence and clinical decision-making related to rehabilitation therapy rather than issues related to or being dependent on organisational issues.

As a consequence, the evidence-based practice recommendations that had been developed with an international perspective can be applied globally for clinical decision-making in stroke rehabilitation. In addition, the knowledge provided can be used in very different health care situations to further structure and adapt regional or local stroke rehabilitation pathways. Last but not least, by providing clinical orientation the practice recommendations can support service development in a way that will eventually achieve effective stroke rehabilitation in areas with limited services so far.

The international practice recommendations for stroke rehabilitation developed by the WFNR are published open access with this book supporting their accessibility and dissemination. May they help to promote effective stroke rehabilitation for those in need.

Greifwald, Germany   Thomas Platz
December 2020

Acknowledgements

All authors dedicated their time and effort to collectively provide evidence-based guidance for clinical decision-making in stroke rehabilitation. In addition, they provided peer review for the other chapters of this book as did the feedback panel members (for reference see Table 1 in Chap. 2). All these contributions are gratefully acknowledged.

The World Federation for NeuroRehabilitation (WFNR) sponsored this book project and made it possible to be published as an open access book. This will largely facilitate its distribution and availability quite independent of financial resources of potential users.

Contents

Neurobiology of Stroke Recovery

Eddie Kane and Nick S. Ward

A stroke occurs somewhere in the world every 2 s adding up to almost 17 million people each year (Feigin et al. 2014). Stroke is one of the most common causes of disability. Over one million people in the UK are currently living with the consequences of stroke, over one-third of whom are dependent on others for their care. Even though stroke mortality is declining (Lackland et al. 2014), the number of people set to live with the consequences of stroke is set to rise over the next 20 years (Patel et al. 2017; Crichton et al. 2016) with huge personal, societal and economic consequences (Patel et al. 2017). Improvement of recovery and long-term outcomes is therefore an urgent clinical and scientific goal, but success is slow to materialize. Understanding the underlying neurobiology of stroke recovery could speed up ways to help improve outcomes.

Care in the hyperacute and acute period after stroke has improved dramatically over the past two decades, but it is widely accepted that our attention must turn to treatments that actively promote recovery. The key treatments for promoting behavioural recovery in motor, language and cognitive domains after stroke are themselves behavioural treatments (loosely grouped under the headings physiotherapy, occupational therapy, speech and language therapy, neuropsychology) that we can consider inputs (into the brain). The consequent change in behaviour can be

E. Kane
Department of Clinical and Motor Neuroscience,
UCL Queen Square Institute of Neurology, London, UK
e-mail: edward.kane.18@ucl.ac.uk

N. S. Ward (✉)
Department of Clinical and Motor Neuroscience,
UCL Queen Square Institute of Neurology, London, UK

The National Hospital for Neurology and Neurosurgery, Queen Square, London, UK

UCL Partners Centre for Neurorehabilitation,
UCL Institute of Neurology, Queen Square, London, UK
e-mail: n.ward@ucl.ac.uk

© The Author(s) 2021
T. Platz (ed.), *Clinical Pathways in Stroke Rehabilitation*,
https://doi.org/10.1007/978-3-030-58505-1_1

1

considered an output (from the brain). It is becoming more accepted that the amount of input (and probably the quality) affects the output (Lohse et al. 2014). For example, significantly higher doses of good quality upper-limb rehabilitation have large beneficial effects, even in chronic stroke (McCabe et al. 2015; Daly et al. 2019; Ward et al. 2019). The input–output relationship can be modulated by brain states, and we think of these states as enhancing the potential for experience dependent plasticity, and it is these brain states that will be the focus of this review.

The early post-stroke phase has been described as a period of 'spontaneous biological recovery' (Krakauer et al. 2012). Spontaneous biological recovery is a behavioural response to underlying biological events occurring in the first few weeks and months after stroke attributable to enhanced post-stroke plasticity mechanisms. Recovery is rapid, occurs at the level of impairment and generalizes beyond the tasks that are used in post-stroke training, which is different to improvements seen in the chronic phase of stroke (Zeiler and Krakauer 2013). This leads to the hypothesis that behavioural interventions will have a quantitative and qualitatively greater effect if delivered in this period compared to outside of this period. This raises two major challenges for the field of stroke rehabilitation. The first is to determine what is the correct form of behavioural training (the input) to take advantage of this critical period. This is not trivial, as has been discussed elsewhere (Krakauer and Carmichael 2017). The second challenge is how (and importantly, when) to augment the biological mechanisms of post-stroke plasticity to enhance or prolong the effects of behavioural training in patients after a stroke. It is important to note that although work in preclinical animal models has been pivotal in highlighting the biological basis of recovery, few benefits have been seen for human stroke patients. This is likely to require the development of human biomarkers to move this field of research into the human arena (Ward 2017). Here, we define biomarkers using the Stroke Recovery and Rehabilitation Roundtable criteria—Indicators of disease state that can be used clinically as a measure reflecting underlying molecular or cellular processes that might be difficult to measure directly in humans, and can be used to predict recovery or treatment response (Bernhardt et al. 2016).

One of the first studies providing behavioural evidence of this post-stroke critical period for recovery-related training was provided by Biernaskie and colleagues (Biernaskie et al. 2004) who found that rats commencing training of the affected forelimb starting at 30 days post-stroke exhibited the same level of improvement as those who received no training. However, those whose treatment commenced at 5–14 days post-stroke had better recoveries. This suggests that there is a time limited effect of the lesion itself on the brain's potential for plasticity. This was supported by Zeiler and colleagues (Zeiler et al. 2015) who showed that intensive motor training of a mouse commenced 7 days after stroke was not able to promote full recovery. However, when the same animal was given a second stroke and training was commenced 2 days later then recovery was substantially enhanced. These results suggest that focal brain damage results in a series of biological events that, when combined with appropriate behavioural training (Krakauer et al. 2012), can support recovery.

1   Changes in Structural Plasticity After Stroke

A substantial amount of work has been undertaken in animal models to define the molecular and cellular processes that occur after stroke. These studies are well described elsewhere (Krakauer and Carmichael 2017; Murphy and Corbett 2009; Carmichael 2016; Cramer and Chopp 2000; Wieloch and Nikolich 2006) and by the nature of the experimental model concern largely sensorimotor recovery rather than other domains that are important in human stroke. Nevertheless, these studies are instructive if we are interested in the capacity of the central nervous system to support recovery. Briefly, focal ischaemic brain damage leads to cell death followed by secondary damage, then to the elements important for recovery, namely regeneration and (partial) repair (Krakauer and Carmichael 2017; Wieloch and Nikolich 2006). The basic elements of neural repair that can be seen in animal models of stroke change over time and include axonal sprouting, dendritic branching, synaptogenesis, neurogenesis and gliogenesis and all can be enhanced in the early post-stroke period. These post-stroke changes also have spatial characteristics, seeming to occur in brain regions connected to the damaged area, including peri-infarct, ipsilesional and contralesional brain and spinal cord networks. Not all these biological responses to injury are necessarily beneficial. For example, only axonal sprouting that links functionally related brain areas is consistently associated with improved post-stroke outcomes (Carmichael et al. 2016). The precise temporal and spatial ordering of the biological events that occur after stroke are likely to be governed by alterations in gene expression and it is often suggested that the biological environment of the post-stroke brain resemble that of the developing brain, and that 'recovery recapitulates ontogeny' (Cramer and Chopp 2000). Recent work however points to this being an over simplification and that in reality there is a unique regenerative molecular program at work with a clear distinction between regenerative and developmental transcriptomes (Li et al. 2010). Furthermore, expression of the regenerative transcriptome is strongly influenced by age at stroke onset, with younger animals expressing growth-promoting molecules earlier and growth-inhibiting molecules later than older animals (Li and Carmichael 2006). Definitive evidence of these restorative processes in humans is scarce, but markers suggestive of neurogenesis (Jin et al. 2006), gliogenesis (Sanin et al. 2013) and axonal sprouting (Jin et al. 2006) have been found in human post-stroke perilesional brain tissue. Consequently, the occurrence of similar biological responses to brain injury in both animals and humans seems probable.

There are a number of approaches to developing pharmacological therapies that aim to promote structural plasticity after stroke in order to enhance outcomes. Firstly, there is successful preclinical work to block extracellular inhibitory signals that counteract regeneration using axonal growth inhibitors (Wahl and Schwab 2014; Benowitz and Carmichael 2010). For example, myelin-associated proteins such as NogoA, myelin-associated glycoprotein (MAG) and myelin-associated oligodendrocyte basic protein have been shown to block neuronal regeneration. Anti-NogoA strategies have been used in preclinical models both of stroke and of spinal cord injury and can lead to improved recovery profiles, probably through both vascular and neural repair mechanisms (Rust et al. 2019). In terms of structural changes to the central nervous system in response to anti-NogoA, axonal sprouting is often seen across the midline, either at the level of brain stem or spinal cord. Lindau and colleagues (Lindau et al. 2014) found that in rats undergoing sensorimotor cortex ablation but then treated with anti-NogoA antibody, intact corticospinal tract had extensively sprouted across the midline into the denervated spinal hemicord, which led to a somatotopic anatomical and functional side switch in the projection of adult corticospinal neurons. The safety of anti-NogoA antibodies has been tested in patients with spinal cord injury (Wahl and Schwab 2014) and amyotrophic lateral sclerosis (Meininger et al. 2014), and anti-MAG has been tested in patients with stroke (Cramer et al. 2013). Many of the antibody molecules are large and it is not clear how well they cross the blood–brain barrier after stroke (when it is damaged). Alternative ways of achieving the same response, through genetic manipulation for example (Rust et al. 2019), are being explored.

Other candidate molecules that inhibit the axonal growth cone, e.g. semaphorins and ephrins, and so block neuronal regeneration are also being investigated. After stroke damage, ephrin-A5 is induced in astrocytes in peri-infarct cortex, which leads to inhibition of axonal sprouting. When ephrin-A5 signalling is blocked, motor training is more liable to promote recovery (Overman et al. 2012).

Axon growth can also be blocked by perineuronal nets (PNNs), a property mediated by chondroitin sulphate proteoglycans. After ischaemic cortical damage, the density of PNNs is reduced in peri-infarct cortex, likely representing one of the mechanisms of spontaneous biological recovery (Allred et al. 2005). This biological environment can be recreated by the enzyme chondroitinase ABC, which can reverse blocking of axonal growth, thereby reinstating critical period plasticity via the inactivation of chondroitin sulphate proteoglycans and therefore PNNs (Pizzorusso et al. 2002). In a rat model of stroke, chondroitinase ABC helped restore motor function after both acute and delayed administration (Gherardini et al. 2015).

Rather than blocking axonal growth inhibitors, the naturally occurring purine nucleoside inosine has been reported to enhance axon growth and improve outcomes in a preclinical model of stroke. Inosine promotes axonal collateral sprouting into areas that have lost their normal innervation, such as the corticospinal tract after stroke (Zai et al. 2009) or hippocampus after experimental traumatic brain injury (Dachir et al. 2014). Furthermore, inosine can augment the effects of anti-NogoA antibody to restore skilled forelimb use after stroke (Zai et al. 2011).

In other classes of drugs, phosphodiesterase (PDE) inhibitors can prevent the degradation of cyclic nucleotides (cAMP and cGMP) which amongst other things promote axonal sprouting. There has been interest in whether drugs such as sildenafil (PDE5 inhibitor) or cilostazol (PDE3 inhibitor) can improve outcomes after stroke (Munshi and Das 2017), but their translation into use in human stroke remains a long way off.

Increasingly, interest has been shown in the use of stem cell therapy to promote recovery after stroke (Kalladka and Muir 2016). The two main lines of stem cell therapies are endogenous (promoting the production of existing neural stem cells) or exogenous (transplanted from another source) (Azad et al. 2016). Over the past few years, research has explored how to reprogram adult human somatic cells to induced pluripotent stem cells thereby producing patient-specific cells for autologous transplantation (Tornero et al. 2013). Rather than restoring lost tissue, stem cells could act as stimulants for trophic factors and modulators of immunological and inflammatory changes after stroke. Trials of exogenous cells in humans have proved safe, and claims have been made for improved clinical outcomes in patients with chronic stroke (Steinberg et al. 2016; Kalladka et al. 2016).

The timing of administration of growth-promoting compounds, both in relation to the initial stroke damage and to the behavioural training itself, will clearly have a major effect on the therapeutic capacity. Whether training is delivered at the same time as growth-promoting molecules or sequentially could influence the type of sprouting that occurs and, consequently, whether behaviour is helped or hindered (Wahl et al. 2014). In addition, the effect that post-stroke behaviour can have on regenerative processes themselves is important to understand. For example, early compensatory use of the contralesional forelimb impairs recovery of the affected limb (Allred et al. 2005), possibly through aberrant synaptogenesis in the perilesional cortex (Kim et al. 2015). Any behaviour, if overtrained, will take advantage of the increased post-stroke potential for experience-dependent plasticity, and so abnormal or compensatory patterns of behaviour can become learned. Once again, this finding highlights the need for an appropriate form of behavioural training that can take advantage of any spontaneous or therapeutically enhanced potential for plasticity.

As well as asking 'when' treatment should be administered and 'where' is probably an equally important question. Most of the compounds discussed have been administered via intravenous or intrathecal routes, but accurate spatial and temporal delivery might both be necessary to achieve the desired outcomes. Advances made in the last few years in tissue engineering (Nih et al. 2016; Memanishvili et al. 2016) and optogenetics (Pendharkar et al. 2016) provide potential methods for precisely delivering regenerative molecules to functionally relevant brain regions. In this case, it might then be preferable to take advantage of the possibility of delivering brain region–specific stem cell therapies (cells that have cortical or basal ganglia-like phenotypes). Given the importance of white matter damage in human stroke (white matter constitutes over 50% of brain volume in humans in comparison to less than 10% in rodents), it is even possible that replacing lost glia is a more successful strategy in some cases, than replacing lost neurons (Tornero et al. 2013; Kokaia et al. 2017).

2   Changes in Functional Plasticity After Stroke

So far, we have concentrated on post-stroke changes in brain structure and how these processes may be therapeutically altered. In addition to these structural changes, focal brain damage also results in alterations in neuronal excitability (Carmichael 2012). Immediately after stroke, signalling by the excitatory neurotransmitter glutamate is excitotoxic and contributes to cell death, whereas signalling by the inhibitory neurotransmitter GABA can counteract this toxicity through cell hyperpolarization (Lai et al. 2014). In the mouse model, the beneficial and detrimental effects of GABA and glutamate signalling seem to reverse after about 3 days post-stroke (Clarkson et al. 2010). This is of potentially great interest, since changes to the cortical excitatory–inhibitory balance have long been known to influence the potential for experience-dependent plasticity and can reopen critical periods of plasticity in the adult brain (Bavelier et al. 2010). The link between changes in so called 'functional plasticity' is that reduced inhibitory tone can lead to facilitation of downstream changes in neuronal structure (Chen et al. 2011). One possibility then is that the altered levels of neuronal activity that result from a change in excitability regulate neurogenesis and the activity of growth factors (such as brain derived neurotrophic factor; BDNF) through epigenetic mechanisms (Felling and Song 2015). Reduced cortical inhibitory mechanisms can also lead to expanded and less specific receptive fields (Alia et al. 2016; Winship and Murphy 2008), enhanced long-term potentiation (Hagemann et al. 1998) and remapping of sensorimotor functions to surviving cortex (Takatsuru et al. 2009) in both hemispheres (Que et al. 1999), all of which is potentially useful when functional reorganization of residual post-stroke brain structures is important for recovery of normal function. Stroke-induced changes in the inhibitory–excitatory balance in surviving brain regions (particularly cortex) could, therefore, be a key event that sets other restorative mechanisms in motion.

One idea is that attenuation of neuronal activity in brain regions connected to the damaged area after stroke might be reversed by a homeostatic increase in neuronal excitability, a process that can last at least several weeks (Murphy and Corbett 2009). Levels of neuronal excitability are determined by the balance in activity between GABA and glutamate, both of which are known to be altered after stroke (Carmichael 2012). For example, enhanced glutamate signalling through AMPA receptors, the major excitatory signalling system in the adult brain, is associated with improved recovery in stroke models due to downstream induction of BDNF (Clarkson et al. 2011). $GABA_A$ receptors, on the other hand, are downregulated (Que et al. 1999; Schiene et al. 1996), and the density of a number of inhibitory interneurons is reduced after focal brain damage (Alia et al. 2016; Zeiler et al. 2013), suggesting a reduction in in phasic (synaptic) inhibition in the first few weeks after injury (Neumann-Haefelin et al. 1995) to increase the likelihood of long-term potentiation (Hagemann et al. 1998). Both increased glutamatergic signalling and reduced phasic GABAergic signalling would be consistent with the idea of a homeostatic restitution of neuronal activity (Murphy and Corbett 2009). However, other work has focussed on tonic GABAergic inhibition, suggesting that there is a dominant increase in perilesional tonic inhibition, mediated by extrasynaptic $GABA_A$ receptors (Clarkson et al. 2010; Lake et al. 2015). Reversing this tonic inhibition (using an α5 subunit that contained an extrasynaptic $GABA_A$-receptor inverse agonist) improved motor outcomes in both mouse (Tornero et al. 2013) and rat (Lai et al. 2014) models of stroke. The increase in tonic inhibitory signalling can persist for more than 1 month (Carmichael 2012) making this therapeutic window attractive.

The interactions between excitatory pyramidal cells and numerous inhibitory interneurons in the cortex are clearly complex and become more complex after stroke (Clarkson 2012). In addition, prolonged ischaemia affects different cell types unequally (Sakuma et al. 2008) and causes alterations in the distribution of receptor subtypes (Kharlamov et al. 2008). Nevertheless, the weight of evidence from animal studies to date suggests that spontaneous biological recovery is either augmented by a homeostatic restitution of cortical activity secondary to reduced phasic GABAergic inhibitory signalling or blocked by excessive tonic GABAergic inhibitory signalling. Beyond the hyperacute period (up to 3 days post-stroke), what follows at a cellular level suggests that alterations in cortical inhibitory and excitatory mechanisms are important in determining the potential for plasticity and downstream structural changes that support recovery. Consequently, components of these inhibitory and excitatory mechanisms represent exciting and novel therapeutic targets for enhancing behavioural training after stroke.

The mechanisms responsible for the alterations in cortical excitatory–inhibitory balance that underlie changes in post-stroke functional plasticity are amenable to pharmacological and non-pharmacological manipulation. There is much interest in the use of selective serotonin reuptake inhibitors (SSRIs) for promoting recovery after stroke. SSRIs can influence structural plasticity, but there is compelling evidence to support a plasticity-modifying effect mediated through the GABAergic system. Chronic doses of fluoxetine can reinstate critical period plasticity in adult rats through a reduction of extracellular levels of GABA and an increase in BDNF expression (Maya Vetencourt et al. 2008). Furthermore, in a mouse model of stroke, Ng and colleagues (Ng et al. 2015) showed that fluoxetine treatment prolonged (but did not reinstate) the critical period of post-stroke plasticity through the reduction of inhibitory interneuron expression in intact cortex (Ng et al. 2015). Serotonin can have inhibitory (via $5HT_{1A}$ receptors) or facilitatory (via $5HT_{2A}$ receptors) effects on pyramidal cells, but most fast-spiking inhibitory interneurons are inhibited by serotonin through $5HT_{1A}$ receptors (Puig et al. 2010). In the cortex, chronic fluoxetine administration induces a reduction in layer II–III inhibitory interneuron activity which facilitates experience-driven structural dendritic remodelling (Chen et al. 2011). A separate study in human primary motor cortex slices demonstrated that fluoxetine-induced reduction of inhibitory tone comes about through suppression of layer II–III monosynaptic excitatory connections from pyramidal cells to inhibitory interneurons, which leaves the monosynaptic output of GABAergic cells unaffected (Komlósi et al. 2012). This layer-specific effect of fluoxetine is interesting in the context of work that demonstrates that early post-stroke 'enriched rehabilitation' is more effective than environmental enrichment or reach training alone as a result of the enhancement of use-dependent plasticity in peri-infarct layer II–III cortex (Clarke et al. 2014). One idea is that fluoxetine (and other pharmacotherapies) might influence training effects by replicating the biological effects of enriched environments.

Fluoxetine has been well studied in human stroke patients. The fluoxetine for motor recovery after acute ischemic stroke (FLAME) study in which 20 mg fluoxetine daily, started 5–10 days after ischaemic stroke and continued for 3 months, enhanced upper-limb motor recovery (Chollet et al. 2011). However, the larger FOCUS study did not show that fluoxetine had an effect on the modified Rankin Scale (FOCUS Trial Collaboration 2019). However, we know that changing the potential for plasticity still requires the appropriate behavioural intervention to take advantage of this new brain state. In FOCUS, no attempt was made to control for or measure the amount of rehabilitation patients received, which makes the results difficult to interpret.

Another approach might be to target the proposed increase in perilesional tonic inhibition. Tonic inhibition can be reversed by antagonists or inverse agonists of the α5-subunit-containing extrasynaptic $GABA_A$ receptor, and compounds for use in humans are currently available and under investigation. Zolpidem is an interesting pharmacological agent that binds with high affinity to α1-containing $GABA_A$ receptors through which it mediates sedative and hypnotic effects. However, zolpidem can also influence tonic inhibition through α5-containing $GABA_A$ receptors in a dose-dependent manner, such that low levels of the drug augment tonic inhibition and high levels reduce it (Prokic et al. 2015). Zolpidem can improve recovery in a mouse model of stroke (Hiu et al. 2015) and has been reported to mediate interesting effects such as the temporary reversal of deficits in language, cognitive and motor function in single patient cases with stroke (Cohen et al. 2004; Hall et al. 2010). However, given the uncertainty over how zolpidem works, the mechanism of recovery in these individuals remains unclear.

The most studied therapeutic option for promoting recovery after stroke is likely to be non-invasive brain stimulation (NIBS). Several systematic reviews suggest that NIBS is able to enhance the effects of behavioural training to a small degree (Hsu et al. 2012; Kang et al. 2015). In a mouse model, direct current stimulation to the brain appeared to augment synaptic plasticity through BDNF dependent mechanisms (Fritsch et al. 2010). However, in human studies, it is not clear how much or how accurately electrical current is delivered to target brain regions, and consequently results are inconsistent and potential mechanisms poorly understood (Bonaiuto and Bestmann 2015; de Berker et al. 2013).

3 Conclusion Regarding the Neurobiology of Stroke Recovery

The rationale for understanding how to optimize the post-stroke brain environment is to maximize the effect of behavioural training—which can take the form of physical, cognitive or speech therapy. The presence of a critical period of plasticity mandates for the delivery of high dose and high intensity behavioural training during this window of opportunity to maximize recovery of function by minimizing impairment (Zeiler and Krakauer 2013). Whilst this idea is strongly supported in animal models as already discussed (Biernaskie et al. 2004; Zeiler et al. 2015), there is as yet no direct evidence of this in human stroke patients. Targeting the mechanisms that underlie early spontaneous biological recovery in humans represents the most-promising path to dramatically improve patients' outcomes (Zeiler and Krakauer

2013) and should be prioritized. The limits of what is possible in stroke recovery have not yet been explored, especially if the delivery of high doses of behavioural therapy in post-acute or reopened critical periods of plasticity becomes possible.

4   Take Home Message for Clinical Practice in Stroke Rehabilitation

This chapter on the neurobiology of stroke recovery portrays the state of the art in research on the structural and functional mechanisms of recovery after stroke. It provides scientific reasoning on how clinical interventions in stroke rehabilitation might work and where potentials for future research in stroke recovery and rehabilitation are seen from a neuroscience perspective. It does, however, not provide clinical evidence for stroke rehabilitation, and hence it is not possible to link clinical practice recommendations directly to this type of reasoning. This information will be given in the remainder of the chapters in this book.

As far as the neuroscience perspective goes, some general take-home messages are nevertheless worthwhile to portray on the basis of the overview given.

Alterations of body functions after acquired brain damage such as motor, perceptual, language or cognitive dysfunctions are results of network activities that are affected by structural brain damage. Complex changes in neural excitability and structural changes that occur over an extended period after brain damage will eventually determine the extent of functional recovery achieved by an individual. These processes can be influenced by rehabilitation treatment most likely if it is based on targeted training of high enough intensity and specificity for the affected brain networks and hence dysfunctions. In addition, the processes related to functional recovery can theoretically be modulated by non-invasive brain stimulation, medication and stem cell therapy as outlined above. It is important to keep in mind that these are not completely independent mechanisms. Rather to consider their (partial) contribution and integration into the complex processes of recovery are conceptually appropriate. Whilst the potential for rehabilitation-mediated recovery seems to be biggest early after stroke and needs to be supported by rehabilitation therapy, strategies to promote recovery in later stages after stroke also need to be entertained as focus on its own.

Declaration The authors declare no competing interests.

References

Alia C et al (2016) Reducing GABAA-mediated inhibition improves forelimb motor function after focal cortical stroke in mice. Sci Rep 6:37823

Allred RP, Maldonado MA, Hsu And JE, Jones TA (2005) Training the 'less-affected' forelimb after unilateral cortical infarcts interferes with functional recovery of the impaired forelimb in rats. Restor Neurol Neurosci 23:297–302

Azad TD, Veeravagu A, Steinberg GK (2016) Neurorestoration after stroke. Neurosurg Focus 40:E2

Bavelier D, Levi DM, Li RW, Dan Y, Hensch TK (2010) Removing brakes on adult brain plasticity: from molecular to behavioral interventions. J Neurosci 30:14964–14971

Benowitz LI, Carmichael ST (2010) Promoting axonal rewiring to improve outcome after stroke. Neurobiol Dis 37:259

Bernhardt J et al (2016) Moving rehabilitation research forward: developing consensus statements for rehabilitation and recovery research. Int J Stroke 11:454–458

Biernaskie J, Chernenko G, Corbett D (2004) Efficacy of rehabilitative experience declines with time after focal ischemic brain injury. J Neurosci 24:1245–1254

Bonaiuto JJ, Bestmann S (2015) Understanding the nonlinear physiological and behavioral effects of tDCS through computational neurostimulation. Prog Brain Res 222: 75–103

Carmichael ST (2012) Brain excitability in stroke: the yin and yang of stroke progression. Arch Neurol 69:161–167

Carmichael ST (2016) Emergent properties of neural repair: elemental biology to therapeutic concepts. Ann Neurol 79:895–906

Carmichael ST, Kathirvelu B, Schweppe CA, Nie EH (2016) Molecular, cellular and functional events in axonal sprouting after stroke. Exp Neurol 287:384. https://doi.org/10.1016/j.expneurol.2016.02.007

Chen JL et al (2011) Structural basis for the role of inhibition in facilitating adult brain plasticity. Nat Neurosci 14:587–594

Chollet F et al (2011) Fluoxetine for motor recovery after acute ischaemic stroke (FLAME): a randomised placebo-controlled trial. Lancet Neurol 10:123–130

Clarke J, Langdon KD, Corbett D (2014) Early poststroke experience differentially alters periinfarct layer II and III cortex. J Cereb Blood Flow Metab 34:630–637

Clarkson AN (2012) Perisynaptic GABA receptors the overzealous protector. Adv Pharm Sci 2012(708428):1

Clarkson AN, Huang BS, Macisaac SE, Mody I, Carmichael ST (2010) Reducing excessive GABA-mediated tonic inhibition promotes functional recovery after stroke. Nature 468: 305–309

Clarkson AN et al (2011) AMPA receptor-induced local brain-derived neurotrophic factor signaling mediates motor recovery after stroke. J Neurosci 31:3766–3775

Cohen L, Chaaban B, Habert M-O (2004) Transient improvement of aphasia with zolpidem. N Engl J Med 350:949–950

Cramer SC, Chopp M (2000) Recovery recapitulates ontogeny. Trends Neurosci 23:265–271

Cramer SC et al (2013) Safety, pharmacokinetics, and pharmacodynamics of escalating repeat doses of GSK249320 in patients with stroke. Stroke J Cereb Circ 44:1337–1342

Crichton SL, Bray BD, McKevitt C, Rudd AG, Wolfe CDA (2016) Patient outcomes up to 15 years after stroke: survival, disability, quality of life, cognition and mental health. J Neurol Neurosurg Psychiatry 87:1091–1098

Dachir S et al (2014) Inosine improves functional recovery after experimental traumatic brain injury. Brain Res 1555:78–88

Daly JJ et al (2019) Long-dose intensive therapy is necessary for strong, clinically significant, upper limb functional gains and retained gains in severe/moderate chronic stroke. Neurorehabil Neural Repair 33(7):523–537. https://doi.org/10.1177/1545968319846120

de Berker AO, Bikson M, Bestmann S (2013) Predicting the behavioral impact of transcranial direct current stimulation: issues and limitations. Front Hum Neurosci 7:613

Feigin VL et al (2014) Global and regional burden of stroke during 1990–2010: findings from the global burden of disease study 2010. Lancet 383:245–254

Felling RJ, Song H (2015) Epigenetic mechanisms of neuroplasticity and the implications for stroke recovery. Exp Neurol 268:37–45

FOCUS Trial Collaboration (2019) Effects of fluoxetine on functional outcomes after acute stroke (FOCUS): a pragmatic, double-blind, randomised, controlled trial. Lancet 393:265–274

Fritsch B et al (2010) Direct current stimulation promotes BDNF-dependent synaptic plasticity: potential implications for motor learning. Neuron 66:198–204

Gherardini L, Gennaro M, Pizzorusso T (2015) Perilesional treatment with chondroitinase ABC and motor training promote functional recovery after stroke in rats. Cereb Cortex 1991(25):202–212

Hagemann G, Redecker C, Neumann-Haefelin T, Freund HJ, Witte OW (1998) Increased long-term potentiation in the surround of experimentally induced focal cortical infarction. Ann Neurol 44:255–258

Hall SD et al (2010) GABA(a) alpha-1 subunit mediated desynchronization of elevated low frequency oscillations alleviates specific dysfunction in stroke—a case report. Clin Neurophysiol 121:549–555

Hiu T et al (2015) Enhanced phasic GABA inhibition during the repair phase of stroke: a novel therapeutic target. Brain 139(Pt 2):468–480. https://doi.org/10.1093/brain/awv360

Hsu W-Y, Cheng C-H, Liao K-K, Lee I-H, Lin Y-Y (2012) Effects of repetitive transcranial magnetic stimulation on motor functions in patients with stroke: a meta-analysis. Stroke J Cereb Circ 43:1849–1857

Jin K et al (2006) Evidence for stroke-induced neurogenesis in the human brain. Proc Natl Acad Sci U S A 103:13198–13202

Kalladka D, Muir KW (2016) Where are we in clinical applications of stem cells in ischaemic stroke? Adv Clin Neurosci Rehabil 16:9–12

Kalladka D et al (2016) Human neural stem cells in patients with chronic ischaemic stroke (PISCES): a phase 1, first-in-man study. Lancet 388:787–796

Kang N, Summers JJ, Cauraugh JH (2015) Transcranial direct current stimulation facilitates motor learning post-stroke: a systematic review and meta-analysis. J Neurol Neurosurg Psychiatry 87:345. https://doi.org/10.1136/jnnp-2015-311242

Kharlamov EA, Downey KL, Jukkola PI, Grayson DR, Kelly KM (2008) Expression of GABA a receptor alpha1 subunit mRNA and protein in rat neocortex following photothrombotic infarction. Brain Res 1210:29–38

Kim SY et al (2015) Experience with the 'good' limb induces aberrant synaptic plasticity in the perilesion cortex after stroke. J Neurosci 35:8604–8610

Kokaia Z, Tornero D, Lindvall O (2017) Transplantation of reprogrammed neurons for improved recovery after stroke. Prog Brain Res 231:245–263

Komlósi G et al (2012) Fluoxetine (prozac) and serotonin act on excitatory synaptic transmission to suppress single layer 2/3 pyramidal neuron-triggered cell assemblies in the human prefrontal cortex. J Neurosci 32:16369–16378

Krakauer JW, Carmichael ST (2017) Broken movement: the neurobiology of motor recovery after stroke. MIT, Cambridge, MA

Krakauer JW, Carmichael ST, Corbett D, Wittenberg GF (2012) Getting neurorehabilitation right: what can be learned from animal models? Neurorehabil Neural Repair 26:923–931

Lackland DT et al (2014) Factors influencing the decline in stroke mortality: a statement from the American Heart Association/American Stroke Association. Stroke J Cereb Circ 45:315–353

Lai TW, Zhang S, Wang YT (2014) Excitotoxicity and stroke: identifying novel targets for neuroprotection. Prog Neurobiol 115:157–188

Lake EMR et al (2015) The effects of delayed reduction of tonic inhibition on ischemic lesion and sensorimotor function. J Cereb Blood Flow Metab 35:1601. https://doi.org/10.1038/jcbfm.2015.86

Li S, Carmichael ST (2006) Growth-associated gene and protein expression in the region of axonal sprouting in the aged brain after stroke. Neurobiol Dis 23:362–373

Li S et al (2010) An age-related sprouting transcriptome provides molecular control of axonal sprouting after stroke. Nat Neurosci 13:1496–1504

Lindau NT et al (2014) Rewiring of the corticospinal tract in the adult rat after unilateral stroke and anti-Nogo-a therapy. Brain J Neurol 137:739–756

Lohse KR, Lang CE, Boyd LA (2014) Is more better? Using metadata to explore dose-response relationships in stroke rehabilitation. Stroke J Cereb Circ 45:2053–2058

Maya Vetencourt JF et al (2008) The antidepressant fluoxetine restores plasticity in the adult visual cortex. Science 320:385–388

McCabe J, Monkiewicz M, Holcomb J, Pundik S, Daly JJ (2015) Comparison of robotics, functional electrical stimulation, and motor learning methods for treatment of persistent upper extremity dysfunction after stroke: a randomized controlled trial. Arch Phys Med Rehabil 96:981–990

Meininger V et al (2014) Safety, pharmacokinetic, and functional effects of the nogo-a monoclonal antibody in amyotrophic lateral sclerosis: a randomized, first-in-human clinical trial. PLoS One 9:e97803

Memanishvili T et al (2016) Generation of cortical neurons from human induced-pluripotent stem cells by biodegradable polymeric microspheres loaded with priming factors. Biomed Mater Bristol Engl 11:025011

Munshi A, Das S (2017) Genetic understanding of stroke treatment: potential role for phosphodiesterase inhibitors. Adv Neurobiol 17:445–461

Murphy TH, Corbett D (2009) Plasticity during stroke recovery: from synapse to behaviour. Nat Rev Neurosci 10:861–872

Neumann-Haefelin T, Hagemann G, Witte OW (1995) Cellular correlates of neuronal hyperexcitability in the vicinity of photochemically induced cortical infarcts in rats in vitro. Neurosci Lett 193:101–104

Ng KL et al (2015) Fluoxetine maintains a state of heightened responsiveness to motor training early after stroke in a mouse model. Stroke J Cereb Circ 46:2951–2960

Nih LR, Carmichael ST, Segura T (2016) Hydrogels for brain repair after stroke: an emerging treatment option. Curr Opin Biotechnol 40:155–163

Overman JJ et al (2012) A role for ephrin-A5 in axonal sprouting, recovery, and activity-dependent plasticity after stroke. Proc Natl Acad Sci U S A 109:E2230–E2239

Patel A et al (2017) Executive summary part 2: burden of stroke in the next 20 years and potential returns from increased spending on research. https://www.stroke.org.uk/sites/default/files/costs_of_stroke_in_the_uk_report_-executive_summary_part_2.pdf (The Stroke Association). Accessed 7th September 2020

Pendharkar AV et al (2016) Optogenetic modulation in stroke recovery. Neurosurg Focus 40:E6

Pizzorusso T et al (2002) Reactivation of ocular dominance plasticity in the adult visual cortex. Science 298:1248–1251

Prokic EJ et al (2015) Cortical oscillatory dynamics and benzodiazepine-site modulation of tonic inhibition in fast spiking interneurons. Neuropharmacology 95:192–205

Puig MV, Watakabe A, Ushimaru M, Yamamori T, Kawaguchi Y (2010) Serotonin modulates fast-spiking interneuron and synchronous activity in the rat prefrontal cortex through 5-HT1A and 5-HT2A receptors. J Neurosci 30:2211–2222

Que M et al (1999) Changes in GABA(a) and GABA(B) receptor binding following cortical photothrombosis: a quantitative receptor autoradiographic study. Neuroscience 93:1233–1240

Rust R et al (2019) Nogo-a targeted therapy promotes vascular repair and functional recovery following stroke. Proc Natl Acad Sci U S A 116:14270–14279

Sakuma M, Hyakawa N, Kato H, Araki T (2008) Time dependent changes of striatal interneurons after focal cerebral ischemia in rats. J Neural Transm 1996(115):413–422

Sanin V, Heeß C, Kretzschmar HA, Schüller U (2013) Recruitment of neural precursor cells from circumventricular organs of patients with cerebral ischaemia. Neuropathol Appl Neurobiol 39:510–518

Schiene K et al (1996) Neuronal hyperexcitability and reduction of GABAA-receptor expression in the surround of cerebral photothrombosis. J Cereb Blood Flow Metab 16:906–914

Steinberg GK et al (2016) Clinical outcomes of transplanted modified bone marrow-derived Mesenchymal stem cells in stroke: a phase 1/2a study. Stroke J Cereb Circ 47:1817–1824

Takatsuru Y et al (2009) Neuronal circuit remodeling in the contralateral cortical hemisphere during functional recovery from cerebral infarction. J Neurosci 29:10081–10086

Tornero D et al (2013) Human induced pluripotent stem cell-derived cortical neurons integrate in stroke-injured cortex and improve functional recovery. Brain J Neurol 136:3561–3577

Wahl A-S, Schwab ME (2014) Finding an optimal rehabilitation paradigm after stroke: enhancing fiber growth and training of the brain at the right moment. Front Hum Neurosci 8:381

Wahl AS et al (2014) Neuronal repair. Asynchronous therapy restores motor control by rewiring of the rat corticospinal tract after stroke. Science 344:1250–1255

Ward NS (2017) Restoring brain function after stroke—bridging the gap between animals and humans. Nat Rev Neurol 13:244–255

Ward NS, Brander F, Kelly K (2019) Intensive upper limb neurorehabilitation in chronic stroke: outcomes from the Queen Square programme. J Neurol Neurosurg Psychiatry 90(5):498–506. https://doi.org/10.1136/jnnp-2018-319954

Wieloch T, Nikolich K (2006) Mechanisms of neural plasticity following brain injury. Curr Opin Neurobiol 16:258–264

Winship IR, Murphy TH (2008) In vivo calcium imaging reveals functional rewiring of single somatosensory neurons after stroke. J Neurosci 28:6592–6606

Zai L et al (2009) Inosine alters gene expression and axonal projections in neurons contralateral to a cortical infarct and improves skilled use of the impaired limb. J Neurosci 29:8187–8197

Zai L et al (2011) Inosine augments the effects of a Nogo receptor blocker and of environmental enrichment to restore skilled forelimb use after stroke. J Neurosci 31:5977–5988

Zeiler SR, Krakauer JW (2013) The interaction between training and plasticity in the poststroke brain. Curr Opin Neurol 26:609–616

Zeiler SR et al (2013) Medial premotor cortex shows a reduction in inhibitory markers and mediates recovery in a mouse model of focal stroke. Stroke 44:483–489

Zeiler SR et al (2015) Paradoxical motor recovery from a first stroke after induction of a second stroke: reopening a Postischemic sensitive period. Neurorehabil Neural Repair 30:794. https://doi.org/10.1177/1545968315624783

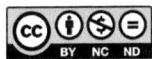

Clinical Pathways in Stroke Rehabilitation: Background, Scope, and Methods

Thomas Platz and Mayowa Owolabi

1   Introduction

Stroke remains the second leading cause of death and disability and one of the leading causes of depression and dementia globally (GBD 2015 Neurological Disorders Collaborator Group 2017; Owolabi et al. 2018). While stroke-related mortality standardized for age decreased over the last decades, the absolute number of new strokes (incidence), stroke-related deaths and stroke survivors living in our societies (prevalence) dramatically increased. From 1990 to 2010, the worldwide stroke prevalence increased by 15% from 435 on average to 502 per 100,000 people (Feigin et al. 2014) and then more recently by 21.8% from 2005 to 2015 for ischemic stroke globally and years lived with stroke-related disability by 22.0% (GBD 2015 Disease and Injury Incidence and Prevalence Collaborators 2016). This "dramatic" increase in stroke-related burden of disease and disability is foreseen to continue in societies around the globe due to ongoing epidemiologic transition and an ageing world population.

T. Platz (✉)
Institute for Neurorehabilitation and Evidence-based Practice ("An-Institute", University of Greifswald), BDH-Klinik Greifswald, Greifswald, Germany

Neurorehabilitation Research Group, University Medical Centre Greifswald (UMG), Greifswald, Germany

Special Interest Group Clinical Pathways, World Federation Neurorehabilitation (WFNR), North Shields, UK
e-mail: T.Platz@bdh-klinik-greifswald.de

M. Owolabi
Department of Medicine, College of Medicine, University College Hospital, University of Ibadan, Ibadan, Nigeria

Blossom Specialist Medical Center, (First Center for Neurorehabilitation in East, West and Central Africa), Ibadan, Nigeria

Special Interest Group Clinical Pathways, World Federation for NeuroRehabilitation, North Shields, United Kingdom

© The Author(s) 2021
T. Platz (ed.), *Clinical Pathways in Stroke Rehabilitation*,
https://doi.org/10.1007/978-3-030-58505-1_2

Fortunately, specialized inter-professional stroke care including rehabilitation can significantly reduce stroke-related disability and prevent the need to receive institutional care among stroke survivors (Stroke Unit Trialists' Collaboration 2013). In the Cochrane review, including 21 RCTs with a total of 39,994 participants, the risk to remain dependent (or die) after stroke could considerably be reduced compared to non-specialized care (OR 0.79, 95% CI 0.68 to 0.90; $P = 0.0007$). Furthermore, there is ample meta-analytic Cochrane evidence that specific interventions developed for stroke rehabilitation reduce impairment and promote activities, examples are arm robot therapy (Mehrholz et al. 2018), treadmill training with partial body-weight support (Mehrholz et al. 2017a), or electromechanical gait training (Mehrholz et al. 2017b) to name a few. Without proper care, stroke survivors are at higher risk to remain dependent on carers, face heavy restrictions in their societal participation, and have to leave their homes and become nursing home residents.

Thus, there is an urgent need to promote, achieve, and sustain multidisciplinary stroke rehabilitation to tame the rapidly increasing burden of stroke-related disability worldwide. This is best performed by a multidisciplinary approach involving specialist doctors, nurses, and therapists from various disciplines with the best available external evidence being implemented in clinical practice.

But how should such teams know the most valid up-to-date evidence and thus take their decisions reliably in the best interest of their patient? How can the knowledge from clinical research be translated to everyday clinical practice so that stroke survivors regain independence with activities of daily living, participate in social life to the best possible degree, and maximize their quality of life?

Clinical pathways can be of great help for this purpose. They are documented tools that provide multidisciplinary teams with recommendations for appropriate care for a medical condition. When they are based on the best available up-to-date and valid evidence, they help to maximize achievement of treatment goals.

2   Clinical Pathways

Clinical pathways (CP) are structured multidisciplinary care plans for a certain condition (Campbell et al. 1998). They declare how in a standardized way multistep managed care of a clinical condition is meant to be performed at a given point of health care provision, i.e. locally. Based on three sentinel articles (Campbell et al. 1998; De Bleser et al. 2006; Vanhaecht et al. 2006), a Cochrane review on CPs identified five characteristic features of CPs: a CP is (1) a structured multidisciplinary plan of care, (2) promoting translation of evidence or guideline to local structures, (3) detailing steps in the course of treatment for a medical condition, (4) with time frames of criteria-based progression, and (5) aiming for standardization of care for a clinical condition (Rotter et al. 2010).

As such, they are suitable for the guidance and implementation of evidence-based interventions for stroke rehabilitation with the involvement of various health care disciplines, for the different clinical target domains (e.g. perception [somatosensory, visual], communication, swallowing, arm activities, mobility, cognition, and emotion) to be addressed during the time course after stroke, [i.e. the acute (up to 7 days), the subacute (first 6 months) and chronic phase], with implications for functional recovery and achievement of therapeutic goals (Bernhardt et al. 2017).

3   The Evidence Gap

The inherent challenge for the generation of evidence-based clinical pathways for such a complex issue as stroke rehabilitation is the very broad and rapidly expanding evidence base that needs to be taken into account. For any individual or health care centre, it is impossible to systematically search and critically appraise the relevant evidence even when one would restrict oneself to only the most relevant and valid research, i.e. randomized controlled trials (RCTs) and systematic reviews (SR) with meta-analytic data synthesis. Even national societies will hardly be able to cover all relevant evidence and perform an explicit critical appraisal when they generate their guidelines for stroke rehabilitation.

Anyone responsible for the generation of (local) stroke rehabilitation CPs will invariably face the following challenges:

While high-quality SR can provide valid and precise estimate of beneficial therapeutic effects, they do so only for a single type of intervention and one target syndrome. Hence, their coverage in stroke rehabilitation is rather restricted. Most frequently, they give no clue on how to decide between the various available therapeutic options when faced with a clinical question. In addition, even for their restricted scope they provide evidence, but refrain from giving explicit clinical practice recommendations. They are meant to provide an evidence synthesis, but do not incorporate the methodological structure to systematically deduce practice recommendations.

Guidelines, on the other hand, are more comprehensive in their coverage, yet have critical limits that may restrict their validity and applicability for CP development outside their primary societal context (Platz 2019). In some countries, recommendations for stroke rehabilitation were embedded in general stroke care guidelines or overall stroke rehabilitation guidelines, yet with a restricted evidence base; this may cause bias by evidence selection. In other countries, guidelines were limited to certain target domains within stroke rehabilitation (e.g. mobility) and thereby had a chance to be systematically evidence-based; here the restriction is their coverage in terms of clinical aspects in stroke rehabilitation. In addition, most of the available guidelines were developed in high-income countries and formulated for their specific national health care systems (Platz 2019). As such, they are not necessarily applicable in other nations, especially not in low- or middle-income countries with quite different health care context and practice settings.

Therefore, the development of valid up-to-date systematically evidence-based stroke rehabilitation CP is daunting. Nevertheless, two initiatives of the World Federation for NeuroRehabilitation (WFNR) might help to better achieve these goals in the future, one being a project on research for the provision of systematic evidence-to-decision knowledge covering both (a) a systematic best evidence synthesis based on systematic reviews and (b) a systematic multistep approach from the evidence to clinical practice recommendations (compare Platz et al. 2020 as an example), and the second being the evidence-based clinical practice recommendations for major topics in stroke rehabilitation provided in this book.

4 International Provision of Practice Recommendations

The evidence-based clinical practice recommendations, as presented in this book and authorized by the WFNR, systematically link best evidence synthesis with specific clinical practice recommendations for various key clinical problems faced in stroke rehabilitation. The recommendations do not go into organizational issues (i.e. how to organize the implementation) except for the final chapter. Any organizational recommendations related to individual clinical problems would likely only be valid for a restricted scope of health care systems. Implementation needs to take regional context and resources into account and is thus better addressed by local clinical pathway development, not international recommendations.

Other aspects integrated in the development of the practice guidelines presented in this book are (a) the coverage of individual chapters by international experts in the respective field, mostly being members of the corresponding Special Interest Groups (SIG) of the WFNR, (b) a multi-professional group of authors, (c) coming from different health care settings around the globe, and (d) a structured review process for the recommendations involving the panel of all book authors, further WFNR experts (non-authors), and stroke survivor representatives.

The rest of this chapter will present the scope, content, and methodology used for the generation of these practice recommendations in greater detail.

5 Scope, Content, and Methodology Used for the Generation of the Practice Recommendations

5.1 Scope of the Evidence-Based Clinical Practice Recommendations

The International Classification of Functioning, Disability, and Health (ICF) (World Health Organization 2001) is based on the biopsychosocial approach used to integrate the biological, individual, and social dimensions of health. The ICF distinguishes three components: (1) body functions and structures; (2) activity and participation; and (3) environmental and personal factors. While the organic brain damage causes deficits of body structures (i.e. of the brain) and function (so-called "impairments" such as paresis), the resulting activity limitations (e.g. reduced mobility) translate into participation restrictions (i.e. handicaps) depending on multiple individual and environmental factors.

Each chapter of this book addresses the assessment and treatment of the specific functional consequences of stroke that are related to breathing, swallowing, consciousness, cognition, emotion, communication, visual perception, motor functions, and activities including arm activities and mobility as well as driving after stroke.

Individual stroke survivors might be affected by one or more functional deficits with high inter-individual variation of degree of functional deficit and remaining functional capacity. Furthermore, these deficits change over time due to spontaneous recovery and therapeutic effects. Therefore, stroke rehabilitation treatment needs to be highly individualized. Most chapters of this book focus on the evidence for treatment effects in a specific dimension of function and provide valuable guidance on treatment decisions. This is to be implemented in the context of an individualized comprehensive rehabilitation care plan.

It is crucial to understand the overall current situation of a stroke survivor, to assess any functional strengths and weaknesses as well as individual goals for rehabilitation. Individualized treatment decisions across functional domains are then taken on that basis. Practice recommendations as provided in this book are not meant to be of a recipe-book character. They are rather subjected to the overall individualized rehabilitation goals and plan and apply whenever the rehabilitation plan addresses the clinical problem covered.

Since stroke rehabilitation works best when team-based (Stroke Unit Trialists' Collaboration 2013) and stroke rehabilitation frequently involves different professions such as neuropsychologists, occupational therapists, physiotherapists, speech and language therapists, sport therapists, nurses, and physicians, an interdisciplinary team is formed whenever possible. Accordingly, goal setting and team approach with the ICF used as framework are important in stroke rehabilitation and are addressed in Chap. 3.

Stroke rehabilitation starts within acute stroke care and remains a life-long endeavor in many cases. It takes place in various health care settings from the intensive care unit, the acute stroke care, and stroke rehabilitation unit, to the outpatient clinic, community-based, and domiciliary settings. These issues are discussed in Chap. 14 on health care settings in neurorehabilitation.

5.2   Target Users of the Practice Recommendations

Target population of the clinical pathways for stroke rehabilitation are physicians treating stroke survivors, especially neurologists and physiatrists, physiotherapists, (neuro)psychologists, nurses, occupational therapists, and speech and language therapists among other health care professionals involved in stroke rehabilitation.

Stroke survivors, their related proxy carer, stroke service providers, and politicians might also benefit from the pathways for their interest and purposes. The language necessary to portray the evidence and recommendations specifically might however not permit an easy understanding for non-professionals, even though the intention was to promote understanding across a broad audience.

5.3   Stakeholder Involvement

5.3.1   Practice Recommendations Developer Group

The practice recommendation development group includes individuals from the various relevant professional groups, i.e. occupational therapists, physicians, physiotherapists, psychologists, and speech and language therapists. In addition, members of the group come from different continents and regions with diverse socioeconomical backgrounds. By these facts, the broadest representation of stroke rehabilitation scenarios by profession, region, and socioeconomical background was sought to be achieved.

For each member of the guideline development group, the following information is provided (see Table 1):

- name,
- discipline/content expertise (e.g. neurologist, physiotherapist),
- institution (e.g. City hospital),
- geographical location (e.g. Nigeria),
- description of the member's role in the guideline development group,
- conflict of interest statement

5.3.2   Integration of Views and Preferences
of the Target Population

We created an feedback panel with all book authors, two neurorehabilitation expert clinicians sharing international responsibility within the WFNR who were not authors of chapters and who come from different socioeconomic backgrounds (the U.S.A. and Mexico), and four representatives of stroke survivor support groups from Germany (Stiftung Deutsche Schlaganfall-Hilfe; www.schlaganfall-hilfe.de/) and Europe (Stroke Alliance for Europe, SAFE is a non-profit organization that represents a range of stroke patient groups from across Europe; www.safestroke.eu/). They all were invited to provide feedback on individual chapters and their recommendations.

Feedback given on individual chapter's recommendations by the panel of all authors, the two independent neurorehabilitation experts, and the representatives of stroke survivor support groups through a structured chapter-by-chapter webpage-based process was used by chapter authors to revise their chapter before it was accepted for publication.

5.4   Methods Used for Evidence Synthesis
and Recommendation Development

5.4.1   General Remarks

The methods for evidence synthesis described below apply to a truly systematic review with critical appraisal of the literature. Given the resource restraints of the author groups, this was not possible for most of the chapters; the aspects fulfilled are

Table 1 Practice recommendations developer group

Name/title	Discipline/content expertise	Institution	Geographical location	Description of the member's role in the guideline development group	Conflict of interest statement
Abiodun E Akinwuntan, Prof. Dr.	Neurorehabilitation	University of Kansas Medical Center, Kansas City	USA	Co-author	Dr. Akinwuntan has nothing to disclose
Jane Burridge, PhD, Prof.	Physiotherapist	University of Southampton, Southhampton	UK	Co-author	Dr. Burridge has nothing to disclose
Amber M. Conn, O.T., Driving Rehabilitation Specialist	Occupational therapist; driving assessment/rehabilitation	University of Kansas Medical Center, Kansas City	USA	Co-author	Ms Conn has nothing to disclose
Hannes Devos, Associate Professor	Physical therapy	University of Kansas Medical Center, Kansas City	USA	Co-author	Dr. Devos received funds from the National Institutes of Health, National Multiple Sclerosis Society, Parkinson's Foundation, and Department of Transportation. He is one of the leading authors on clinical trials and observational studies related to driving with a neurological condition
Markus Ebke, Dr. med.	Neurologist	NRZ Bad Salzuflen-MEDIAN-Kliniken, Bad Salzuflen	Germany	Feedback panel member	Dr. Ebke has nothing to declare
Klemens Fheodoroff, MD	Neurologist	Gailtal-Klinik Hermagor, Neurorehabilitation, Hermagor	Austria	Co-author	Dr. Fheodoroff has nothing to disclose

(continued)

Table 1 (continued)

Name/title	Discipline/content expertise	Institution	Geographical location	Description of the member's role in the guideline development group	Conflict of interest statement
Gerard E. Francisco, MD; Professor of PM&R	Physiatrist	Department of PM&R, McGovern Medical School, University of Texas Health Science Center – Houston, and TIRR Memorial Hermann, Houston, TX	USA	Corresponding author	Dr. Francisco reports grants and other from Allergan, grants from Ipsen, grants and other from Merz, grants from Revance, grants from Indego, grants from Microtransponder, grants from Ottobock, grants from ReWalk, other from Shionogi, other from Sword Health, outside the submitted work.
Jorge Hernández-Franco, MD	Rehabilitation medicine, certified in neurological rehabilitation	Instituto Nacional de Neurología y Neurocirugía (INNN), Mexico City	Mexico	Feedback panel member	Dr. Hernández-Franco has nothing to disclose
David Good, MD, Professor of Neurology	Neurologist	Penn State Milton S. Hershey Medical Center, Hershey, Pennsylvania	USA	Feedback panel member	Dr. Good reports grants from National Institutes of Health, outside the submitted work; and President elect, World Federation for Neurorehabilitation
Carol Hawley, Dr	Psychologist	Warwick Medical School, University of Warwick, Warwick	UK	Corresponding author	Dr. Hawley has nothing to disclose
Georg Kerkhoff, Prof. Dr. phil.	Neuropsychologist	Saarland University, Clinical Neuropsychology, Neuropsychological Outpatient Unit, Saarbrücken	Germany	Corresponding author	Dr. Kerkhoff has nothing to disclose

Won-Seok Kim, MD PhD, Prof.	Physiatrist	Seoul National University College of Medicine, Seoul National University Bundang Hospital, Seongnam	South Korea	Co-author	Dr. Kim has nothing to disclose
Matilde Leonardi, MD	Neurologist, Pediatrician, Child Neurologist	Fondazione IRCCS Istituto Neurologico Carlo Besta	Italy	Co-author	Dr. Leonardi has nothing to disclose
Sheng Li, MD, PhD Professor	Physiatrist	PM&R Dept. McGovern Med School, University of Texas Health Science Center – Houston, Houston, TX	USA	Co-author	Dr Li reports personal fees from consultation for Saol Therapeutics. Outside his contribution to the chapter—post-stroke spasticity
Giorgio Maggioni, Dr.	Neurorehabilitation	ICS Maugeri IRCCS Veruno (NO)	Italy	Corresponding author	Dr. Maggioni has nothing to disclose
Shawn Marshall, Professor, Dr.	Physiatrist	University of Ottawa/Ottawa Hospital Research Institute/Bruyere Research Institute, Ottawa	Canada	Co-author	Dr. Marshall has nothing to disclose
Mayowa Owolabi, MD, Dr. med.	Neurologist	University of Ibadan, Blossom Center for Neurorehabilitation, Ibadan	Nigeria	Co-author	Dr. Owolabi has nothing to disclose
Nam-Jong Paik, MD PhD, Professor	Rehabilitation Medicine	Seoul National University College of Medicine, Seoul National University Bundang Hospital, Seongnam	South Korea	Corresponding author	Dr. Paik has nothing to disclose
Rebecca Palmer, Dr	Speech and language therapist	University of Sheffield, School of Health and Related Research, Sheffield	UK	Co-author	Dr Palmer reports personal fees from Pro-Ed publication of the Frenchay Dysarthria Assessment 2, outside the submitted work

(continued)

Table 1 (continued)

Name/title	Discipline/content expertise	Institution	Geographical location	Description of the member's role in the guideline development group	Conflict of interest statement
Apoorva Pauranik, Dr. M.D., D.M.	Neurologist	Pauranik Academy of Neurology, Indore	India	Co-author	Dr. Pauranik has nothing to disclose
Caterina Pistarini Prof. MD	Physician, Neurorehabilitation	ICS Maugeri IRCCS, Genoa	Italy	Co-author	Dr. Pistarini has nothing to disclose
Thomas Platz, Prof. Dr. med	Neurologist	BDH Klinik Greifswald, Universitätsmedizin Greifswald, Greifswald	Germany	Editor, corresponding author, co-author	Dr. Platz reports and conducted clinical trials and other clinical research on arm rehabilitation, especially the arm ability training and arm basis training that were sponsored by the German research agency (DFG) and the German Ministry of Health (BMBF) with grants for the research. TP provides educational courses for these arm rehabilitation techniques.
Marcus Pohl, Prof. Dr. med.	Neurologist	VAMED Klinik Schloss Pulsnitz, Pulsnitz	Germany	Corresponding author	Dr. Pohl has nothing to disclose
Hariklia Proios, Prof. Dr.	Speech Pathologist/ Neuropsychologist	Stroke Alliance for Europe, and University of Macedonia, Thessaloniki	Greece	Feedback panel member	Dr. Proios reports grants and non-financial support from Boehringer Ingelheim International GmbH, outside the submitted work
Gary Randall, PhD	Psychologist/Patient representative	Stroke Alliance for Europe, Brussels	Belgium	Feedback panel member	Dr. Randall has nothing to disclose
Sybille Roschka, M.Sc. (Research)	Occupational therapist	Universitätsmedizin Greifswald, Institut für Community Medicine, Greifswald	Germany	Co-author	Ms Roschka has nothing to disclose

Name	Role	Affiliation	Country	Authorship	Disclosure
Linda Schmuck, Dr. med.	Physician, resident	Universitätsmedizin Greifswald, department for psychiatry and psychotherapy, Greifswald	Germany	Co-author	Dr. Schmuck has nothing to disclose
Mervyn Singer, M.D., Professor of Intensive Care Medicine	Internal Medicine, Intensive Care Medicine	Bloomsbury Institute of Intensive Care Medicine, University College London, London	UK	Co-author	Dr. Singer has nothing to disclose
Nirmal Surya, Dr.	Neurologist	Bombay Hospital Institute of Medical Sciences, Mumbai	India	Co-author	Dr. Surya has nothing to disclose
Caroline van Heugten, Prof. Dr.	Neuropsychologist	Maastricht University, Maastricht	Netherlands	Corresponding author	Dr. Van Heugten has nothing to disclose
Markus Wagner, Dr., MPH	Biologist	German Stroke Foundation, Gütersloh	Germany	Feedback panel member	Dr. Wagner reports grants from Pfizer, grants from Boehringer, outside the submitted work
Nick Ward, Professor of Clinical Neurology and Neurorehabilitation	Neurologist	UCL Queen Square Institute of Neurology, London	UK	Author	Dr. Ward has nothing to disclose
Sabahat Asim Wasti, Dr	Consultant Neurorehabilitation	Cleveland Clinic Abu Dhabi, Abu Dhabi	United Arab Emirates	Corresponding author	Dr. Wasti has nothing to disclose
Barbara A. Wilson, Ph.D.	Neuropsychologist	The Oliver Zangwill Centre for Neuropsychological Rehabilitation, Ely, Cambridgeshire; St. George's Hospital, London	UK	Co-author	Dr. Wilson has nothing to disclose
Jörg Wissel, Prof. Dr. med.	Neurologist	Neurologische Rehabilitation und Physikalische Therapie, Vivantes Klinikum Spandau, Berlin	Germany	Co-author	Dr. Wissel reports personal fees from Allergan, personal fees from Ipsen, personal fees from Merz, personal fees from Richter, personal fees from Medtronic, personal fees from Shionogi, outside the submitted work

given in individual chapters. The methods presented here, nevertheless, describe the "gold standard".

In terms of the rules to assess the level of evidence of references, the quality of evidence, and the grading of recommendations, the methodology as described below was applied in all clinical chapters of this book.

5.4.2   Systematic Search

Details of the strategy used to search for evidence should be provided including search terms used, sources consulted, and dates of the literature covered. Sources included electronic databases (e.g. MEDLINE, EMBASE, CINAHL) and databases of systematic reviews (e.g. the Cochrane Library, DARE) and published conference proceedings. Other guidelines (e.g. the US National Guideline Clearinghouse, the German Guidelines Clearinghouse) could be used for comparison.

The information provided should include:

- named electronic database(s) or evidence source(s) where the search was performed (e.g. MEDLINE, EMBASE, PsycINFO, CINAHL),
- time periods searched (e.g. January 1, 2008 to April 30, 2018),
- search terms used (e.g. text words, indexing terms, subheadings),
- and may include the full search strategy (e.g. located in supplementary online material).

5.4.3   Criteria and Methods for Evidence Selection and Data Extraction

Criteria for including/excluding evidence should be provided. For example, some chapter authors decided to only include evidence from randomized clinical trials and to exclude articles not written in English. A description of the inclusion criteria included the target population (patient, public, etc.) characteristics, type of study design, intervention(s), comparison(s), outcome(s), language, and context, using an extended PICO schema (Lichtenstein et al. 2009).

Two independent assessors should perform evidence selection and data extraction. A consensus process should be in place to resolve any disagreement.

5.4.4   Critical Appraisal, Level of Evidence, Evidence Synthesis, and Grading its Quality

The following steps were taken from search for and critical appraisal of evidence to formulation of recommendations (Platz 2017, 2021) and are described in greater detail below.

I. For each source (original paper, systematic review, and meta-analysis)
   1. evaluation of the methodology (internal validity, e.g. study design, risk of bias)
   2. classification of evidence level of each source (1a to 5 according to the CEBM, for explanation see Table 1) (CEBM 2009)

3. summarizing the results and their relevance for clinical practice based on individual sources.

II. For the collated data from all sources for a specific therapeutic intervention (original papers, systematic reviews, and meta-analyses)

4. assessment of the quality of evidence for the sources included, i.e. the resulting confidence in the estimate of the therapeutic effect strength (Schünemann et al. 2013) and.

5. formulating and grading of the derived recommendation (Schünemann et al. 2013; Platz 2017).

Ad (I)

Accordingly, for each reference and the body of literature for a given therapeutic intervention, the level of evidence was described (for details see Table 2).

Apart from data extraction and level of evidence classification, various aspects of trial validity should be critically appraised as presented in Table 3 for individual evaluation studies.

For systematic reviews, questions that are suggested to be addressed are given in Table 4. The criteria were adapted from AMSTAR 2 (A Measurement Tool to Assess Systematic Reviews) (Shea et al. 2017).

The *characteristics of an individual study/systematic review* together with the results of the critical appraisal, the main study results, and any clinical implications of that piece of information should be documented in an evidence table. There, the conclusion for individual references should specifically take into consideration the clinical relevance of the outcome measure(s), the magnitude and precision of the effect documented, the benefit-harm ratio, and the intervention's acceptability; methodological weaknesses/risk of bias; in case of meta-analyses subgroup analyses and heterogeneity; and finally, the relevance of findings for clinical practice.

Ad (II)

For any intervention-related recommendation, the quality of the *evidence collated across all studies and systematic reviews* included was assessed according to

Table 2 Level of Evidence Classification

1a	1b	2b	3	4	5
Systematic review (with homogeneity) of RCTs	Individual RCT (with narrow confidence interval)	Individual cohort study or low-quality RCT (e.g. <80% follow-up)	Individual case-control study	Case series (and poor-quality cohort and case control studies)	Expert opinion without explicit critical appraisal, or based on physiology, bench research, or "first principles"

Levels of evidence for Therapy, Prevention, Aetiology and Harm 1a to 5 according to the "Oxford Center for Evidence-Based Medicine—Levels of Evidence", presented in table is the version from March 2009, retrieved from https://www.cebm.net/2009/06/oxford-centre-evidence-based-medicine-levels-evidence-march-2009/) (CEBM 2009). Alternatively, the classification from 2011 may be used (https://www.cebm.net/wp-content/uploads/2014/06/CEBM-Levels-of-Evidence-2.1.pdf)

Table 3 Critical appraisal of individual evaluation studies

1. Clear definition of eligibility criteria.
2. Clear definition and adequate assessment of study outcomes.
3. Reporting of side effects and acceptability.
4. Adequate follow-up assessment (long-term effects).
5. Clear definition and description of experimental and control condition.
6. Were participants randomly allocated (selection bias)?
7. Allocation concealment (selection bias).
8. Comparability of experimental and control groups at baseline (selection bias).
9. Blinded staff and patients during intervention and comparable treatment of randomized groups aside from investigated effects (performance bias).
10. Blinded outcome assessment (detection bias).
11. No selective reporting (reporting bias).
12. (Almost) Complete outcome data (attrition bias).
13. Intention-to-treat analysis reported.
14. Do the results sufficiently support the conclusions reported?
Answers can be: yes (y), no (n), or not clear (nc).

Table 4 Critical appraisal of systematic reviews and meta-analyses

1. Were review methods established prior to the conduct of the review (written protocol)?
2. Were research questions clearly phrased, e.g. did selection criteria for the review include the components of PICO, and clinically meaningful?
3. Was the study design selection of included trials adequate for the research question?
4. Did the review authors use a comprehensive literature search strategy (data bases, key words, justify search restrictions [e.g. language])?
5. Were all processes (screening, selection, assessment risk of bias, data extraction) performed in duplicate?
6. Did the review authors describe the included studies in adequate detail (compare PICO)?
7. Did the review authors use a satisfactory technique for assessing the risk of bias (RoB) in individual studies that were included in the review?
8. If meta-analysis was performed, did the review authors use appropriate methods for statistical combination of results, and was it meaningful to combine the studies selected for meta-analyses?
9. Have all clinically relevant effects of the intervention(s) of interest (benefit, including long-term effects; harm; acceptability) been addressed?
10. Did the review authors assess the potential impact of RoB in individual studies and of publication bias on the results of the meta-analysis or other evidence synthesis and discuss the implications of the findings of their assessment on the estimates of therapeutic effects as reported?
11. Did the review authors provide a satisfactory explanation for and discussion of any heterogeneity observed in the results of the review?
12. Did the review authors report any potential sources of conflict of interest (CoI), including any funding they or the authors of included studies received for conducting the review or their studies? If a risk that CoI might have influenced the review's result is not unlikely, was its management described (for the review or the trials included) and adequate?
13. Do the results sufficiently support the conclusions drawn?
Answers can be:
yes (y), partially yes (py) [not all, but "essential features" yes], no (n), not clear (nc), or not applicable (na).

Table 5 GRADE definition for quality of evidence

Quality of evidence category	Description	Examples
High	We are very confident that the true effect lies close to that of the estimate of the effect	Evidence from high-quality RCTs or meta-analyses of RCTs
Moderate	We are moderately confident in the effect estimate: The true effect is likely to be close to the estimate of the effect, but there is a possibility that it is substantially different	Evidence from RCTs or meta-analyses of RCTs with serious limitations Evidence from observational studies with special strengths
Low	Our confidence in the effect estimate is limited: The true effect may be substantially different from the estimate of the effect	Evidence from observational studies Evidence from RCTs or meta-analyses of RCTs with multiple serious or very serious limitations
Very low	We have very little confidence in the effect estimate: The true effect is likely to be substantially different from the estimate of effect	Evidence from observational studies with serious limitations Good clinical practice/expert opinion

The quality of evidence according to the GRADE approach (Grading of Recommendations, Assessment, Development, and Evaluation) reflects the extent to which our confidence in an estimate of therapeutic effect is adequate to support a particular recommendation (left and middle column) (Schünemann et al. 2013). The right column provides examples how the categories were applied in the context of this book and its chapters.

the GRADE approach (Grading of Recommendations, Assessment, Development, and Evaluation) (Schünemann et al. 2013). The quality of evidence reflects the extent to which our confidence in an estimate of therapeutic effect is adequate to support a particular recommendation. The corresponding quality of evidence categories are presented in Table 5.

Randomized trials (and meta-analyses based on RCTs) without serious limitations provide high-quality evidence; observational studies without special strengths or serious limitations provide low-quality evidence. Limitations (risk of bias, inconsistency, indirectness, imprecision, and publication bias) or special strengths (e.g. large magnitude of effect or dose-response gradient) can, however, modify the quality of the evidence of both randomized trials and observational studies. For a more detailed explanation of risk of bias and other factors modifying the quality of the evidence, see the GRADE Handbook (Schünemann et al. 2013) and the Cochrane Handbook for Systematic Reviews of Interventions (Higgins et al. 2019; Schünemann et al. 2019).

5.4.5   Synthesis of Evidence-Based Recommendations

Recommendations were based on evidence for interventions and certain outcomes across studies and when available across systematic reviews. A recommendation reflects the extent to which the group developing the recommendation is confident that desirable effects of an intervention outweigh undesirable effects in case of a positive recommendation, or that undesirable effects of an intervention outweigh desirable effects in case of a negative recommendation.

GRADE specifies two categories of strength of recommendation, i.e. a weak or a strong recommendation in favour or against an intervention (Schünemann et al. 2013). For a strong recommendation, it is necessary to be certain about the various factors that influence the strength of recommendation and to have the information at hand that supports a clear balance towards either the desirable or the undesirable effects of an intervention. When the information is such that the desirable effects of an intervention probably outweigh the undesirable effects (or vice versa), but appreciable uncertainty exists, a weak recommendation for (or against) an intervention is warranted. In a first approach, high-quality evidence qualifies for a strong, moderate-quality evidence for a weak recommendation.

In rehabilitation as in other medical fields, we frequently have some positive, yet low- or even very low-quality evidence favouring an intervention that strictly speaking is not yet sufficient to qualify for a weak recommendation. Nevertheless, this could still be the best available evidence and relevant for clinical guidance. Therefore, a third category of recommendation was introduced indicating a therapeutic "option" (Muche-Borowski et al. 2012; Platz 2017, 2021).

Furthermore, apart from the quality of evidence, other factors influence the grading of recommendations such as the clinical relevance of outcomes assessed, the value attributed by stroke survivors and the acceptability of a therapeutic option, the feasibility of its implementation, and the corresponding resource use. When such other factors contribute substantially to a recommendation's category, this was specifically indicated. Table 6 gives an overview of the recommendation categories used with the corresponding verbal descriptors for the text and the symbols used.

5.4.6 Dissemination, Implementation, Monitoring, and Auditing

This book is published under an open access schema. Thereby, it is accessible globally free of charge as electronic version and with a flat rate in print version. Being authorized by the WFNR, an umbrella organization for the national societies of neurological rehabilitation as well as for individuals working in countries without their own national society, a wide dissemination through national member societies

Table 6 Categories for recommendations

Recommendation category	Verbal description (as used in text) for positive/negative recommendation	Symbol
Strong	"Ought to"/"ought not to"	A+/A−
Weak	"Should"/"should not"	B+/B−
Option	"Can"	0

GRADE specifies two categories of strength of recommendation, i.e. a weak or a strong recommendation in favour or against an intervention, mainly for high- or moderate-quality evidence (Schünemann et al. 2013). A third category of recommendation was introduced indicating a therapeutic "option", mainly based on low- or very low-quality evidence (Muche-Borowski et al. 2012; Platz 2017, 2021) and key stakeholders worldwide is foreseen. While written in the "universal" language English, a language barrier for dissemination still needs to be taken into account. It is therefore intended to translate these practice recommendations into other languages to enhance their dissemination.

As stated above, contextualization, implementation, monitoring, and auditing of these practice recommendations relies on local initiatives. For instance, the recommendations can easily be used as building blocks for generating clinical pathways while taking the local health care settings into account. With their structured format they support both the formulation of local clinical pathways and can help to develop the regional health care architecture in a way that supports evidence-based stroke rehabilitation. Contextualized implementation cycles are suggested that engage all stakeholders such as providers (personnel, clinicians, healthcare workers), policymakers, patients, populace (communities), partners, and payers (Owolabi et al. 2016). This will motivate stakeholders, overcome the obstacle that guidelines developed in high-income countries are not easily applicable in low-and middle-income countries (Platz 2019), and create an enabling environment for the implementation of the evidence-based solutions presented. An illustration is given that addresses the interaction between WFNR-authorized practice recommendations and continuous quality improvement by use of contextualized clinical pathways, their communication, implementation, evaluation, and adjustment (compare Fig. 1).

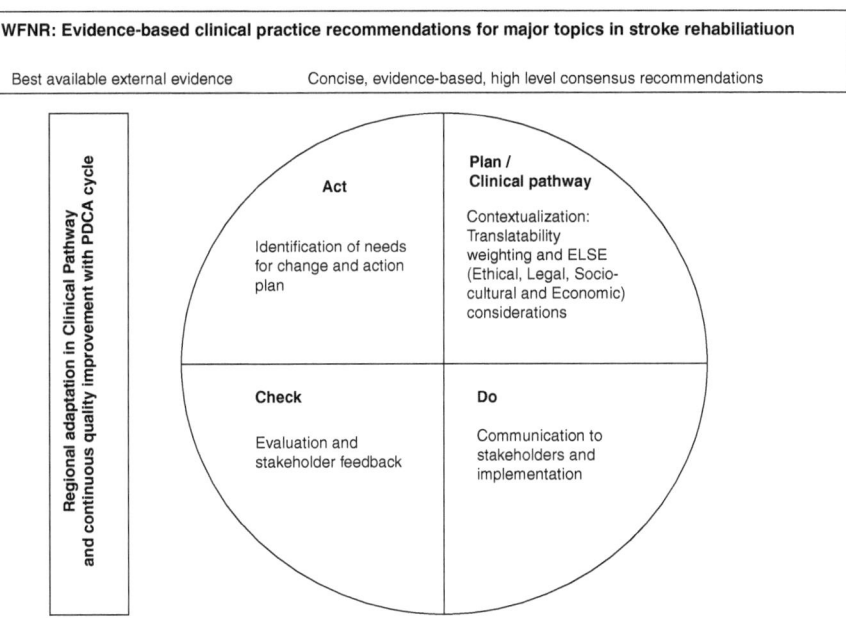

Fig. 1 Illustration of the interaction between WFNR-authorized practice recommendations and continuous quality improvement by use of contextualized clinical pathways, their communication, implementation, evaluation, and adjustment based on the plan-do-check-act (PDCA) cycle

5.4.7   Process of Updating the Clinical Practice Recommendations

The practice recommendations are considered valid for 5 years from their time of publication and are intended to be updated thereafter.

5.4.8   Funding of the Work

The WFNR Research and Education Foundation sponsored the publication charges of this book under an open access schema. Thereby, its universal accessibility was supported. Other sources of funding that might apply for individual book chapters are noted in the respective acknowledgements. Funding did not involve commercial sources.

---

6   Conclusions

Stroke-related disability of any given stroke survivor is a consequence of a highly individual combination of various possible sensory, motor, cognitive impairments, emotional disorders, and associated activity limitations. Stroke rehabilitation aims to reduce disability and promote participation, while improving quality of life and sense of meaning and purpose in life (stroke recovery cycle) (Owolabi 2013). Related therapeutic goals are addressed by patient-tailored combinations of rehabilitation interventions that address specific stroke-related clinical problems. Evidence-based practice recommendations help to take clinical decisions related to these problems in a way that gives the best changes to promote functional recovery and to regain capacities to perform activities of daily living.

The evidence-based practice recommendations provided by the WFNR in this book are premised on a search for the best available valid up-to-date evidence, its critical appraisal, the collation of the evidence across trials, and systematic reviews in a clinical problem- and outcome-centred way. By knowing the evidence and judging its (un)certainty as well as other relevant aspects such as acceptability, feasibility, and resource implications, weak or strong recommendations (or therapeutic options) could be formulated both in favour or against an intervention of concern.

The degree of systematic search and critical appraisal varied across chapters in the book (as indicated in individual chapters) secondary to resources available for the work. The same methodology for classifying the level of evidence, grading the quality of evidence, and any recommendation given as outlined above was, however, used throughout this book.

Expert author groups provided both a best evidence synthesis and recommendations as draft versions for each clinical problem addressed. The recommendations were regarded as final and ready to be published after the contributions and feedback of the panel of all authors, further experts, and the representatives of stroke survivor support groups were incorporated.

These stroke rehabilitation practice recommendations are published under an open access schema (sponsored by the WFNR Research and Education Foundation) and distributed through the many national member societies for neurorehabilitation ensuring global dissemination. Together with knowledge about the regional health care settings, they can directly be used for the development of evidence-based clinical pathways for stroke rehabilitation locally. Their development was free of commercial funding. It is intended to provide an update 5 years after publication.

Acknowledgements This work was supported by the BDH Bundesverband Rehabilitation e.V. (charity for neuro-disabilities) by a non-restricted personal grant to TP. The sponsor had no role in the decision to publish or any content of the publication.

References

Bernhardt J, Hayward KS, Kwakkel G, Ward NS, Wolf SL, Borschmann K, Krakauer JW, Boyd LA, Carmichael ST, Corbett D, Cramer SC (2017) Agreed definitions and a shared vision for new standards in stroke recovery research: the stroke recovery and rehabilitation roundtable taskforce. Int J Stroke 12:444–450

Campbell H, Hotchkiss R, Bradshaw N, Porteous M (1998) Integrated care pathways. J Integr Care Pathw 316:133–137

CEBM (2009) "Oxford Center for Evidence-Based Medicine—Levels of Evidence", last version from March 2009. https://www.cebm.net/2009/06/oxford-centre-evidence-based-medicine-levels-evidence-march-2009/

De Bleser L, Depreitere R, De Waele K, Vanhaecht K, Vlayen J, Sermeus W (2006) Defining pathways. J Nurs Manag 14:553–563

Feigin VL, Forouzanfar MH, Krishnamurthi R, Mensah GA, Connor M, Bennett DA, Moran AE, Sacco RL, Anderson L, Truelsen T, O'Donnell M, Venketasubramanian N, Barker-Collo S, Lawes CM, Wang W, Shinohara Y, Witt E, Ezzati M, Naghavi M, Murray C, Global Burden of Diseases, Injuries, and Risk Factors Study 2010 (GBD 2010) and the GBD Stroke Experts Group (2014) Global and regional burden of stroke during 1990–2010: findings from the global burden of disease study 2010. Lancet 383:245–254

GBD 2015 Disease and Injury Incidence and Prevalence Collaborators (2016) Global, regional, and national incidence, prevalence, and years lived with disability for 310 diseases and injuries, 1990–2015: a systematic analysis for the global burden of disease study 2015. Lancet 388:1545–1602

GBD 2015 Neurological Disorders Collaborator Group (2017) Global, regional, and national burden of neurological disorders during 1990–2015: a systematic analysis for the global burden of disease study 2015. Lancet Neurol 16:877–897

Higgins JPT, Savović J, Page MJ, Elbers RG, Sterne JAC (2019) Chapter 8: Assessing risk of bias in a randomized trial. In: Higgins JPT, Thomas J, Chandler J, Cumpston M, Li T, Page MJ, Welch VA (eds) Cochrane handbook for systematic reviews of interventions. 2nd edition. Chichester (UK): John Wiley & Sons, 205–228

Lichtenstein AH, Yetley EA, Lau J (2009) Application of systematic review methodology to the field of nutrition: nutritional research series, vol 1. Agency for Healthcare Research and Quality (US), Rockville, MD. 2009 Jan. (technical reviews, no. 17.1.) 2, methods. https://www.ncbi.nlm.nih.gov/books/NBK44075/

Mehrholz J, Thomas S, Elsner B (2017a) Treadmill training and body weight support for walking after stroke. Cochrane Database Syst Rev (8):CD002840

Mehrholz J, Thomas S, Werner C, Kugler J, Pohl M, Elsner B (2017b) Electromechanical-assisted training for walking after stroke. Cochrane Database Syst Rev (5):CD006185

Mehrholz J, Pohl M, Platz T, Kugler J, Elsner B (2018) Electromechanical and robot-assisted arm training for improving activities of daily living, arm function, and arm muscle strength after stroke. Cochrane Database Syst Rev (9):CD006876

Muche-Borowski C, Selbmann HK, Müller W et al. (2012) Das AWMF-Regelwerk Leitlinien 1. Aufl.; AWMF; http://www.awmf.org/leitlinien/awmf-regelwerk

Owolabi MO (2013) Consistent determinants of post-stroke health-related quality of life across diverse cultures: Berlin-Ibadan study. Acta Neurol Scand 128:311–320

Owolabi MO, Miranda JJ, Yaria J, Ovbiagele B (2016) Controlling cardiovascular diseases in low and middle income countries by placing proof in pragmatism. BMJ Glob Health 1(3):e000105

Owolabi M, Johnson W, Khan T, Feigin V, for Operations Committee of the Lancet Neurology on Stroke (2018) Effectively combating stroke in low- and middle-income countries: placing proof in pragmatism—the lancet neurology commission. J Stroke Med 1:65–67

Platz T (2017) Practice guidelines in neurorehabilitation. Neurol Int Open 01(03):E148–E152. https://doi.org/10.1055/s-0043-103057

Platz T (2019) Evidence-based guidelines and clinical pathways in stroke rehabilitation—an international perspective. Front Neurol 10:200. https://doi.org/10.3389/fneur.2019.00200

Platz T, Vetter N, Falk M (2020) Treatment of neurovisual disorders post stroke – from systematic review evidence to clinical practice recommendations. PROSPERO CRD42020157933. Available from: https://www.crd.york.ac.uk/prospero/display_record.php?ID=CRD42020157933

Platz T (2021) Evidenzbasierte Leitlinienentwicklung der Deutschen Gesellschaft für Neurologie (DGN) und der Deutschen Gesellschaft für Neurorehabilitation (DGNR) - Methodik für die systematische Evidenzbasierung. Fortschritte der Neurologie – Psychiatrie, in press

Rotter T, Kinsman L, James EL, Machotta A, Gothe H, Willis J, Snow P, Kugler J (2010) Clinical pathways: effects on professional practice, patient outcomes, length of stay and hospital costs. Cochrane Database Syst Rev (3):CD006632

Schünemann H, Brożek J, Guyatt G, Oxman A (2013) GRADE handbook for grading quality of evidence and strength of recommendations. The GRADE Working Group. Updated October 2013. guidelinedevelopment.org/handbook

Schünemann HJ, Higgins JPT, Vist GE, Glasziou P, Akl E, Skoetz N, Guyatt GH (2019) Chapter 14: Completing 'Summary of findings' tables and grading the certainty of the evidence. In: Higgins JPT, Thomas J, Chandler J, Cumpston M, Li T, Page MJ, Welch VA (eds) Cochrane handbook for systematic reviews of interventions. 2nd edition. Chichester (UK): John Wiley & Sons, 375–402

Shea BJ, Reeves BC, Wells G, Thuku M, Hamel C, Moran J, Moher D, Tugwell P, Welch V, Kristjansson E, Henry DA (2017) AMSTAR 2: a critical appraisal tool for systematic reviews that include randomised or non-randomised studies of healthcare interventions, or both. BMJ 358:j4008

Stroke Unit Trialists' Collaboration (2013) Organised inpatient (stroke unit) care for stroke. Cochrane Database Syst Rev (9):CD000197

Vanhaecht K, De Witte K, Depreitere R, Sermeus W (2006) Clinical pathway audit tools: a systematic review. J Nurs Manag 14:529–537

World Health Organization (2001) International classification of functioning, disability and health. World Health Organization, Geneva

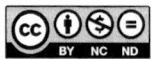

Goal Setting with ICF (International Classification of Functioning, Disability and Health) and Multidisciplinary Team Approach in Stroke Rehabilitation

Matilde Leonardi and Klemens Fheodoroff

1 Introduction

Stroke is among the leading causes for adult disability. The impairments associated with a stroke display a wide variety of clinical signs and symptoms. Therefore, an interdisciplinary team approach with different experts working cohesively and closely together has been identified as fundamental for effective stroke rehabilitation programs (Teasell et al. 2016a). There is high-confidence evidence on the benefits of the stroke care units and moderate-confidence evidence that integrated, multidisciplinary care teams improve stroke outcome. Within this team approach, coordination and cooperation appear to be key factors for reaching best results within the limitations imposed by stroke-related impairments as well as by contextual factors such as limited time for in-patient rehabilitation or limited resources in community-based rehabilitation programs (see chap.14).

The long-term and transversal nature of care and treatment for stroke have all served to confound hospital traditional, fragmented and top-down led responses. Meanwhile, it became apparent that stroke patients, like all patients with chronic health conditions, are in special need of continuous care, requiring a longitudinal, integrated and multidisciplinary network approach linking health and social care (paradigm shift). Policies, system and services, including payment systems, should be able to cope with care provided in more than one setting. To address the issue of fragmentation and overcome treatment gaps from a health services delivery perspective, it is necessary to 'optimize care and rationalize costs'. There is a need for a healthcare system transformation based on shared-vision and a practical roadmap

M. Leonardi (✉)
Fondazione IRCCS Istituto Neurologico Carlo Besta, Milan, Italy
e-mail: Matilde.Leonardi@istituto-besta.it

K. Fheodoroff
Gailtal-Klinik, Hermagor, Austria

© The Author(s) 2021
T. Platz (ed.), *Clinical Pathways in Stroke Rehabilitation*,
https://doi.org/10.1007/978-3-030-58505-1_3

to implementation of a coordinated system at national and regional level (WHO and UNESCO 2010).

In such a system early diagnosis, treatment and rehabilitation are seen as one seamless process of actions across different healthcare professionals and complementary disciplines (e.g. hospitals, specialists care, primary care, community care, homecare, institutional care or nursing home, pharmacies) that should work together according to a team-based approach in order to deliver patient care and improve health outcomes.

To ensure the continuity of care from the very beginning after a stroke, early intervention is key for optimal management of the disease and for achieving better clinical outcomes. A large body of research links early intervention to measurable health gains such as improved survival rates, reduced disability and complication rates, better quality of life and lower treatment costs (Stroke Unit Trialists 2013).

Optimizing healthcare processes with an outcome-based approach achieving high value for patients is the overarching goal of healthcare delivery, with value defined as the health outcomes achieved per money spent. Treatment is based on the needs of the patient ('demand') instead of on the offer/supply of treatment structures. Each age group according to disease stage has specific needs to be addressed along the care process (biological, psychological, healthcare services, social needs). Care for persons with stroke usually involves multiple specialties and numerous interventions, with final outcomes determined by interventions across the full cycle of care. Measuring, reporting and comparing outcomes are essential to improve outcomes and make informed choices about how to optimize healthcare and rationalize costs (Teasell and Hussein 2016).

Goal setting has been recognized as a core process in managing complex situations, which are challenging service providers in daily routine. Nevertheless, agreed standards on goal setting and evaluation still need to be defined. Many factors such as types and number of goals, the impact of patient involvement in the goal setting and evaluation process or the influence of goal attainment on adherence, self-efficacy and health-related quality of life (HR-QoL) have not been evaluated in the context of stroke rehabilitation in a rigorous way including randomized controlled trials (RCTs). (Rosewilliam et al. 2011; Sugavanam et al. 2013). Currently only low-to-moderate evidence on effectiveness of goal setting and evaluation practice on psychosocial factors (HR-QoL, emotional status and self-efficacy) is available (Levack et al. 2015).

For years, neurorehabilitation has been searching for an agreed framework suitable for interdisciplinary documentation. The International Classification of Functioning, Disability and Health (ICF), (WHO 2001) based on a biopsychosocial model of health and disability, offers such a framework. ICF is helpful in establishing a common language between different professionals and different stakeholders such as stroke patients, caregivers, administrative and health policy providers. It might also serve as the basis for a shared documentation system. Disability in ICF is defined as the interaction of health condition with hindering or facilitating environmental factors.

In this chapter, we highlight some aspects with relevance for multidisciplinary team building and coordination and for using the ICF in the context of stroke rehabilitation; in detail, how to describe individual levels of functioning and to set treatment goals as well as to identify barriers and facilitators to functioning and health.

2   Methodological Considerations

This chapter fulfils an educational purpose by introducing concepts and their application in stroke rehabilitation related to the ICF (WHO 2001) as a common language to describe individual functioning in a given context, multidisciplinary team building and coordination as well as goal setting. As such, it is primarily heuristic and not evidence-driven.

Hence, a systematic search for evidence is not the basis for this chapter. The most up-to-date relevant evidence is nevertheless reported.

The recommendations given in this chapter follow the same rules as outlined in chapter "Clinical Pathways in Stroke Rehabilitation: Background, Scope, and Methods" (see chap. 2): The level of evidence that served as basis for a recommendation is provided according to the 'Oxford Center for Evidence-Based Medicine - Levels of Evidence' (CEBM 2009) ranging from 'expert opinion' ('5') to 'systematic review (with homogeneity) of RCTs' ('1a'). The quality of the evidence is rated with the GRADE approach (Grading of Recommendations, Assessment, Development and Evaluation) (Schünemann et al. 2013) reflecting our confidence in an estimate of therapeutic effect that can range from very low to high. In addition, GRADE specifies two categories of strength of recommendation, i.e. a weak ('B', 'should') or a strong ('A', 'ought to') recommendation in favour ('+') or against ('−') an intervention, mainly for high- or moderate-quality evidence (Schünemann et al. 2013). A third category of recommendation was introduced indicating a therapeutic 'option' ('0', 'can'), mainly based on low- or very low-quality evidence (Platz 2017). Deviations are indicated by their reason, e.g. when upgrading a recommendation that is supported by low quality of evidence only to a 'week recommendation' instead of formulating an 'option': 'B+ [clinical reasoning]'.

3   Multidisciplinary Team Building and Coordination

Organized stroke care has been identified as an important factor for better overall outcomes for individuals with stroke (Teasell et al. 2016b).

3.1   Improving Quality of Stroke Care

Stroke is a leading cause of disability and death among adults. It is the second cause of death worldwide and the first cause of acquired disability. Despite improvements in care, around one-third of the 1.3 million people who have a stroke in Europe each year will not survive. One-third will make a good recovery, but one-third will live with long-term disability. Furthermore, stroke might lead to post-stroke dementia, depression, epilepsy and falls that cause substantial morbidity and economical costs. Strokes are more likely to occur with ageing with 75% of strokes happening to people older than 65 years. However, 25% of strokes still occur in younger people of working age, resulting in a significant loss of productivity.

Care for stroke patients starts before a stroke has happened (primary prevention) with the identification of people at risk for stroke, modification of lifestyle patterns and treatment of vascular risk factors in the primary care setting. It then focuses on optimal treatment of acute stroke in stroke units and on avoiding further vascular events (secondary prevention), ideally delivered through a comprehensive stroke service (Stroke units Trialists 2013). The effect of acute treatment is dependent on the time from stroke onset. Every step of the patient trajectory from symptom onset to the start of treatment within the hospital should be optimized in order to save time and to offer all opportunities for minimizing brain tissue damage. A shorter delay from onset of symptoms to treatment with intravenous thrombolysis (IVT) and thrombectomy can make the difference between being independent or dependent on help from others. During and after the acute phase, targeted rehabilitation is needed to reduce the remaining deficits to a minimum, to optimize the level of individual functioning and to reintegrate stroke victims into normal life.

3.2   Low Access to Rehabilitation

Many stroke survivors experience impairments making them dependent on others for their daily tasks. As stated in article 26 of the UN Convention on the Rights of Persons with Disability, rehabilitation aims to 'enable persons with disabilities to attain and maintain maximum independence, full physical, mental, social and vocational ability, and full inclusion and participation in all aspects of life. To that end, States Parties shall organize, strengthen and extend comprehensive habilitation and rehabilitation services and programmes, particularly in the areas of health, employment, education and social services...' (UN 2007). The early rehabilitation process after stroke is best initiated in a stroke units. However, it is rarely complete when it is time to leave hospital, impacting on goal pursuit and goal adaption (Brands et al. 2014). Although it has been shown that continued rehabilitation after discharge during the first year after stroke reduces the risk of disability, only very few clinical trials have been conducted in this field. Therefore, many of the recommendations for treatment in this field are weak, and investment in research in this area is essential.

Improving the access to timely and effective rehabilitation is a crucial point for stroke patients. Access to timely and individualized rehabilitation should be available to all stroke patients, through development of stroke units linked with rehabilitation services matched to patient needs, from community-based early supported discharge up to comprehensive inpatient rehabilitation units.

To address the complex disabilities arising from stroke, an interdisciplinary group of professionals with complementary skills is essential. Team composition and size may vary in different settings. Core disciplines in most stroke rehabilitation units include neurology and rehabilitation medicine, nursing, occupational therapy (OT), physiotherapy (PT), speech and language therapy (SLT) and case management/social work. (Teasell et al. 2016b). While frequently not available, a neuropsychologist would be important to integrate in teams given the high prevalence of cognitive and emotional disorders post-stroke and their relevance for disability (Ayerbe et al. 2013; Wagle et al. 2011).

Strasser (Strasser et al. 2005, 2008) demonstrated relations between team processes—how a team deals with coordinating and communicating its work, and the attitudes and perceptions expressed by its members—and patient outcomes. If patients were treated by more structured teams that made greater use of patient outcome data, patients experienced greater functional gains. Regular meetings to discuss patients' progress and plan treatment are the main process by which multidisciplinary teams operate and coordinate. Tyson developed—and subsequently tested—a framework of features for successful team meetings, including pre-meeting preparation of participants, setting an agenda, skilled chairing, using a structured documentation and the formal use of standardized measurement tools. Following implementation, all aspects of meeting quality improved by 5%–58% without loss of staff productivity or additional resources. In a longitudinal follow-up design, they found a greater increase in Barthel Index score after implementation, indicating greater functional recovery (Tyson et al. 2014a, 2015) (Fig. 1).

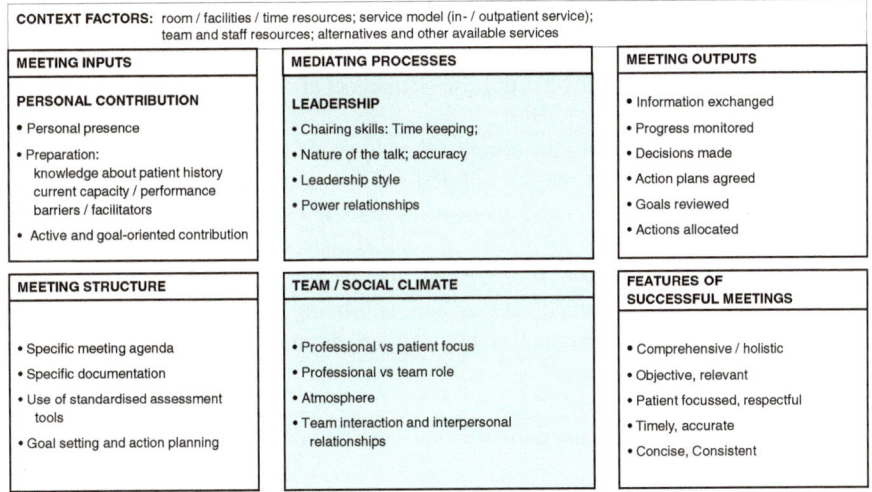

Fig. 1 Conceptual framework for multidisciplinary team meetings in stroke rehabilitation. (Modified from Tyson et al. 2014a)

3.3   The Chronic Care Model for Stroke Patients

From an international perspective, the paradigm shift is leading to the transformation of health care and illustrates one or perhaps the most applied strategy for improving the quality of care for people with chronic conditions such as many brain disorders which is the Multimorbidity Chronic Care Model (Palmer et al. 2018). This care model is of particular interest for the management of stroke and its high complexity. This complexity must be better understood if people's needs are to be properly addressed. The EU joint action JA-CHRODIS (2013–16) identified best practices and effective interventions for management of chronic diseases and developed this Multimorbidity Chronic Care Model (MCCM). To develop it, first, the five components from the Chronic Care Model (Wagner 1998) and the Innovative Care for Chronic Conditions Model (Epping-Jordan et al. 2004) were identified: self-management support; delivery system design; decision support; clinical information systems and interaction with community partners. The aim of MCCM is to meet patient's needs and transform daily care for patients with chronic diseases from a system that is essentially reactive—responding mainly when a person is sick—to one that is proactive and focused on patient-oriented care. It is designed to accomplish these goals through a combination of effective team care and planned interactions with the patients; self-management support; patient registries and other supportive information technology such as digital solutions allowing better exchange of information.

These elements are designed to work together to strengthen the healthcare providers–patient relationship and improve health outcomes. MCCM could be the model for better stroke patients' management and care and summarizes the basic elements for improving care in health systems at the community, organization, practice and patient levels.

Another important concept for the organization of care is emerging with the principle of 'patient-centred care': a person living with stroke has needs that evolve according to the stage of his/her disease (Brands et al. 2012, 2014):

- biological needs (mainly the relief of the physical symptoms, as pain),
- psychological needs (need for tailored information, e.g. on treatment options, evolution of the disease; and need for psychological support to deal with emotions such as fear, frustration, depression and distress),
- need and implementation of care plans may be an additional support to coordinate medical care, paramedical care and well-being,
- ongoing support in areas such as housing, employment, social relationships and community participation.

The reorganization of care delivery requires a paradigm shift and the adoption of three intertwined principles, namely: patient-centred care, improved hospital efficiency and interventions in an optimal setting, either in hospitals, at home or in communities. All these developments underpin the need to address the integration between the different healthcare providers and the different settings.

Efforts to empower stroke patients to be engaged in responding to their health needs may improve health outcomes, adherence to treatment and has the potential for patients to make more informed decisions with regard to their health.

By overcoming fragmentation and by creating linkages between services along the full continuum of care improved quality, continuity and efficiency in the delivery of services may be realized and ultimately improved health outcomes secured.

In stroke rehabilitation, a holistic view on functioning and disability of the individual beyond impairments is necessary to establish an individualized and comprehensive treatment program. Information on personal factors such as education, work and employment, recreation and leisure as well as information on environment such as housing, support and relationship should be available to all members of the interdisciplinary team responsible for the patient. Furthermore, a capacity check in different areas of interest, such as swallowing, mobility, self-care and interpersonal interactions, is necessary for setting goals and planning appropriate interventions.

The World Health Organization's *International Classification of Functioning, Disability and Health* (ICF) (WHO 2001) based on an integrative model of health provides a holistic, multidimensional and interdisciplinary understanding of health and health-related conditions. According to the ICF, the problems associated with a disease may concern *body functions* and *body structures* and *activities and participation* in life situations. Health states and the development of disability are modified by contextual factors, including environmental factors and personal factors, these latter not classified in the ICF.

Increasingly, countries are enhancing their data about functioning and disability using the ICF. The ICF is an international standard for health and disability information—key for collecting valid, reliable and comparable health and disability data. To be a standard for harmonization and comparability, however, the ICF has to be applied consistently around the world by all users. Therefore, the aims and rationale of the ICF, and the specific skills needed to use it, must be taught in an accessible and standardized manner (Raggi et al. 2010; Tempest et al. 2012, 2013).

The ICF comprises 1424 categories from the components: *body functions*, *body structures*, *activities and participation* and *environmental factors*, which are organized in a hierarchical structure (Fig. 2). Categories are divided into chapters, which constitute the first level of specification. High-level categories (e.g. second, third or fourth level) are more detailed.

An ICF category is coded by the component letter and a suffix of 1 to 5 digits. The letters **b, s, d** and **e** refer to the components: *body functions* (b), *body structures* (s), *activities and participation* (d) and *environmental factors* (e). This letter is followed by a one-digit number indicating the chapter, the code for the second level (2 digits), and the codes for the third and fourth levels (1 digit each). The component letter with the suffixes of 1, 3, 4 or 5 digits corresponds to the code of the ICF categories. Within each component, the categories are arranged in a stem/branch/leaf scheme. This scheme indicates that a more detailed, high-level category covers all the aspects applicable for the low-level category, of which it is a member, but not vice versa. Numerous reports on the use of the ICF have been published both in theoretical and clinical context (Cerniauskaite et al. 2011; Maribo et al. 2016). There is a trend towards development of ICF-based assessment tools through identification of relevant categories. The most common ICF-derived generic assessment

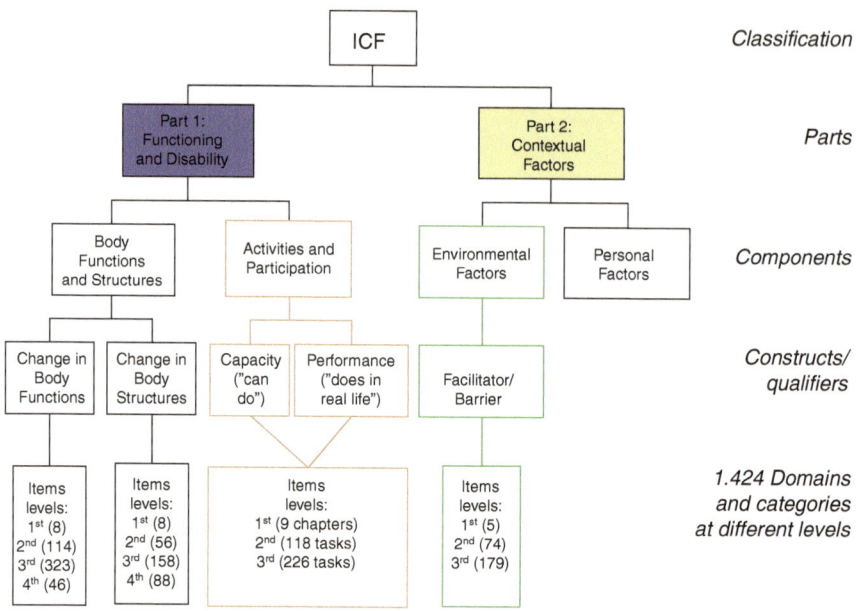

Fig. 2 Structure of the World Health Organization's International Classification of Functioning, Disability and Health (ICF)

tool is the WHO DAS 2.0 Disability Assessment Schedule (Ustun et al. 2010; Garin et al. 2010; Schlote et al. 2009). For stroke, a disease-specific core set was released in 2004 (Geyh et al. 2004).

4 ICF-Based Common Language in Reporting and Documentation Along the Care Pathway of Stroke Patients

Using the ICF as the common language to describe clinical findings at different time points and between different specialists makes it easy to establish a shared reporting system avoiding ambiguities and inconsistencies arising from sectoral reports (i.e. 'transferring oneself' might be labelled as 'mild activity limitation' by one and 'moderate activity limitation' by another team member). Here it is noteworthy to separate description of clinical findings from description of interventions, which arise as a consequence to findings at different time points. A classification of interventions is currently under development by WHO to provide a common tool for reporting and analysing health interventions for statistical purposes. The International Classification of Health Interventions (ICHI) is built around three axes: Target (the entity on which the action is carried out), Action (a deed done by an actor to a target) and Means (the processes and methods by which the action is carried out) (WHO 2017).

Establishing such a shared reporting system is helpful to monitor progresses from admission to discharge travelling through milestones (in terms of progress or setbacks) in a reasonable way minimizing reporting efforts. Prior to that, a common understanding on reasons for and content of reporting as well as a common understanding of the basic concepts of the framework should have been elaborated within the rehabilitation team (Raggi et al. 2010; Tempest et al. 2012, 2013). Having achieved an agreement on individual responsibilities for reporting, a shared ICF-based documentation system can be established easily, fulfilling all legal requirements for traceability.

4.1   ICF-Based Scales and Assessments

Standardized measurement tools support and inform clinical decision-making and communication with others (Tyson et al. 2010; Rosewilliam et al. 2011; Brown et al. 2013; Plant et al. 2016). Also, feedback on progresses to patients and relatives are much more likely to be understood if standardized assessments are used (Tyson et al. 2014b; Levack et al. 2015). To enhance comparability of health information collected in different settings, linking rules are available to serve as a basis for evidence-based decision-making across all levels of health systems (Cieza et al. 2004, 2016). The Academy for Neurologic Physiotherapy (ANPT) published a review on a total of 54 outcome measures in the ICF categories. Most of them are linked to body function (mostly musculoskeletal and sensation) and Mobility and Self-Care Activities and participation codes (ANPT 2015).

4.2   ICF-Based Goal Setting

In a systematic review of the ICF, Yen and colleagues found benefits for integrating the ICF into goal-setting practice. They concluded that the use of the ICF in healthcare goal-setting provides clinicians and patients with specific steps to follow when attempting to set goals collaboratively (Yen et al. 2014).

5   Theoretical Background in Goal-Setting Practice

5.1   Goal-Setting Theory (Locke and Latham)

According to goal-setting theory, three types of goals are to be distinguished: outcome goals (winning), performance goals (doing well by your own standards) and process-oriented or learning goals (learning skills for improving performance). This triad, originally developed in sports, might also be useful in rehabilitation.

- **Outcome goals** play an important role, where goal attainment depends on the performance of competitors. Within the context of neurorehabilitation, this type of goals has not been investigated so far but might play a role in group settings when patients compare among themselves.

- **Performance goals** prompt individuals to use routines or strategies that they have previously acquired and which are effective in performing the task. Individual ability is a key factor, and key questions are: How often, how well, under which circumstances will you act?
- In contrast, **process/learning/mastery goals** frame the goal instructions in terms of knowledge or skill acquisition (e.g. discover effective strategies to cope with impairments). Consequently, a learning goal draws attention away from a specific end result towards discovering and acquiring appropriate strategies, processes or procedures necessary to perform a given task. The key questions are: How will you achieve it? What can you do?

Stretch goals are intentionally set at levels that are 'seemingly unattainable with present resources'. Stretch goals have been used in business units as a supplement to 'required' or 'minimally acceptable' goals. Their purpose is to stimulate creative, 'outside-the-box' thinking with the intent to generate new ideas for improving business units' performance. (Kerr and Lepelley 2013). In the context of neurorehabilitation, stretch goals may not be applicable for individual goal setting but for team development. Furthermore, if individuals self-set their goals at an unrealistic level, it might be helpful to label them as *stretch goals* and put in relation individuals' importance with experts' views of difficulty to achieve this stretch goal, alongside a number of sub-goals including goals related to 'perceiving and appreciating individual's task capacity/performance' and 'managing risk behaviour'. Furthermore, it will be helpful to establish a commitment on short-time sub-goals, which mediate the relationship between actual performance and self-efficacy.

Already in 1967, Locke has demonstrated a clear linear relationship between the degree of goal difficulty and performance, if set within the limit of the individual's ability. This has been confirmed in several studies since then. (Locke and Latham 2002). Goal setting was found to have a greater positive effect on tasks that were straightforward (uncomplicated and easy to do) and on tasks that people already had the knowledge and skills to perform well.

Approach-oriented goal statements ('mind obstacles') induce self-efficacy and search-for-information behaviour, whereas avoidance-oriented goal statements ('avoid falls') are associated with reduced goal adherence (Wood et al. 2013). Furthermore, a positive relationship between goal specificity, goal importance and goal commitment has been demonstrated. Therefore, wording of goals and instructions might impact on goal commitment and adherence. Here, the acronym: RUMBA (relevant, understandable, measurable, behavioural, achievable) has turned out to be an appropriate mnemonic (Braun et al. 2010).

5.2   Goal Setting and Action Planning (Scobbie)

Scobbie et al. (2011, 2013) developed and implemented theory-based Goal setting and Action Planning framework (G-AP, Fig. 3) suitable for in-patient and community-based stroke rehabilitation. The framework is based on three main pillars: the Goal-Setting Theory (Locke and Latham 1990, 2013a), the Social Cognitive Theory (Bandura 2010, 2013) and the Health Action Process Approach (Sniehotta et al. 2005, 2016).

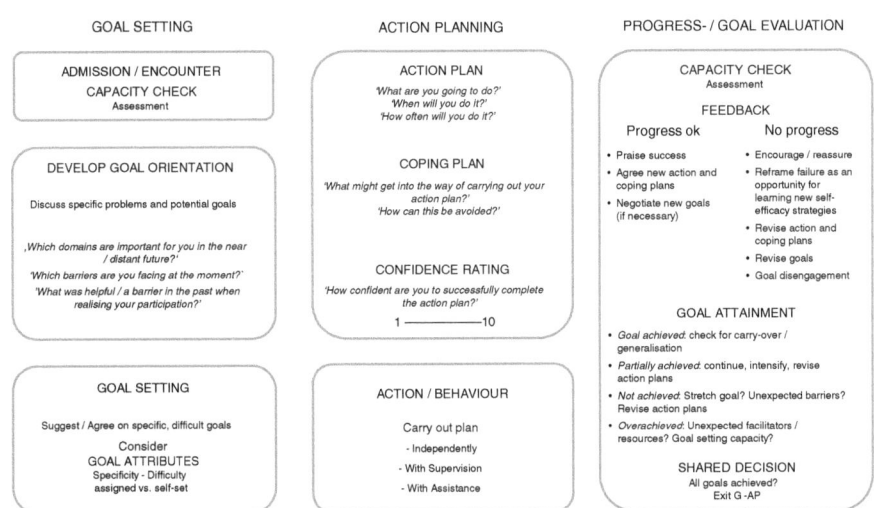

Fig. 3 Goal setting—action planning framework. (Modified from Scobbie et al. 2011)

The framework starts with a capacity check in relevant life domains (with/without assistance/devices) to identify a baseline level and develop possible goal intentions. Here, the beneficial effects of legitimate authorities/experts and a supportive leadership must not be underestimated (Locke and Latham 2013b). Nevertheless, active engagement of the stroke survivors in goal setting and treatment planning appears to be a central factor for developing self-management skills and for social participation after stroke (Woodman et al. 2014).

Having established specific, attractive, difficult and agreed goals, the next step—setting up action plans and reviewing coping strategies with respect to individual's confidence to accomplish a task successfully—forces us to think about treatment strategies which patients are likely to follow. To optimize self-regulation, planning has proven useful (Sniehotta et al. 2005). This planning can be divided into two sub constructs serving different purposes. The first sub construct, action planning, specifies the intended action in terms of when, where, and how to act (implementing intentions to act). The second sub construct, coping planning, refers to coping strategies to prioritize the intended behaviour over the habitual responses when obstacles or barriers are faced.

Successful engagement in everyday activities is influenced by feedback from others, usually accepted persons such as family, friends and experts. Cianci and colleagues found that healthy individuals with learning goal instructions performed better after negative feedback but worse after positive feedback, whereas performance declined when negative feedback was combined with performance goals (Cianci et al. 2010).

Feedback also has affective consequences. Individuals feel joy or disappointment based in part on feedback regarding their success or failure to attain a goal. As feedback represents attention from a (usually accepted) person in the environment, a social component may also play an important role. Simply knowing that someone cares and is attending to the individual's progress may motivate him or her (Ashford and de Stobbeleir 2013).

5.3 Goal Achievement and Goal Attainment Scaling

Outcome measurement is required to determine the effectiveness of rehabilitation interventions. Goal achievement has been considered to be an important outcome measure (Hurn et al. 2006). It depends on two things: the patient's ability to achieve their goals and the clinician's ability to predict outcome, which requires knowledge and experience (Turner-Stokes 2009). Within the G-AP framework, evaluation of goal achievement (appraisal and feedback) is a distinct and important intervention aiming to enhance self-efficacy and set the basis for (guided) self-management, marking the transition from 'therapy' (receptive) to 'training' (active, self-set).

If goals are 'achieved as expected', interventions usually come to an end and patients should have gained a higher level of independence. If goals are 'partially achieved', further treatment and/or changes of action plans might be required. Goals will be 'not achieved', if individuals (self-)set their goals at an unrealistic level. Allowing difficult stretch goals alongside, 'realistic' goals during goal negotiation might be helpful to increase insight into and acceptance of limited recovery.

One way of quantifying the achievement of goals for statistical and research purposes beyond simply recording achievement as a 'pass' or 'fail' is through goal attainment scaling (Kiresuk and Sherman 1968). Goal attainment scaling (GAS) is a method of scoring the extent to which patient's individual goals are achieved in the course of intervention. When using goal attainment scaling, tasks are individually identified and set around current and expected levels of performance. In effect, each individual has its own outcome measure, but this is scored in a standardized way as to allow statistical analysis. (Turner-Stokes 2009). If goal performance at baseline is rated −1 (some activities, could worsen), an initial T-score around 35–40 (depending on the number of goals) will result. If all goals are achieved as expected (rating 0), a T-score of 50 will be achieved. An overachievement of goals leads to a value above, an under or partial achievement below 50.

Concerns about GAS have been raised about non-linearity of the scaling and lack of uni-dimensionality (Tennant 2007). Multiple variations on the original GAS approach have been published such as using a different number of levels of goal achievement (from −3 to +3) (Turner-Stokes and Williams 2010) and a different scoring system than was originally proposed, involving greater patient participation in goal selection and having the treating therapist rather than an independent third-party select and re-evaluate the GAS goals (Cytrynbaum et al. 1979; Turner-Stokes 2009). Finally, there is no agreed approach to goal setting (McPherson et al. 2014; Wade 2009). Some authors have proposed the development of standardized goals or 'item banks'. (Tennant 2007). Nevertheless, there is growing evidence that goal attainment scaling is a good person-centred outcome measure for rehabilitation (Hurn et al. 2006; Ashford and Turner-Stokes 2006; Turner-Stokes et al. 2009), although GAS is not a measure of outcome per se, but a measure of achievement of intention. It depends on the quality of goal setting as well as on the quality of treatment. Hence, it does not replace standardized measures at the moment until validity of GAS has been demonstrated by studies investigating correlations with standardized measures. Finally, important but difficult (stretch)goals likely to be 'not achieved' will lead to lower T-scores, if counted. Therefore, no added value arises from calculating individual T-scores in clinical practice, as patients and clinicians prefer words to numbers.

5.4   Examples on ICF-Based Goal Setting

ICF-based goal statements usually denominate a task/an action (what?) followed by modifiers describing circumstances (how?) for successfully accomplishing the task (such as time, number repetitions and contextual factors such as aids and devices, assistance).

In early phases of stroke rehabilitation, gaining or improving functioning and establishing independence is in the center of all attempts (Wood et al. 2010). In ICF terminology, most relevant goals are about mobility (d4) and self-care (d5). After discharge home, stroke survivors are confronted with the remaining impairments of several body function impacting on their usual activities (d6 domestic life, d7 interactions and relations and d9 social and civic life). Usually these areas are not very likely to be covered by initial goal setting, such is not 'handling stress and other psychological demands' (d240). Especially in persons with several impairments causing severe disability, goals related to interactions and relations such as 'making/holding eye contact—for a few minutes in quiet/lively environment' or 'signalling discomfort/agreement/dissent—spontaneously/after being asked...' are very useful to guide caregivers and the team to work towards the same goal. The classification of environmental factors allows also to define what facilitates or hinders the functioning of the patients.

Currently, only a few attempts have been made to develop standardized goals or 'item banks'. Here, the ICF offers an agreed framework for goal areas, which easily can be adopted for individual goal setting. Examples are given in Table 1.

6   Goal Setting in Stroke Patients in Practice

In a Cochrane review on goal setting and strategies to enhance goal pursuit in neuro-rehabilitation, Levack et al. (2015) found 39 studies published before December 2013, involving a total of 2846 participants receiving rehabilitation in a variety of countries and clinical situations. They identified at least 12 different approaches to goal setting with a lot of variations regarding goal identification, selection, prioritizing, goal characteristics, the use for intervention planning, etc. Yet, they identified two common features in goal setting: having measurable goals and involving patients in goal setting. The review found an increase in health-related quality of life or self-reported emotional status (8 studies, 446 participants; standardized mean

Table 1 ICF-based goal examples—setting up a goal agreement document

d1	Learning and applying knowledge	Context (how?)
	Observing obstacles	Spontaneous/on advice/in quiet/lively environment—Despite hemianopia/neglect…
	Observing the left side of space	Spontaneous/on advice/in quiet/lively environment—Despite hemianopia/neglect…
	Recognising danger (at home)	Spontaneous/after feedback/with cues/under supervision …
	Recognising own capabilities (potential)	With regard to … Spontaneous/after feedback/with support …
	Focussing attention up to … mins	In in quiet/lively environment/with distractors…
	Solving (simple/complex) problems	Spontaneous/with advice/feedback/assistance …
	Taking decisions regarding …	Spontaneous/with advice/feedback/assistance …
	…	
d2	General tasks and demands	Context (how?)
	Using means of orientation, memory, …	Spontaneous/with advice/cues/assistance …
	Using swallowing strategies (chin down…)	Spontaneous/with advice/cues/assistance …
	Performing stretching/strengthening exercises	Spontaneous/with advice/cues/assistance …
	Planning and conducting daily routine	Independently/with assistance/considering own level of resources…
	Taking breaks before overtiredness, pain attacks	Spontaneous/with advice/cues/assistance …
	Using pain control strategies (breathing, muscle relaxation, …)	Spontaneous/with advice/cues/assistance …
	Fixing wheelchair brakes before standing up	Spontaneous/with advice/cues/assistance …
	…	
d3	Communication	Context (how?)
	Understanding short/long messages	After first hearing/after one repetition/in quiet/lively environment …
	Starting/sustaining/ending a conversation with one person/several persons	Spontaneously, about familiar/current topics; with/without help from communication partner …
	Participating in a conversation with (more than) one person(s)	With - w/o help from a familiar partner/despite word finding difficulties
	Communicating ones needs and wishes	Verbally/with gestures/by signing/writing …
	Using communication devices (e.g. phone, text, emails …)	Independently/with the help of a familiar person in a protected environment
	…	

Table 1 (continued)

d4	Mobility	Context (how?)
	Getting out of bed; standing up; sitting down...	Independently/with a rail/supervised/guided/with help of (un-)skilled person...
	Sitting, standing, squatting, kneeling	For # mins., independently/holding on a rail/supervised/with help of (un-)skilled person... With additional activity, in quiet/lively environment
	Getting up from the floor	Spontaneously, without help, with layperson's/professional help, ...
	Walking in house/out of the house/for short – Long distance	Independently/with an orthosis/cane/wheeled walker Supervised/with help of (un-)skilled person... On slopes, on grass/snow/gravel ...
	Grasping, lifting and carrying objects such as a pencil/a coin/a glass/...	With one hand/both hands; up to ... kg, while sitting/standing ...
	Opening water bottles	With both hands, despite reduced strength, with eye-hand-control ...
	Manipulating small objects such as coins, needles, buttons, ...	With both hands, spontaneously, after instruction ....
	...	
d5	Self-care	Context (how?)
	Washing face/arm/chest/legs/oneself	Independently/prepared utensils/final control/supervised/guided/with help of (un-) skilled person, in adequate time/in customized/unexperienced environment...
	Dressing oneself	Independently/prepared clothes/final control/supervised/guided/with help of (un-) skilled person, in adequate time/in customized/unexperienced environment...
	Showering/bathing	Independently, prepared utensils ...
	Brushing one's teeth, combing, shaving ...	Independently, prepared utensils ...
	Eating/drinking (food/drink consistency to be defined according level of functioning)	Independently/supervised/with help of (un-)skilled person; with -w/o swallowing strategy, adapted cutlery, drinking straw; ...
	Taking care for the paretic arm	Independently/with reminder/supervised/guided In customized /unexperienced environment...
	Taking one's medicine	Independently/with reminder/supervision/help...
	...	
d6	Domestic life	Context (how?)
	Shopping	With a shopping list, by using an 'aphasia id', independently/supervised/with the help of ...,
	Preparing simple/complex meals	Independently/supervised/with the help of ..., By using aids such as ..., in adequate time ....
	Cleaning the kitchen/the bath/... Using a vacuum cleaner ...	Independently/supervised/with the help of ..., By using aids such as ..., in adequate time ....
	Washing/drying one's clothes/hanging up clothes/ironing	Independently/with reminder/supervision/help...
	Carrying out garden work (using a shovel/rake/shears ...)	For ... mins./taking pauses after .... mins., Independently/with reminder/supervision/help...
	Looking after the (grand-)children, animals...	For ... hours, ...
	....	

(continued)

Table 1 (continued)

d7	Interpersonal interactions and relationships	Context (how?)
	Making eye contact/holding eye contact	For ... mins., in quiet/lively environment, after having been told ...
	Signalling discomfort/agreement/dissent...	Spontaneously/after having been asked, ...
	Showing respect/warmth/appreciation (to familiar/unknown persons, in a group of peers, ...)	Spontaneously, with cues, on advice, with (un-) structured feedback, with help...
	Maintaining social distance (gender related, in a group of peers, towards staff members...)	Spontaneously, with cues, on advice, with (un-) structured feedback, with help...
	Accepting help (for walking/eating/toileting ...)	Spontaneously, with cues, on advice, with (un-) structured feedback, ...
	Sticking to agreements/rules (regarding walking/eating/toileting ...)	Spontaneously, with cues, on advice, with (un-) structured feedback, ...
	Getting in touch/maintain contact with peers (Parkinson, Aphasia, MS ...)	After preparation, with an escort, ...
	...	
d8	**Major life areas**	**Context (how?)**
	Working on a computer	Independently, for ... mins., with adapted keyboard, in quiet/noisy environment ...
	Conducting voluntary work	For up to # hrs/week, with guidance/supervision/help of ...
	Taking part in a professional retraining course	Independently/with help, ...
	Paying one's bills	Independently/with the help of ...,
	Conducting one's bank affairs	Independently/with the help of ...,
	...	
d9	**Community, social and civic life**	**Context (how?)**
	Participating in family/social life	Spontaneously/with help, for ... hrs/day, with familiar people/strangers, ...
	Visiting friends	...
	Playing cards/chess/boards games ...	Independently, with familiar people, ...
	Going swimming/horse riding/climbing/cycling ...	Independently/with help, regularly, ...
	Voting in elections	Independently ...
	....	

First column: to denominate goal agreement status (agreed with patient/relatives/significant others)
Second column: to denominate the task/action (what task?)
Third column: to denominate the context/circumstances (how will it work?)
Fourth column: level of goal attainment at date of follow-up (achieved—partially—not achieved—overachieved) (not included here)

difference (SMD) 0.53, 95% confidence interval (CI) 0.17 to 0.88; quality of evidence very low) and self-efficacy (3 studies, 108 participants; SMD 1.07, 95% CI 0.64 to 1.49; quality of evidence very low) when some form of goal setting (plus or minus strategies to enhance goal pursuit) was used in comparison to no goal setting. No consistent evidence was found that goal setting impacts on impairments. There was insufficient information whether goal setting increases or reduces the risk of adverse events or justifies additional costs for goal setting and action planning. Because of the variety of approaches to studying goal setting in rehabilitation and because of limitations in the design of many studies completed to date, the authors expect that 'it is very possible that future studies could change the conclusions of this review' (Levack et al. 2015).

Two reviews of goal setting within the context of stroke rehabilitation concluded that active patient participation in goal setting appeared to be something that patients value and that structured methods of goal setting seem to increase patients' perceptions of their level of involvement in clinical decision-making (i.e. enhancing a sense of self-determination); however, the effects of a patient-centred goal-setting practice in stroke rehabilitation have been studied mostly with weak methodologies (Rosewilliam et al. 2011; Sugavanam et al. 2013).

Plant and colleagues reviewed barriers and facilitators to goal setting during stroke rehabilitation. Nine qualitative papers were selected, involving 202 participants in total: 88 patients, 89 healthcare professionals and 25 relatives of participating patients (Plant et al. 2016). The main barriers to goal setting during stroke rehabilitation were: a mismatch between patients' and staff's perspective; lack of confidence by the staff to manage patient expectations; patients' stroke-related impairments and lack of time and ineffective organizational systems. The main facilitators were: early, frequent, active communication with patient and family; individually tailoring the goal-setting process; effective, confident and encouraging staff; education of patients and families; providing support and educational materials and adequate resources. They concluded that current methods of goal setting during stroke rehabilitation are not fit for purpose.

7 Recommendations for Multidisciplinary Team Approach and ICF-Based Goal Setting in Stroke Rehabilitation

If possible, stroke rehabilitation should be delivered by interdisciplinary teams with specific training and experience in the field (level of evidence 1a, quality of evidence moderate, B+).

The early rehabilitation process after stroke should be initiated in a stroke units (level of evidence 1a, quality of evidence moderate, B+).

Since the rehabilitation process after stroke will rarely be complete when it is time to leave hospital, rehabilitation should be continued after discharge especially during the first year after stroke to reduce the risk of disability and may individually be needed at later stages (level of evidence 5, quality of evidence very low, B+ [clinical relevance]0).

For delivering high-quality healthcare for stroke survivors, the integration (in contrast with fragmentation) of care providers (e.g. specialists, general practitioners and other healthcare providers such as pharmacists, nurses, psychologists, physiotherapists) and close coordination (multidisciplinary care) of their activities across levels of care and multiple sites is warranted, all of which can be optimally embedded within a system that promotes patient empowerment (level of evidence 5, quality of evidence very low, 0).

Heightened attention should be spent to evaluate team processes related to assessing/reporting of clinical findings and to goal setting and action planning processes. This includes to review the structure of team meetings, encourage the use of standardized measurement tools and assessments for clinical status and progress monitoring and the explicit method used for goal setting and action planning. (Level of evidence 2b, quality of evidence low, B+ [clinical relevance]).

All domains, including the body functions and structures (impairment), the activity and participation as well as the environmental factors domain of the ICF, can be used as a common language for professionals when setting goals in a semi-structured, 'guided' manner. Using the main ICF activity and participation domain as broad goal categories will prevent from missing important goal areas, such as, interactions and relations and social and civic life. (Level of evidence 5, quality of evidence very low, 0).

Heightened attention can be spent to the goal syntax (starting with a verb, denominating a task, followed by modifiers, denominating the circumstances to accomplish the task). Patient's perceptions/appraisal of goal importance, goal difficulty, self-efficacy and emotional stability can be checked, as they will mainly impact on individual goal choice and ranking and how to avoid goal conflicts. Evaluation of goal achievement (appraisal and feedback) can be used as a distinct and important intervention aiming to enhance self-efficacy and set the basis for (guided) self-management, marking the transition from 'therapy' (receptive) to 'training' (active, self-set). (Level of evidence 5, quality of evidence very low, 0).

8   Summary

Here, we highlight the importance of developing a common understanding of the basic concepts for reporting clinical findings at different time points and in the different setting of the care pathways as well as for goal setting using the ICF and its biopsychosocial model as an agreed language and framework.

Overcoming fragmentation by a person-centred approach in line with the Multimorbidity Chronic Care Model supports a fact-based identification of individual goals to be pursued and reached in each specific phase of the care and rehabilitation process. Goal setting and action planning processes are described alongside the underlying theoretical assumptions.

Goal setting has become a central component of effective rehabilitation practice, both as a part of the communication and decision-making process and as a person-centred outcome measure for stroke rehabilitation. The evidence regarding the individual contribution of specific components of the goal setting process (e.g. levels of patient involvement, levels of goal difficulty) remains inconclusive. Therefore, agreed standards on goal setting and evaluation are still lacking and current methods of goal setting in stroke rehabilitation are still quite arbitrary. This chapter provides the rationale for a more organized process along all the care pathway of stroke patients, from acute event to social reintegration and inclusion, having an ICF-based methodology that will allow the definition of all the steps.

Translating the evidence from the huge research body on goal-setting theory into clinical practice will lead to a higher impact and a more structured approach in utilizing the power of individual goal setting and action planning in the future.

References

ANPT (2015) ANPT outcome measures recommendations (EDGE) [online]. Academy of Neurologic Physical Therapy, Alexandria, VA. http://www.neuropt.org/professional-resources/. Accessed 14 Jan 2019

Ashford SJ, de Stobbeleir KEM (2013) Feedback, goal setting, and task performance revisited. In: Locke EA, Latham GP (eds) New developments in goal setting and task performance, 1st edn. Routledge, New York, London

Ashford S, Turner-Stokes L (2006) Goal attainment for spasticity management using botulinum toxin. Physiother Res Int 11:24–34

Ayerbe L, Ayis S, Wolfe CD, Rudd AG (2013) Natural history, predictors and outcomes of depression after stroke: systematic review and meta-analysis. Br J Psychiatry. 202(1):14–21. https://doi.org/10.1192/bjp.bp.111.107664.

Bandura A (2010) Self-efficacy: the exercise of control. Freeman, New York

Bandura A (2013) The role of self-efficacy in goal-based motivation. In: Locke EA, Latham GP (eds) New developments in goal setting and task performance, 1st edn. Routledge, New York, London

Brands IM, Wade DT, Stapert SZ, Van Heugten CM (2012) The adaptation process following acute onset disability: an interactive two-dimensional approach applied to acquired brain injury. Clin Rehabil 26:840–852

Brands I, Stapert S, Kohler S, Wade D, Van Heugten C (2014) Life goal attainment in the adaptation process after acquired brain injury: the influence of self-efficacy and of flexibility and tenacity in goal pursuit. Clin Rehabil 29:611–622

Braun JP, Mende H, Bause H, Bloos F, Geldner G, Kastrup M, Kuhlen R, Markewitz A, Martin J, Quintel M, Steinmeier-Bauer K, Waydhas C, Spies C, NEQUI (2010) Quality indicators in intensive care medicine: why? Use or burden for the intensivist. Ger Med Sci 8:Doc22

Brown M, Levack W, McPherson KM, Dean SG, Reed K, Weatherall M, Taylor WJ (2013) Survival, momentum, and things that make me "me": patients' perceptions of goal setting after stroke. Disabil Rehabil 36:1020–1026

Cerniauskaite M, Quintas R, Boldt C, Raggi A, Cieza A, Bickenbach JE, Leonardi M (2011) Systematic literature review on ICF from 2001 to 2009: its use, implementation and operationalisation. Disabil Rehabil 33:281–309

Cianci AM, Schaubroeck JM, Mcgill GA (2010) Achievement goals, feedback, and task performance. Hum Perform 23:131–154

Cieza A, Ewert T, Ustun TB, Chatterji S, Kostanjsek N, Stucki G (2004) Development of ICF core sets for patients with chronic conditions. J Rehabil Med:9–11

Cieza A, Fayed N, Bickenbach J, Prodinger B (2016) Refinements of the ICF linking rules to strengthen their potential for establishing comparability of health information. Disabil Rehabil:1–10

Cytrynbaum S, Ginath Y, Birdwell J, Brandt L (1979) Goal attainment scaling:a critical review. Eval Q 3:5–40

Epping-Jordan JE, Pruitt SD, Bengoa R, Wagner EH (2004) Improving the quality of health care for chronic conditions. Qual Saf Health Care 13:299–305

Garin O, Ayuso-Mateos J, Almansa J, Nieto M, Chatterji S, Vilagut G, Alonso J, Cieza A, Svetskova O, Burger H, Racca V, Francescutti C, Vieta E, Kostanjsek N, Raggi A, Leonardi M, Ferrer M, CONSORTIUM, M (2010) Validation of the "World Health Organization disability assessment schedule, WHODAS-2" in patients with chronic diseases. Health Qual Life Outcomes 8:51

Geyh S, Cieza A, Schouten J, Dickson H, Frommelt P, Omar Z, Kostanjsek N, Ring H, Stucki G (2004) ICF core sets for stroke. J Rehabil Med:135–141

Hurn J, Kneebone I, Cropley M (2006) Goal setting as an outcome measure: a systematic review. Clin Rehabil 20:756–772

Kerr S, Lepelley D (2013) Stretch goals: risks, possibilities, and best practices. In: Locke EA, Latham GP (eds) New developments in goal setting and task performance, 1st edn. Routledge, New York, London

Kiresuk TJ, Sherman RE (1968) Goal attainment scaling: a general method for evaluating comprehensive community mental health programs. Community Ment Health J 4:443–453

Levack WM, Weatherall M, Hay-Smith EJ, Dean SG, McPherson K, Siegert RJ (2015) Goal setting and strategies to enhance goal pursuit for adults with acquired disability participating in rehabilitation. Cochrane Database Syst Rev 7:CD009727

Locke EA, Latham GP (1990) A theory of goal setting & task performance. Prentice Hall, Englewood Cliffs, NJ

Locke EA, Latham GP (2002) Building a practically useful theory of goal setting and task motivation. A 35-year odyssey. Am Psychol 57:705–717

Locke EA, Latham GP (2013a) Goal setting theory: the current state. In: Locke EA, Latham GP (eds) New developments in goal setting and task performance, 1st edn. Routledge, New York, London

Locke EA, Latham GP (2013b) New developments in goal setting and task performance. London, Routledge, New York

Maribo T, Petersen KS, Handberg C, Melchiorsen H, Momsen AM, Nielsen CV, Leonardi M, Labriola M (2016) Systematic literature review on ICF from 2001 to 2013 in the Nordic countries focusing on clinical and rehabilitation context. J Clin Med Res 8:1–9

McPherson K, Kayes N, Kersten P (2014) MEANING as a smarter approach to goals in rehabilitation. In: Siegert RJ, Levack WMM (eds) Rehabilitation goal setting: theory, practice and evidence. Taylor & Francis Group, London

Oxford Centre for Evidence-Based Medicine (2009). Levels of Evidence (March 2009). Centre for Evidence-Based Medicine. https://www.cebm.ox.ac.uk/resources/levels-of-evidence/oxford-centre-for-evidence-based-medicine-levels-of-evidence-march-2009. Accessed 20.09.2020.

Palmer K, Marengoni A, Forjaz MJ, Jureviciene E, Laatikainen T, Mammarella F, Muth C, Navickas R, Prados-Torres A, Rijken M, Rothe U, Souchet L, Valderas J, Vontetsianos T, Zaletel J, Onder G, Joint Action on Chronic, D. & Promoting Healthy Ageing Across the life, C (2018) Multimorbidity care model: recommendations from the consensus meeting of the joint action on chronic diseases and Promoting healthy ageing across the life cycle (JA-CHRODIS). Health Policy 122:4–11

Plant SE, Tyson SF, Kirk S, Parsons J (2016) What are the barriers and facilitators to goal-setting during rehabilitation for stroke and other acquired brain injuries? A systematic review and meta-synthesis. Clin Rehabil 30:921–930

Platz T (2017). Practice guidelines in neurorehabilitation. Neurology International Open. 1(3): E148–E152. https://doi.org/110.1055/s-0043-103057

Raggi A, Leonardi M, Cabello M, Bickenbach JE (2010) Application of ICF in clinical settings across Europe. Disabil Rehabil 32(Suppl 1):S17–S22

Rosewilliam S, Roskell CA, Pandyan AD (2011) A systematic review and synthesis of the quantitative and qualitative evidence behind patient-centred goal setting in stroke rehabilitation. Clin Rehabil 25:501–514

Schlote A, Richter M, Wunderlich MT, Poppendick U, Möller C, Schwelm K, Wallesch CW (2009) WHODAS II with people after stroke and their relatives. Disabil Rehabil 31:855–864

Schünemann H, Brożek J, Guyatt G, Oxman A, editors (2013) GRADE handbook for grading quality of evidence and strength of recommendations. Updated October 2013. The GRADE Working Group. Available from www.guidelinedevelopment.org/handbook

Scobbie L, Dixon D, Wyke S (2011) Goal setting and action planning in the rehabilitation setting: developed and implemented a theory-based Goal setting and Action Planning framework. Clin Rehabil 25:468–482

Scobbie L et al (2013) Implementing a framework for goal setting in community based stroke rehabilitation: a process evaluation. BMC Health Serv Res 13(1):190

Sniehotta FF, Schwarzer R, Scholz U, Schüz B (2005) Action planning and coping planning for long-term lifestyle change: theory and assessment. Eur J Soc Psychol 35:565–576

Sniehotta FF, Presseau J, Allan J, Araujo-Soares V (2016) "you Can't always get what you want": a novel research paradigm to explore the relationship between multiple intentions and behaviours. Appl Psychol Health Well Being 8(2):258–275

Strasser DC, Falconer JA, Herrin JS, Bowen SE, Stevens AB, Uomoto J (2005) Team functioning and patient outcomes in stroke rehabilitation. Arch Phys Med Rehabil 86:403–409

Strasser DC, Falconer JA, Stevens AB, Uomoto JM, Herrin J, Bowen SE, Burridge AB (2008) Team training and stroke rehabilitation outcomes: a cluster randomized trial. Arch Phys Med Rehabil 89:10–15

Stroke Unit Trialists C (2013) Organised inpatient (stroke unit) care for stroke. Cochrane Database Syst Rev 2013(9):CD000197

Sugavanam T, Mead G, Bulley C, Donaghy M, Van Wijck F (2013) The effects and experiences of goal setting in stroke rehabilitation—a systematic review. Disabil Rehabil 35:177–190

Teasell R, Hussein N (2016) Background concepts in stroke rehabilitation. In: Teasell R, Foley N, Hussein N, Speechley M (eds) Evidence-based review of stroke rehabilitation, 17th edn. London, Ontario, Canada, Sockit Solutions

Teasell R, Foley N, Hussein N, Cotoi A (2016a) The efficacy of stroke rehabilitation. In: Teasell R, Richardson M, Allen L, Hussein N (eds) Evidence-based review of stroke rehabilitation, 17th edn. London, Sockit Solutions

Teasell R, Foley N, Hussein N, Speechley M (2016b) The elements of stroke rehabilitation. In: Teasell R, Foley N, Hussein N, Speechley M (eds) Evidence-based review of stroke rehabilitation, 17th edn. London, Ontario, Canada, Sockit Solutions

Tempest S, Harries P, Kilbride C, De Souza L (2012) To adopt is to adapt: the process of implementing the ICF with an acute stroke multidisciplinary team in England. Disabil Rehabil 34:1686–1694

Tempest S, Harries P, Kilbride C, De Souza L (2013) Enhanced clarity and holism: the outcome of implementing the ICF with an acute stroke multidisciplinary team in England. Disabil Rehabil 35:1921–1925

Tennant A (2007) Goal attainment scaling: current methodological challenges. Disabil Rehabil 29:1583–1588

Turner-Stokes L (2009) Goal attainment scaling (GAS) in rehabilitation: a practical guide. Clin Rehabil 23:362–370

Turner-Stokes L, Williams H (2010) Goal attainment scaling: a direct comparison of alternative rating methods. Clin Rehabil 24:66–73

Turner-Stokes L, Williams H, Johnson J (2009) Goal attainment scaling: does it provide added value as a person-centred measure for evaluation of outcome in neurorehabilitation following acquired brain injury? J Rehabil Med 41:528–535

Tyson S, Greenhalgh J, Long AF, Flynn R (2010) The use of measurement tools in clinical practice: an observational study of neurorehabilitation. Clin Rehabil 24:74–81

Tyson SF, Burton L, McGovern A (2014a) Multi-disciplinary team meetings in stroke rehabilitation: an observation study and conceptual framework. Clin Rehabil 28:1237–1247

Tyson SF, Burton LJ, McGovern A, Sharifi S (2014b) Service users' views of the assessment process in stroke rehabilitation. Clin Rehabil 28:824–831

Tyson SF, Burton L, McGovern A (2015) The effect of a structured model for stroke rehabilitation multi-disciplinary team meetings on functional recovery and productivity: a phase I/II proof of concept study. Clin Rehabil 29:920–925

UN (2007) Convention on the rights of persons with disabilities and optional protocol. United Nations, New York

Ustun TB, Chatterji S, Kostanjsek N, Rehm J, Kennedy C, Epping-Jordan J, Saxena S, Von Korff M, Pull C, Project, W. N. J (2010) Developing the World Health Organization disability assessment schedule 2.0. Bull World Health Organ 88:815–823

Wade DT (2009) Goal setting in rehabilitation: an overview of what, why and how. Clin Rehabil 23:291–295

Wagner EH (1998) Chronic disease management: what will it take to improve care for chronic illness? Eff Clin Pract 1:2–4

Wagle J, Farner L, Flekkøy K, Wyller T, Sandvik L, Fure B, et al (2011). Early post-stroke cognition in stroke rehabilitation patients predicts functional outcome at 13 months. Dementia and geriatric cognitive disorders 31;379–387. https://doi.org/10.1159/000328970

WHO (2001) International classification of functioning, disability and health: ICF. World Health Organization, Geneva

WHO (2017) International Classification of Health Interventions (ICHI) - Beta [online]. World Health Organisation (WHO), Geneva. http://www.who.int/classifications/ichi/en/. Accessed 11 Dec 2018

WHO & UNESCO (2010) Community-based rehabilitation: CBR guidelines. World Health Organization, Geneva

Wood JP, Connelly DM, Maly MR (2010) 'Getting back to real living': a qualitative study of the process of community reintegration after stroke. Clin Rehabil 24:1045–1056

Wood RE, Whelan J, Sojo V, Wong M (2013) Goals, goal orientations, strategies, and performance. In: Locke EA, Latham GP (eds) New developments in goal setting and task performance, 1st edn. Routledge, New York, London

Woodman P, Riazi A, Pereira C, Jones F (2014) Social participation post stroke: a meta-ethnographic review of the experiences and views of community-dwelling stroke survivors. Disabil Rehabil 36:2031–2043

Yen T-H, Liou T-H, Chang K-H, Wu N-N, Chou L-C, Chen H-C (2014) Systematic review of ICF core set from 2001 to 2012. Disabil Rehabil 36:177–184

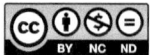

Disorders of Consciousness

Caterina Pistarini and Giorgio Maggioni

1   Introduction

Consciousness is defined as the state of awareness of the self and environment with appropriate arousal or wakefulness (Giacino et al. 2018a, b). Disorders of Consciousness (DoC) are a wide spectrum of correlates of brain's disruptions of arousal and awareness that may result from altered functional neural activities from cortico-cortical connectivity to subcortico-cortical and global connectivity of all networks such as default mode network (DMN) and others (Giacino et al. 2014; Hodelìn-Tablada 2016).

The mentioned neural networks that define consciousness are primarily assessed by clinical means (i.e., scale like CRS-r—Coma Recovery Scale revised) to detect patient's behavior and capability to have and show conscious experience; these are the only validated means, while some critics recently arose (Bayne et al. 2017; Seel et al. 2010).

Arousal is clinically assessed by evidence of eye opening and brain stem reflexes and is defined by a spectrum of conditions from sleep to complete wakefulness.

Awareness may be clinically evaluated by the examination of motor and communication behaviors assessing visual pursuit, localization to noxious stimulation, command following, intelligible verbalization, and object recognition in order to define the perceiving of the external environment and the voluntary interaction with it (Laureys et al. 2004).

C. Pistarini
Department of NeuroRehabilitation Medicine,
ICS Maugeri SB, Institute of Genova Nervi, Genoa, GE, Italy
e-mail: caterina.pistarini@icsmaugeri.it

G. Maggioni (✉)
NeuroRehabilitation Unit, Department of NeuroRehabilitation Medicine,
IRCCS ICS Maugeri Veruno SB, Institute of Veruno, Gattico-Veruno, NO, Italy
e-mail: giorgio.maggioni@icsmaugeri.it

© The Author(s) 2021   57
T. Platz (ed.), *Clinical Pathways in Stroke Rehabilitation*,
https://doi.org/10.1007/978-3-030-58505-1_4

Perturbations of arousal and awareness depict different clinical syndromes of DoC including coma, different sleep stages, drug anesthesia, vegetative state, minimally conscious state, and emerging state (Blume et al. 2015).

Coma, defined by the absence of arousal and consciousness, sleep stages and drug-induced alterations are not at center of our interest while we refer to the other mentioned syndromes on a rehabilitation point of view.

DoC are defined on the basis of assessment of motor and communication behaviors; a coma lasting more than 28 days may lead to different DoC, starting from vegetative state (VS) or otherwise named "unresponsive wakeful syndrome" (UWS): in this case, patients are unaware but awake showing eye opening (both spontaneously or induced) and reflexive movements (Giacino et al. 2018a, b; Laureys et al. 2010).

In case the VS (UWS) clinical condition will last more than 1 month, it should be classified as "persistent" and not as "permanent."

When patients show voluntary behavior, usually beginning with visual pursuit, they are in the clinical condition of the minimally conscious state (MCS) with inconsistent but reproducible behavior demonstrating awareness of external or internal world (Giacino et al. 2014).

Recently, the complexity of behavioral responses allows to classify MCS patients in "plus or minus" (MCS −/MCS +): in the first case, patients show interactions with external environment only through motor behavior and in the latter also some preserved language function. Any functional object use or evidence of accurate and functional communication will define the emerging state from MCS (EMCS) (Bruno et al. 2011; Giacino et al. 2014).

We refer to Table 1 and to the cited articles for detailed description of DoC conditions.

Table 1 Different features of clinical presentation of DoC (adapted from: Eapen et al. 2017; Giacino et al. 2014)

	Sleep–wake cycle	Arousal	Awareness	Motor purposeful behavior[a]	Preserved language function[b]
Coma	Absent	Absent	Absent	Absent/ reflexives	Absent
VS/UWS	Present, altered, intermittent	Present	Absent	Absent/ reflexives	Absent
MCS−	Present	Present	Present	Present	Absent
MCS+	Present	Present	Present	Present	Present
Emerging state	Present	Present	Present	Present	Present: Reliable communication; use of functional object

[a]Motor purposeful behavior: visual pursuit, localization to noxious stimulation, simple command following
[b]Preserved language function: intelligible verbalization, object recognition, command following

While the definition and our understanding of the pathomechanisms of DoC improved in recent years, we are still facing the difficulty of correct diagnosis and related procedures such as appropriate assessment of awareness and alertness and partially as a consequence have limited valid evidence regarding beneficial treatment options including rehabilitation or medication (Bender et al. 2015; Bodien et al. 2017).

Recent data on the annual incidence of VS/UWS in the US is 4200 persons/year with reported prevalence rates ranging from 5000 to 42,000 (112,000–280,000 for MCS); while prevalence on a world basis of UWS/VS is 0.2–6.1/100,000 inhabitants (Giacino et al. 2018a, b; Van Erp et al. 2014).

The repeatedly cited 42% rate of misdiagnosis is now decreasing to a 37% minimum but has yet to be precisely defined (Bender et al. 2015; Peterson et al. 2015; Wade 2018).

In fact, the proper means and clinical algorithm to perform a correct diagnosis of UWS/VS and MCS are still a matter of debate (Giacino et al. 2013).

Nontraumatic coma (NTC) is primarily caused by stroke (6–54%) when compared to post-anoxic or metabolic injuries; but it is still difficult to describe DoC while the patients is in the acute hospital ward and only the presence of a coma lasting more than 28 days may depict the consciousness impairment as a steady disorder such as UWS/VS or MCS and not as a transient event (Woimant et al. 2014).

The available literature relates to either traumatic (TBI) or nontraumatic (nTBI) DoC mainly. Few studies consider cerebrovascular accidents (CVA) specifically and fewer discriminate cerebral infarction, parenchymal hemorrhage, and subarachnoidal bleeding; a recent systematic review could not describe more precisely DoC in stroke alone (Horsting et al. 2015).

Evidence is lacking regarding diagnosis and natural history in nTBI MCS patients while four studies with nTBI VS patients note a survival rate of 80% on average (95% confidence interval, 95% CI "67% to 93%") at 3 months (Hannawi et al. 2015; Horsting et al. 2015; Kondziella et al. 2016; O'Donnel et al. 2019). Little is known about any differentiation between CVA, cardiac arrest, and metabolic DoC.

While a systematic approach to the rehabilitation of DoC exists since almost 30 years, many problems related to clinical diagnosing, assessments, and treatment remain unsolved (De Tanti et al. 2015; Kondziella et al. 2016; Giacino et al. 2018a, b). As one example, the use of the reliable and valid assessment tools is essential to properly define the clinical pattern, to plan the care process adequately, and ensure a precise prognosis (Di Perri et al. 2014; Eapen et al. 2017; Giacino et al. 2014).

This chapter reviews the available evidences regarding DoC after a stroke and as a whole.

Topics for our evidence synthesis and practice recommendations are: (1) DoC assessment including technical diagnostic tools and clinical assessments; (2) general DoC rehabilitation; (3) specific DoC treatment options including drug therapy, technology-based treatment, music therapy, surgical therapies, and noninvasive brain stimulation (NIBS).

2   Methods

We systematically searched for guidelines, reviews, and clinical trials that provide evidence and clinical decision guidance for DoC assessment including technical diagnostic tools and clinical assessments; general DoC rehabilitation; or specific DoC treatment options. Exclusion criteria were: non-English papers, commentaries, case series, case reports, book chapters, and conference reports.

We, in January 2019, searched for articles published from 1997 to January 2019 in the PubMed, Cochrane Library using medical subject heading (MeSH) keywords and the search algorithm "(rehabilitation OR stroke OR cerebral hemorrhage OR cerebral infarction) AND (disorders of consciousness OR persistent vegetative state OR vegetative state OR minimally conscious state)," and in the EMBASE via the EMTREE with following keywords and algorithm "(Cerebrovascular accident) AND (disorders of consciousness OR persistent vegetative state OR vegetative state OR minimally conscious state)."

We found a total of 862 articles: two independent raters screened the 862 articles, solving disagreement by discussion.

Systematic reviews ($n = 11$), nonsystematic reviews ($n = 13$), RCT ($N = 2$), observational studies ($N = 12$) were selected together with two guidelines for full-text review to critically appraise and collate the evidence, to rate the overall quality of evidences, and to provide recommendations.

Two clinical evidence and practice guidelines (GL) were found (De Tanti et al. 2015; Giacino et al. 2018a, b).

The level of evidence used for recommendations was categorized according to the Oxford Centre for Evidence-Based Medicine Levels of Evidence (CEBM, 2009 version).

Further, the quality of the evidence was rated with four categories according to "GRADE" ("Grades of Recommendation, Assessment, Development, and Evaluation") (Owens et al. 2010):

- High quality: further research is unlikely to affect our confidence in the estimation of the (therapeutic) effect;
- Medium quality: further research is likely to affect our confidence in the estimation of the (therapeutic) effect and may alter the estimate;
- Low quality: further research will most likely influence our confidence in the estimation of the (therapeutic) effect and will probably change the estimate;
- Very low quality: any estimation of the (therapy) effect or prognosis is very uncertain.
- The grading of the recommendations was performed in accordance with GRADE with the categories "ought to" (A) (strong recommendation), "should" (B) (weak recommendation) (Schünemann et al. 2013). As a third category had been introduced "can" (0) (option) (Platz 2017).

3   DoC Assessment: Clinical Behavioral and Instrumental Diagnostic Tools

3.1   Clinicals and Behavioral Tools for DoC Assessments

A systematic review of the main assessment behavioral means for clinical practice identified 13 DoC scales and reported on their inter-rater reliability (IRR), internal consistency (IC), and test–retest reliability (TRR) qualities (Seel et al. 2010).

Authors of this review also studied other features of assessment scales such as existent guidelines for their application, their power to detect DoC, i.e., VS and MCS, to differentiate between the two syndromes and their feasibility to be used in clinical practice. Considered scales were: the Coma Recovery Scale-revised (CRS-r), Sensory Stimulation Assessment Measure (SSAM), Wessex Head Injury Matrix (WHIM), Western Neuro Sensory Stimulation Profile (WNSSP), Sensory Modality Assessment Technique (SMART), Disorders of Consciousness Scale (DoC), Coma/Near-Coma Scale (CNC), Full Outline of UnResponsiveness Score (FOUR), Comprehensive Levels of Consciousness Scale (CLOCS), Innsbruck Coma Scale (INNS), Glasgow-Liege Coma Scale (GLS), Loewenstein Communication Scale (LOEW), and the Swedish Reaction Level Scale-1985 (RLS85).

CRS-r was considered superior to the other scales while review states that many unproven features still remain; in Table 2 are summarized diagnostic features of all mentioned scales.

Overall diagnostic validity of the assessment scales was unproven; in particular, the prognostic and the diagnostic validity of CRS-r are not proven. The only scale with a good predictive power for good recovery at 30 days was FOUR (Wolf et al. 2007). Systematic review conducted to define the American Academy of Neurology guidelines found little evidences with no recommendation possible: a study considered 43 patients and found CRS-r as an independent predictor of recovery with wide CIs limit (95% CI "1.05 to 11643.58") of interpretation (Estraneo et al. 2013; Luauté et al. 2010).

Recommendation:

Clinical assessment of DoC, i.e., VS and MCS should be performed with standardized assessment tools in patients with prolonged DoC (CEBM classification: level 1a, GRADE moderate; recommendation B+). The CRS-r appears to have advantages concerning its psychometric properties; its use is suggested (CEBM classification: level 1a, GRADE moderate; recommendation B+).

3.2   Instrumental Diagnostic Tools for DoC Assessment

One systematic review (SR), following established recommendations for conducting SR including Preferred Reporting Items for Systematic review and Meta-Analysis protocols (PRISMA) and checklist for SR such as the Quality Assessment

Table 2 Summary of clinical features evidence for DoC behavioral assessment scales (adapted from Seel et al. 2010)

Scales	Standardization of Scoring	Content Validity	Reliability—IC	Reliability—IRR	Reliability—TRR	Criterion/Construct validity	Diagnostic validity	Prognostic validity
CRS-r	Acceptable	Excellent	Good—Class 1a	Good—Class 2b	Excellent—Class 3a	Unproven	Unproven	Unproven
SMART	Acceptable	Good	Na	Excellent—Class 2c	Excellent—Class 2b	Unproven	Unproven	Unproven
WNSSP	Acceptable	Good	Excellent—Class 2b	Unproven	Unproven	Unproven	Unproven	Unproven
SSAM	Acceptable	Good	Unproven	Unproven	Unproven	Unproven	Unproven	Unproven
WHIM	Acceptable	Good	Unproven	Unproven	Unproven	Unproven	Unproven	Unproven
DOCS	Acceptable	Acceptable	Good—Class 2b	Unproven	Unproven	Construct valid—Class 2b	Unproven	Unproven
CNC	Acceptable	Acceptable	Unacceptable	Unproven	Unproven	Unproven	Unproven	Unproven
CLOCS	Unacceptable	Acceptable	Good—Class 2b	Unproven	Unproven	Strong—Class 3b	Unproven	Unproven
LOEW	Unacceptable	Acceptable	Unproven	Excellent—Class 2b	Unproven	Unproven	Unproven	Unproven
RLS85	Unacceptable	Acceptable	Na	Unproven	Unproven	Strong—Class 3b	Unproven	Unproven
FOUR	Unacceptable	Unacceptable	Excellent—Multiple class 1b	Good—Class 2b	Unproven	Unproven	Unproven	Probably not predictive—Class 1b
INNS	Unacceptable	Unacceptable	Acceptable—Class 1b	Unproven	Unproven	Unproven	Unproven	Possibly not predictive—Class 3b
GLS	Unacceptable	Unacceptable	Unproven	Unacceptable	Unproven	Unproven	Unproven	Possibly predictive—Class 3b

Abbreviations: multiple class are stated in accordance to the CEBM levels following the Oxford Centre for Evidence-Based Medicine Levels of Evidence (CEBM, 2009 version) of Diagnostic Accuracy Studies-2 (QUADAS-2), analyzed the usefulness of neurophysiological recordings to assess DoC patients, focusing on electroencephalography (EEG), electromyography (EMG), Event-related Potentials (ERP), and Mismatch Negativity (MMN) (Hauger et al. 2017; Kable et al. 2012; Mother et al. 2015).

Results in this SR are not conclusive: specificity rates of different methods were highly variable from 0% to 100%, with a high rate of false-positive classifications. Two studies report a rate of 17% and 33% of false-positive classifications of UWS instead of MCS (King et al. 2013; Sitt et al. 2014).

An SR and meta-analysis considered 20 clinical studies with a total sample of 470 MCS patients and 436 VS patients studied with quantitative method EEG (qEEG), ERP, functional magnetic resonance imaging (fMRI): qEEG showed the highest sensitivity (90% on average; 95% CI "69% to 97%") and high specificity (80% on average with 95% CI "66% to 90%") compared to ERP and fMRI; the sensitivity of fMRI was 44% on average (95% "CI 19% to 72%") and specificity 67% on average (95% CI "55% to 77%"), while the sensitivity of ERP was 59% on average (95% CI "26% to 85%") and specificity 75% on average (95% CI "51% to 90%") (Bender et al. 2015).

A third SR included 36 studies with 687 patients (10.3% with ischemic stroke and 6.6% with intracerebral hemorrhage and 2.7% with subarachnoid hemorrhage) studied with fMRI, fluorodeoxyglucose (FDG)-positron emission tomography (PET), single-photon emission computed tomography (SPECT) with different tracers (Hannawi et al. 2015). These approaches could detect reduced activity in several brain areas and may be useful in clinical DoC diagnosis, in particular considering modifications of the Default Mode Network (DMN); but the heterogeneity observed in study results and the meta-analysis conducted in 13 studies (272 patients and 259 controls) showed that the small number of studies that reported increased functional connectivity limited the importance of results with little support in clinical practice (Hannawi et al. 2015).

An SR included 1041 patients from 44 originals articles (54.1% VS and 45.9% MCS; 25% of all DoC patients had CVA) to study EEG, fMRI (ERP were excluded in this SR) to detect consciousness with active and passive paradigms such as the cortical functional connectivity or resting-state studies, and on same sample of patients a meta-analysis was performed on 37 studies: researchers failed to indicate a diagnostic superiority for the analysis of active and passive paradigms considering both command–no command following and cortical–no cortical connectivity on an fMRI motor imagery task to distinguish MCS and VS compared to EEG: Odds ratio (OR) of EEG versus fMRI were 0.73 (95% CI "0.50 to 1.07") in the active paradigms and 1.78 (95% CI "1.16 to 2.74") in the passive paradigms; the authors concluded that EEG protocols were two times more likely to be interpreted as compatible with preserved consciousness compared to fMRI (Kondziella et al. 2016).

A study on EEG mainly showed that MCS patients had less abnormal EEG findings (61%, 95% CI "41% to 78%") compared to VS patients (25%, 95% CI "7% to 59%") with a sensitivity for MCS diagnosis of 61% (95% CI "39% to 80%") (Casarotto et al. 2016).

There is, however, no evidence available to support EEG as a diagnostic tool to distinguishing VS from MCS on an individual basis.

There is insufficient evidence that electromyography (EMG) may support the diagnostic value of the presence of EMG activity to a command: a study considered 38 DoC patients and in only one VS patient and three MCS patients an EMG response to command was found (sensitivity for MCS 21%, 95% CI "5% to 51%", and specificity 90% 95% CI "56% to 100%") (Habbal et al. 2014).

In conclusion, the accuracy in diagnostic approach of neurophysiological and other technical tools is limited. (1) EEG evaluation seems to be the best method, with good balance between rates for sensitivity and specificity; (2) ERP may help to detect reactivity to few sensory stimuli; (3) fMRI may be useful to specifically study the activity of different functional networks; and (4) EMG may be only of little help to distinguish MCS from VS patients with reference to voluntary movements.

Recommendation:

Assessment of DOC with qEEG can be performed in patients with prolonged DOC as a supplementary diagnostic approach (CEBM classification: level 1, GRADE moderate; recommendation 0). For all other approaches, i.e., EMG, ERP, and fMRI the evidence is too weak to give a recommendation for their routine diagnostic use in prolonged DOCs (CEBM classification: level 1, GRADE moderate).

---

4   DoC Rehabilitation

The complex approach of rehabilitation for DoC patients, though it is highly recommended, is difficult to appraise critically. There are only very few randomized controlled trials (RCT) available.

RCTs are of course difficult to perform in DoC patients because of the control groups required, long-lasting follow-up, little acceptance to participate while caregivers are easily reluctant to consent to trials limiting treatment options if not as "last option" that might induce a lack of valid samples for studies (Giacino et al. 2013).

A small number of studies have evaluated issues related to the early rehabilitation phase of DoC (Pistarini and Maggioni 2018). Seel made, based on a single-center retrospective study, six recommendations for a better ER management but little evidences arise (Seel et al. 2013). Authors studied data on CRS-r scale scores pre–post rehabilitation and discharge disposition in a sample of 210 patients with DoC (VS and MCS) and 53% of patients showed at least one or more signs of emergence into full consciousness (26% emerged from MCS in 2 CRS-r criteria and 27% in 1 of CRS-r criteria (Seel et al. 2013).

Rehabilitation methods used range from stretching exercises, postures (early mobilization/verticalization), splinting, casting, range of motion mobilization, but no RCT studied them. Only case studies, observational studies, and nonsystematic reviews are available (Giacino et al. 2013).

Previous systematic and nonsystematic reviews stated that structured sensory stimulation could not positively be recommended, if it was to be based on relevant clinical evidence (Georgiopoulos et al. 2010; Lombardi et al. 2002).

One systematic review retrieved 157 articles with 18 studies investigating MCS/VS patients with spasticity (Martens et al. 2017). Three prospective studies reported an occurrence of spasticity in DoC patients. Six articles focused only on spasticity treatments as primary outcome: 2 were clinical trials, 2 case reports, and last 2 were reviews. The rehabilitation methods studied were splinting and acupuncture, but no outcome differences were elicited when comparing splinting to physiotherapy sessions, and the hypothesis of decreasing overexcitability in muscle hypertonia induced by acupuncture is not yet validated (Thibaut et al. 2015).

Available treatments for spasticity range from the use of drugs such as phenol, botulinum toxin, baclofen, tizanidine, dantrolene sodium, diazepam to physical treatments, in particular passive range of motion and stretching, splinting orthoses, casting, positioning, to surgical approaches such as intrathecal baclofen therapy and selective posterior rhizotomy. All available studies show little evidences of efficacy with a low-GRADE quality scoring. Other nine reports (2 clinical trials, 1 open-label study, 4 case reports, and 2 reviews) observed and studied spasticity treatments as secondary outcome, including deep brain stimulation to induce Cortical Activation by Thalamic Stimulation (CATS) and intrathecal baclofen (ITB) pump: no RCT among all selected studies are existing (Magrassi et al. 2016; Margetis et al. 2014). All studies analyzed could not depict any evidence for differential treatment effects.

While no evidence is available to support specific forms of rehabilitation treatment in DoC patients, the experience from clinical practice indicates that an interdisciplinary rehabilitation approach that addresses the various therapeutic needs of DoC patients should be stated as early as possible and continued for a reasonable time to promote functional recovery including recovery of arousal and awareness as well as of emerging motor and communication functions.

At a later stage, such interdisciplinary rehabilitation treatment might be repeated to reevaluate the potential for functional recovery.

Recommendation:

Complex interdisciplinary rehabilitation should be provided by a team experienced with patients with prolonged DOCs, started in an early phase, as soon as the clinical condition allows, with an individualized approach (CEBM classification: level 5, GRADE quality: very low [expert opinion], recommendation grade: B+). It should be continued for a reasonable time to ensure that a potential for gradual recovery has a chance to evolve under specialized treatment and might be repeated at later stages to reevaluate the potential for recovery (CEBM classification: level 5, GRADE quality: very low [expert opinion], recommendation grade: B+).

5 Pharmacological Therapies for DoC

Several drugs have been used in the therapy of patients with DoCs. Most frequently used were centrally acting drugs including dopamine and GABA agonists. Among the first mentioned class are bromocriptine, levodopa, and apomorphine. Most frequently used GABA agonists are zolpidem and baclofen (both oral and intrathecal—ITB). Among most used drugs are then amantadine and methylphenidate.

Studies on dopamine agonists either have considerable methodological restrictions or used very small samples; they often do not consider effects of spontaneous recovery and/or do not describe correctly clinical conditions with reference to comorbidities: neither results nor any suggestions may then be reported from those studies (Gosseries et al. 2014).

Only studies on amantadine report results that provide sufficient evidence for clinical decision-making. Specifically, an RCT compared the effects of a prescription of amantadine versus placebo over a treatment course of 4 weeks in 184 DoC (only traumatic DoC in VS-MCS) patients (Giacino et al. 2012).

The outcomes were disability measured with the Disability Rating Score scale (DRS) and clinical DOC assessment with the CRS-r.

Results showed a significantly faster recovery in the treatment group (mean difference 0.24 DRS point per week 95% CI "0.07% to 0.4%"). At 2 weeks, after washout, the difference decreased while remaining significant and at 6 weeks follow-up, the DRS scores were similar between control and treatment group with no significant difference (mean difference—0.7 DRS point per week 95% CI "−2 to 10.7"). No significant differences in result arose when considering the analysis of CRS-r.

Data available on zolpidem are conflicting. In a non-randomized, placebo-controlled trial only one out of 15 DoC (12 VS and 3 MCS) patient showed improvement in CRS-r scoring, being able to open her eyes sustainably (Whyte and Myers 2009).

All other studies reviewed are not of high quality (no RCT); while it has been reported in at least 6 studies and 23 clinical reports that zolpidem may induce EEG activation, may enhance BOLD signal in different brain regions, and activate metabolic and neuronal activity studied with PET scans, M-EEG, Magnetoencephalography, and MRI imaging, a clinically relevant beneficial therapeutic effect of zolpidem on DOC had not been shown with an appropriate clinical trial to address this question (Gosseries et al. 2014).

No RCTs are available on ITB: few clinical reports support that the use of ITB, mainly for spasticity treatment purposes, may facilitate recovery; these articles are mainly clinical reports on a small sample and do not provide sufficient evidence for clinical decision-making process (Francois et al. 2001; Shrestha et al. 2011; Thibaut et al. 2015).

Recommendation.

A course of amantadine treatment over a couple of weeks can be used in the beginning of the rehabilitation treatment of stroke survivors with DoC (VS-MCS) to promote recovery in the disability domain (CEBM classification: level 1b, GRADE quality: moderate, recommendation grade: 0 [indirectness of evidence]).

The evidence is too limited to guide clinical decision-making with respect to long-term use and discontinuation of amantadine, or the prescription of other drugs to treat DoC in stroke survivors.

6 Other Specific Therapies for DoC

One RCT enrolled 44 out of 50 initially considered patients with DoC (14 VS and 30 MCS) and analyzed the results from the use of a tilt table therapy compared to tilt therapy integrated with a stepping device (product Erigo® by Hocoma, Switzerland); both groups received 1 h sessions over a course of 3 weeks (Krewer et al. 2015).

The primary outcome was the improvement rate of CRS-r scores after treatment, and the secondary outcome was the difference in the Modified Ashworth Scale (MAS) again after treatment. Both control and treatment group improved, and the intervention effect for the stepping device was less when changes scores from baseline to week 6 were analyzed (median (25%–75% percentile): Erigo® 4 (−1–6); tilt table: 9 (5–10); U-Test = 122.0; $z = -2.824$, $p = 0.005$, $r = -0.42$). Changes in MAS scoring did not significantly differ between the two patient groups.

A case series investigated the effects on CRS-r scoring and electrophysiological criteria in response to the use of deep brain stimulation (DBS) in 21 VS patients with an increase odd of recovery (OR 88.0; 95% CI "5.4 to 1219.0") (Yamamoto et al. 2010). No control group was considered and the sample was very small.

Other specific therapies used to treat DoC that were investigated are music therapy, noninvasive brain stimulation (NIBS) such as 20 Hz repetitive transcranial magnetic stimulation (rTMS) and transcranial direct current stimulation (tDCS) (Bai et al. 2017; He et al. 2018; Rollnik and Altenmuller 2014).

Only clinical studies on a small sample basis are available. Few considerations are reported in nonsystematic reviews like the targeting of the left dorsolateral prefrontal cortex in DoC when using tDCS or rTMS, but no evidence that would be sufficient for clinical decision-making process (Hodelìn-Tablada 2016; Pignat et al. 2015).

Recommendation:

The evidence is too limited to guide clinical decision-making for therapies such as tilt therapy with integrated stepping device, rTMS, or tDCS when used with the intention to treat DoC in stroke survivors. Their use is discouraged for routine clinical practice with the therapeutic goal to improve DoC in stroke survivors (CEBM classification: level 4 to 1b, GRADE quality: very low to moderate, recommendation grade: B−).

References

Bai Y, Xia X, Kang J, Yang Y, He J, Li X (2017) TDCS modulates cortical excitability in patients with disorders of consciousness. NeuroImage Clin 15:702–709

Bayne T, How J, Owen AM (2017) Reforming the taxonomy in disorders of consciousness. Ann Neurol 82(6):866–872

Bender A, Jox RJ, Straube A, Lulé D (2015) Persistent vegetative state and minimally conscious state. A systematic review and meta-analysis of diagnostic procedures. Dtsch Arztebl Int 112:235–242

Blume C, del Giudice R, Wislowska M, Lechinger J, Schabus M (2015) Across the consciousness continuum—from unresponsive wakefulness to sleep. Front Hum Neurosci 9:105

Bodien YG, Chatelle C, Edlow BL (2017) Functional networks in disorders of consciousness. Semin Neurol 37(5):485–502

Bruno MA, Vanhaudenhuyse TA, Moonen G, Laureys S (2011) From unresponsive wakefulness to minimally conscious PLUS and functional locked-in syndromes: recent advances in our understanding of disorders of consciousness. J Neurol 258(7):1373–1384

Casarotto S, Comaducci A, Rosanova M (2016) Stratification of unresponsive patients by an independently validated index of brain complexity. Ann Neurol 80:718–729

De Tanti A, Zampolini M, Pregno S, on behalf of the CC3 Group (2015) Recommendations for clinical practice and research in severe brain injury in intensive rehabilitation: the Italian consensus conference. Eur J Rehabil Med 51:89–103

Di Perri C, Stender J, Laureys S, Gosseries O (2014) Functional neuroanatomy of disorders of consciousness. Epilepsy Behav 30:28–32

Eapen BC, Georgekutty J, Subbarao B, Bavishi S, Cifu DX (2017) Disorders of consciousness. Phys Med Rehabil Clin N Am 28:245–258

Estraneo A, Moretta P, Loreto V, Lanzillo B, Cozzolino A, Saltalamacchia A, Lullo F, Santoro L, Trojano L (2013) Predictors of recovery of responsiveness in prolonged anoxic vegetative state. Neurology 80:464–470

Francois B, Vacher P, Roustan J, Salle JY, Vidal J, Moreau JJ, Vignon P (2001) Intrathecal baclofen after traumatic brain injury: early treatment using a new technique to prevent spasticity. J Trauma 50:158–161

Georgiopoulos M, Katsakiori P, Kafalopoulou Z, Ellul J, Chroni E, Constantoyannis C (2010) Vegetative state and minimally conscious state: a review of the therapeutic interventions. Stereotact Funct Neurosurg 88:199–207

Giacino JT, Whyte J, Bagiella E, Kalmar K, Child N, Khademi A, Eifert B, Long D, Katz DI, Cho S, Yablon SA, Luther M, Hammond FM, Nordenbo A, Novak P, Mercer W, Maurer-Karattup S, Sherer M (2012) Placebo controlled trial of amantadine for severe traumatic brain injury. N Engl J Med 366:819–826

Giacino JT, Katz DI, Whyte J (2013) Neurorehabilitation in disorders of consciousness. Semin Neurol 33:142–156

Giacino JT, Fins JJ, Laureys S, Schiff ND (2014) Disorders of consciousness after acquired brain injury: the state of the science. Nat Rev Neurol 10(2):99–114

Giacino JT, Katz DI, Schiff ND, Whyte J, Ashman EJ, Ashwal S, Barbano R, Hammond F, Laureys S, Ling GSF, Nakase-Richardson R, Seel RT, Yabloon S, Getchius TSD, Gronseth GS, Armstrong MJ (2018a) Practice guideline update recommendations summary: disorders of consciousness. Neurology 91(10):450–460

Giacino JT, Katz DI, Schiff ND, Whyte J, Ashman EJ, Ashwal S, Barbano R, Hammond F, Laureys S, Ling GSF, Nakase-Richardson R, Seel RT, Yabloon S, Getchius TSD, Gronseth GS, Armstrong MJ (2018b) Comprehensive systematic review update summary: disorders of consciousness. Arch Phys Med Rehabil 99:1710–1719

Gosseries O, Charland-Verville V, Thonnard M, Bodard O, Laureys S, Demertzi D (2014) Amantadine, Apomorphine and Zolpidem in the treatment of disorders of consciousness. Curr Pharm Des 20:4167–4184

Habbal D, Gosseries O, Noirhomme Q (2014) Volitional electromyografic responses in disorders of consciousness. Brain Inj 28:1171–1179

Hannawi Y, Lindquist MA, Caffo BS, Sair HI, Stevens RD (2015) Resting brain activity in disorders of consciousness. A systematic review and meta-analysis. Neurology 84:1272–1280

Hauger SL, Schanke A-K, Andersson S, Chatelle C, Schnakers C, Løvstad M (2017) The clinical diagnostic utility of electrophysiological techniques in assessment of patients with disorders of consciousness following acquired brain injury: a systematic review. J Head Trauma Rehabil 32(3):185–196

He F, Wu M, Meng F, Hu Y, Gao J, Chen Z, Bao W, Liu K, Luo B, Pan G (2018) Effects of 20 Hz repetitive transcranial magnetic stimulation on disorders of consciousness: a resting-state electroencephalography study. Neural Plast 25:5036184

Hodelìn-Tablada R (2016) Minimally conscious state: evolution of concept, diagnosis and treatment. MEDICC Rev 18(4):43–46

Horsting MWB, Franken MD, Meulenbelt J, van Klei WA, de Lange DW (2015) The etiology and outcome of non-traumatic coma in critical care: a systematic review. BMC Anesthesiol 15:65

Kable AK, Pich J, Maslin-Prothero SE (2012) A structured approach to documenting a search strategy for publication: a 12-step guideline for authors. Nurse Educ Today 32(8):878–886

King J, Faugeras F, Gramfort A (2013) Single-trial decoding of auditory novelty responses facilitates the detection of residual consciousness. Neuroimage 83:726–738

Kondziella D, Friberg CK, Frokjaer VG, Fabricius M, Møller K (2016) Preserved consciousness in vegetative and minimal conscious states: systematic review and meta-analysis. J Neurol Neurosurg Psychiatry 87:485–492

Krewer C, Luther M, Koenig E, Müller F (2015) Tilt table therapies for patients with severe disorders of consciousness: a randomized, controlled trial. PLoS One 10(12):e0143180

Laureys S, Owen AM, Schiff ND (2004) Brain function in coma, vegetative state, and related disorders. Lancet Neurol 3(9):537–546

Laureys S, Celesia GG, Cohadon F, Lavrijsen J, Léon-Carrion J, Sanita WG, Sazbon L, Schmutzhard E, von Wil KR, Zeman A, Dolce G (2010) Unresponsive wakefulness syndrome: a new name for the vegetative state or apallic syndrome. BMC Med 8:68

Lombardi F, Taricco M, De Tanti A, Telaro E, Liberati A (2002) Sensory stimulation for brain injured individuals in coma or vegetative state. Cochrane Database Syst Rev 2002(2):CD001427

Luauté J, Maucort-Boulch D, Tell L (2010) Long-term outcomes of chronic minimally conscious and vegetative state. Neurology 75:246–252

Magrassi L, Maggioni G, Pistarini C, Di Perri C, Bastianelle S, Zippo AG, Iotti GA, Biella GE, Imberti R (2016) Results of a prospective study (CATS) on effects of talami stimulation in minimally conscious and vegetative state patients. J Neurosurg 125(4):972–981

Margetis K, Korfias SI, Gatzonis S, Boutos N, Stranjalis G, Boviatsis E, Sakas DE (2014) Intrathecal baclofen associated with improvements of consciousness disorders in spasticity patients. Neuromodulation 17:699–704

Martens G, Laureys S, Thibaut A (2017) Spasticity management in disorders of consciousness. Brain Sci 7(12):E162

Mother D, Shamseer L, Clarke M (2015) Preferred reporting items for systematic review and meta-analysis protocols (PRISMA-P). Syst Rev 4:1

Owens D, Lohr K, Atkins D, Treadwell JR, Reston JT, Bass EB, Chang S, Helfand M (2010) AHRQ Series Paper 5: Grading the strength of a body of evidence when comparing medical interventions: AHRQ and the Effective Health Care Program. J Clin Epidemiol 63: 513–523

O'Donnel JC, Browne KD, Kilbaugh TJ, Chen HI, Whyte J, Cullen DK (2019) Challenges and demand for modeling disorders of consciousness following traumatic brain injury. Neurosci Biobehav Rev 98:336–346

Peterson A, Cruse D, Naci L, Weijer C, Owen AM (2015) Risk, diagnostic error, and the clinical science of consciousness. NeuroImage Clin 7:588–597

Pignat JM, Johr J, Diserens K (2015) From disorders of consciousness to early Neurorehabilitation using assistive technologies in patients with severe brain injury. Curr Opin Neurol 28:587–594

Pistarini C, Maggioni G (2018) Early rehabilitation od disorders of consciousness (DOC): management, neuropsychological evaluation and treatment. Neuropsychol Rehabil 28(8): 1319–1330

Platz T (2017) Practice guidelines in neurorehabilitation. Neurol Int Open 01(03):E148–E152. https://doi.org/10.1055/s-0043-103057

Rollnik JD, Altenmuller E (2014) Music in disorders of consciousness. Front Neurosci 8:190

Schünemann H, Brożek J, Guyatt G, Oxman A (2013) GRADE handbook for grading quality of evidence and strength of recommendations. The GRADE Working Group. Updated October 2013. www.guidelinedevelopment.org/handbook

Seel TR, Sherer M, Whyte J, Katz DI, Giacino JT, Rosenbaum AM, Hammond FM, Kalmar K, Pape TLB, Zafonte R, Biester RC, Kaelin D, Kean J, Zaslr N (2010) Assessment scales for disorders of consciousness: evidence-based recommendations for clinical practice and research. Arch Phys Med Rehabil 91(12):1795–1813

Seel TR, Douglas J, Dennison AC, Heaner S, Harris K, Rogers C (2013) Specialized early treatment for persons with disorders of consciousness: program components and outcomes. Arch Phys Med Rehabil 94(10):1908–1923

Shrestha P, Malla H, Pant B, Taira T (2011) Intrathecal baclofen therapy in severe brain injury, first time in Nepal, a technique suitable for underdeveloped countries. Asian J Neurosurg 6:49–51

Sitt JD, King JR, Karoui IEI (2014) Large scale screening of neural signature of consciousness in patients in a vegetative state or minimally conscious state. Brain J Neurol 137(8):2258–2270

Thibaut A, Deltombe T, Wannez S, Gosseries O, Ziegler E, Dieni C, Deroy M, Laureys S (2015) Impact of soft splints on upper limb spasticity in chronic patients with disorders of consciousness: a randomized single-blind, controller trial. Brain Inj 29:830–836

Van Erp WS, Lavrijsen JCM, van de Laar FA, Vos PE, Laureys S, Koopmans RTCM (2014) The vegetative state/unresponsive wakefulness syndrome: a systematic review of prevalence studies. Eur J Neurol 21(11):1361–1368

Wade DT (2018) How often is the diagnosis of the permanent vegetative state incorrect? A review of the evidence. Eur J Neurol 25:619–625

Whyte J, Myers R (2009) Incidence of clinically significant responses to zolpidem among patients with disorders of consciousness: a preliminary placebo-controlled trial. Am J Phys Med Rehabil 88(5):410–418

Woimant F, Biteye Y, Chaine P, Crozier S (2014) Severe stroke: which medicine for which results? Annales Francaises d'Anesthésie et de Réanimation 33:102–109

Wolf CA, Wijdicks EFM, Bamlet WR, McClelland RL (2007) Further validation of the FOUR score coma scale by intensive care nurses. Mayo Clin Proc 82:435–438

Yamamoto T, Katayama Y, Kobayashi K, Oshima H, Fukaya C, Tsubokawa T (2010) Deep brain stimulation for the treatment of vegetative state. Eur J Neurosci 32(7):1145–1151

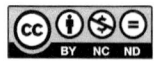

Airway and Ventilation Management

Marcus Pohl and Mervyn Singer

1 Introduction

More patients with severe neurological deficits are surviving because of improvements in the management of stroke, traumatic brain injury, resuscitation, and sepsis. Advances in neurology and neurosurgery enable survival for many patients with malignant ischemic stroke (when more than two-thirds of the area supplied by a cerebral artery is affected), intracerebral haemorrhage, or other intracranial masses. These patients are often so severely affected that they require mechanical ventilation and cannot be successfully weaned from ventilation during their stay at the acute admitting hospital (Rollnik et al. 2017).

While this book focusses on stroke, we have chosen to write this chapter with a broader perspective as critically ill patients with stroke share similarities and risks with patients having other neurological conditions. In Europe, neurological-neurosurgical early rehabilitation (NNER) centres provide care for such patients by bundling neurological, neurosurgical, intensive care, and neurorehabilitation expertise (Rollnik et al. 2017). These NNER centres have successfully proven themselves as a link between acute medical intensive care and rehabilitation and are also established as weaning centres for these severely neurologically ill patients (Rollnik et al. 2017; Pohl et al. 2016).

Patients relocated to weaning centres have been ventilated on average for more than 3 weeks in their primary care acute hospital (Oehmichen et al. 2012a). Their average age is older and they often have significant and multiple

M. Pohl (✉)
VAMED Klinik Schloss Pulsnitz GmbH, Pulsnitz, Germany
e-mail: Marcus.Pohl@vamed-gesundheit.de

M. Singer
Bloomsbury Institute of Intensive Care Medicine,
University College London, London, UK
e-mail: m.singer@ucl.ac.uk

© The Author(s) 2021   71
T. Platz (ed.), *Clinical Pathways in Stroke Rehabilitation*,
https://doi.org/10.1007/978-3-030-58505-1_5

morbidities (Oehmichen et al. 2012a). Ventilation for this duration leads to muscular weakness in non-neurological patients through inactivity (disuse atrophy) and through pathologies such as critical illness neuropathy (CIP) or myopathy (CIM) (Oehmichen et al. 2012b; Prange 2004; Ponfick et al. 2014). Neurologic-neurosurgical early rehabilitants often show significant immobility and nursing dependency. They may have a centrally induced paralysis or neuromuscular disease that may considerably complicate the weaning process. In addition, these patients also suffer neurological or neurosurgical complications, e.g. increased intracranial pressure or epileptic seizures, that requires ongoing involvement of neurological-neurosurgical expertise in the early rehabilitation process. These patients thus require a special setting, such as that provided in neurological weaning and rehabilitation centres. Through the possibilities of neurologically oriented multi-professional rehabilitation, the goal of the best possible interaction can be achieved.

With regard to the technical processes of weaning and the pathophysiology of weaning failure, reference is made to guidelines on "prolonged weaning" (Schönhofer et al. 2014). These do not differentiate between weaning of neurological patients compared to non-neurological patients, e.g. those with primary pulmonary disease. Differences between these specialist weaning centres can be seen, however, both in terms of staffing (multi-professional rehabilitation team, neurological, and neurorehabilitation expertise) and the therapies used.

2 Clinical Evidence and Reasoning

There is no strong evidence base as to how a prolonged weaning stroke patient should be best managed. The few studies involving stroke patients have examined heterogeneous groups of patients and a small proportion of neurological or neuromuscular disorders. Neurological patients are often excluded from automated weaning programs by some ventilator manufacturers (Neumann and Schmidt 2018). Basically, three different methods are used (Schönhofer et al. 2014):

- Gradual reduction of pressure support.
- Combination of full and partial relief with phases of full load.
- Increasing phases of full load.

Which of these three methods, or a combination thereof, most benefit stroke patients is unclear (Ladeira et al. 2014). The use of so-called weaning protocols has not been studied in randomized controlled trials. In a recent PubMed search, the combination of terms *"weaning from mechanical ventilation"* AND *"stroke"* identified only 71 matches while the combination of *"prolonged weaning"* AND *"stroke"* identified only 28 matches. None however provided any evidence of optimal approach.

Thus, all the following recommendations are derived from guidelines or the experience of the authors in the context of good clinical practice.

2.1 Weaning of Neurological Patients

Weaning from mechanical ventilation generally takes between 40–50% of total mechanical ventilation time (Schönhofer et al. 2014). The duration of mechanical ventilation is associated with an increase in mortality and complication rates (Boles et al. 2007; Schönhofer et al. 2014). While the underlying condition of the patient obviously plays an important part, there is a significant iatrogenic contribution from ventilator-induced volu barotrauma, cardiovascular sequelae and hemodynamic, and immunosuppressive side effects of sedative agents. Safe and rapid withdrawal from the ventilator is therefore a top priority. According to an international consensus conference of 2005, a distinction is made between simple, difficult, and prolonged weaning (Boles et al. 2007, Schönhofer et al. 2014). Patients who need to be intubated and ventilated due to a neurological condition usually require prolonged weaning according to this definition (Rollnik et al. 2017).

Among patients with prolonged weaning, the initial reason for mechanical ventilation is an acute illness in more than half of the cases (Schönhofer et al. 2014). The cause of ongoing ventilation is however multifactorial, most commonly respiratory tract disorders, oxygenation problems, oxygen distribution disorders, and respiratory pump failure (Schönhofer et al. 2014). Respiratory muscle weakness is often related to critical illness polyneuropathy (CIP) and/or myopathy (CIM). These are diagnosed in one-third of patients with ARDS, one quarter of those who have ventilation duration of more than seven days, and more than two-thirds of patients with sepsis who require prolonged ventilation and hospitalization (Oehmichen et al. 2012b; Ponfick et al. 2014; Oehmichen and Ragaller 2012). In addition to these weakness syndromes acquired in the intensive care unit (ICU), other neurological and psychological consequences of intensive care management (e.g. delirium, post-traumatic stress disorder) also have an unfavourable influence on weaning (Oehmichen and Ragaller 2012; Rollnik et al. 2017).

Primary neurological conditions are also a frequent cause of prolonged weaning (Oehmichen and Ragaller 2012; Oehmichen et al. 2012a; Rollnik et al. 2010; Bertram and Brandt 2013). Twenty-seven percent of ventilated patients with underlying neurological-neurosurgical disorders were reported as experiencing "weaning failure" (Coplin et al. 2000; Oehmichen et al. 2012a).

Such patients may benefit from relocation to specialized facilities (weaning centres) (Rollnik et al. 2017; Schönhofer et al. 2014). In a retrospective study of 1486 patients enrolled in seven neurological weaning centres in 2009, the underlying causes of long-term ventilation were neurological in 69.2% of cases (52.6% central nervous, 45.2% peripheral neurological, 2.2% mixed), pulmonary in 22.8% of cases, and cardiac disorders in 3% (Oehmichen et al. 2012a). Neurological patients who could not be weaned from mechanical ventilation in primary care require a seamless continuation of rehabilitation measures in secondary care, taking into account an ongoing requirement for intensive care. These specialized NNER weaning centres fulfil specific tasks and requirements for the care of these long-term ventilated patients in order to ensure a parallel and early rehabilitation during their ongoing weaning process.

2.2   Existing Studies on Weaning Success

Uncontrolled studies in NNERs reported that prolonged weaning from mechanical ventilation is often successful (Oehmichen et al. 2012a; Rollnik et al. 2010; Hoffmann et al. 2006; Pohl et al. 2016). However, comparative studies examining, for example weaning of neurological patients with and without the intervention of NNER, are hard to achieve. In many countries, this would conflict with the right to rehabilitation guaranteed in social legislation.

The published literature mainly deals with descriptions of the approach to weaning, or provides expert opinions and conceptual representations (Bertram and Brandt 2013; Oehmichen and Ragaller 2012), retrospective data collections (Pohl et al. 2016; Oehmichen et al. 2012a; Rollnik et al. 2010), concepts of weaning (Oehmichen et al. 2013), or presentations of results for weaning in the context of neurological-neurosurgical early rehabilitation (Hoffmann et al. 2006; Bertram and Brandt 2007).

Table 1 shows results in various NNER weaning centres. Comparison of weaning rates to pneumological weaning centres is particularly difficult due to different admission criteria, inconsistent definition of a primary end point, and the therapeutic goal being sought (Oehmichen et al. 2012a; Rollnik et al. 2017). Comparability of results between different weaning centres can only be achieved if a consistent interdisciplinary dataset is developed. Process and result data must therefore be precisely defined. In our opinion, there is a pressing need for clarification, e.g. for a uniform allocation of essential treatment phases for hospital or rehabilitation treatment, a description of inclusion or rejection criteria for admission, criteria to

Table 1 Results from weaning studies in the field of neurological-neurosurgical early rehabilitation

Patient no.	Discharged weaned (%)	Discharged mechanically ventilated (%)	Mortality (%)	Author
193	66.8	20.2	12.9	Hoffmann et al. (2006)
133	78.2	5.3[a]/?[b]	?	Bertram and Brandt (2007)
82	68.3	6.1[a]/19.5[b]	6.1	Rollnik et al. (2010)
1486	64.9	11.3[a]/7.1[b]	16.6	Oehmichen et al. (2012a)
644	59.5	9.8[a] (8.2[c]/1.6[d])/7.8[b]	23.0	Oehmichen et al. (2013)
192	65.1	8.3[a]/5.2[b]	21.4	Pohl et al. (2016)

[a]To extended supply
[b]Refer to hospital
[c]Invasive mechanical ventilation
[d]Patients with non-invasive ventilation

describe disease severity, a precise definition of weaning, and evaluation of results in relation to the therapeutic goal.

2.3 Difficulties in the Weaning Process

In prolonged weaning of neurological patients, the weakened "respiratory muscle pump" (resulting from peripheral and/or central paresis) and/or a respiratory drive disorder (from brain stem dysfunction) are of primary relevance (Rollnik et al. 2017). In addition to these primary neurological conditions, there may also be development of an ICU-acquired weakness syndrome (Ponfick et al. 2014; Pohl and Mehrholz 2013). Both may lead to pronounced weakness thereby complicating the weaning process (Rollnik et al. 2017). A third of patients transferred to an NNER facility had a main diagnosis of CIP or CIM (Oehmichen et al. 2012a; Pohl et al. 2016). The average age of patients in these centres was 63.7 years (Oehmichen et al. 2012a), thus relevant comorbidities are likely. As mentioned earlier, this particular study classified 22.8% of cases as having an underlying pulmonary cause for mechanical ventilation and 3% a cardiac cause (Oehmichen et al. 2012a).

2.4 Weaning Strategies

Weaning strategies are used with a combination of synchronized intermittent mandatory ventilation (SIMV) and/or pressure support ventilation (PSV) and/or progressively extended spontaneous breathing phases (Rollnik et al. 2017). However, it is known that respiratory muscle recovery does not occur through pressure-assisted ventilation or SIMV and that assisted spontaneous breathing modes may be more of a burden on the breathing pump due to ineffective triggering (Rollnik et al. 2017). Therefore, especially in cases of respiratory muscle pump weakness, weaning strategies with intermittent spontaneous breathing alternating with controlled mechanical ventilation should be used (Rollnik et al. 2017).

The question as to whether one ventilation mode is superior to another in weaning neurological/neurosurgical patients is currently uncertain due to a lack of studies. This question is also controversial in non-neurological patients or in unselected patient groups. Sample sizes are generally small and the use of now outdated technical equipment means that ventilation modes were not used in a way that would have allowed an exact separation between assisted spontaneous breathing and controlled ventilation. In more recent investigations, combinations of assisted spontaneous breathing (ASB) and controlled ventilation (assist-control ventilation and BIPAP) were used during the phases of controlled ventilation (Rollnik et al. 2017).

The aim of weaning in neurological patients is independent breathing, without equipment support. Non-invasive ventilation is used as a de-escalation therapy in patients with good swallowing function and persisting respiratory pump insufficiency (Rollnik et al. 2017). To summarize, during prolonged weaning of neurological patients, weaning strategies can be used that incorporate progressively expanded spontaneous breathing phases, taking into account the underlying pathology and a constant re-evaluation of patient response. With disturbances in neuromuscular transmission, additional pressure support may be useful during the spontaneous breathing phases. Weaning in patients with central respiratory dysregulation disorders should be individualized, taking into account their underlying injury and regular adjustment according to patient response.

2.5   Weaning Protocols and Special Ventilation Techniques

Protocols are generally recommended when weaning long-term mechanically ventilated patients (Rollnik et al. 2017; Schönhofer et al. 2014). These should include a gradual extension of spontaneous breathing attempts. During spontaneous breathing, the patient is disconnected from the ventilator for temporary periods; this is intended to achieve recovery of respiratory muscles with replenishment of energy stores. Such weaning protocols are therefore used in all patients in neurological weaning centres, regardless of whether the patients are suffering from a central nervous disorder, a neuromuscular weakness, a primary hypoxic disorder due to pulmonary insufficiency, or a combination thereof.

Oehmichen et al. described in detail standardized extensions of spontaneous respiration phases (Oehmichen et al. 2013). The documentation of compliance with the protocol (i.e. individual steps in the development of spontaneous breathing phases) is made by the nursing staff. The medical team monitors protocol compliance (per daily documentation) and sets different individualised plans. They reported that this protocol was followed in 86% of ventilator-weaned patients. The authors thus concluded that the use of this spontaneous breathing protocol is well suited to successful weaning of neurological intensive care patients requiring prolonged weaning.

The central notion of all protocol-based weaning strategies is to check respiratory status daily and to continually adjust the plan for the next weaning steps. Whether such a procedure is the subject of a formal treatment protocol led by caregivers, or whether the process is ensured by a structured medical visit, seems to be of minor importance for the outcome but more dependent on the particular circumstances of an intensive care unit.

There is no evidence of superiority to the discontinuous cessation approach described above for continuous weaning in modes such as SIMV or BiLevel ventilation with a gradual reduction of pressure support (Bertram and Brandt 2013; Jubran et al. 2013).

Pressure-assisted spontaneous breathing—inspiratory pressure support of spontaneous breathing (IPS), assisted spontaneous breathing (ASB), pressure support ventilation (PSV)—is another spontaneous breathing mode suitable for weaning of neurological patients with an intact respiratory drive, for example those with severe damage to the peripheral nervous system such as Guillain-Barré syndrome. Without disconnection periods, the muscular respiration pump can be trained by gradually reducing inspiratory pressure, i.e. a gradual "transfer" of ventilation to the patient takes place (Jubran et al. 2013). It is an alternative process to the discontinuous weaning protocols.

Adaptive support ventilation (ASV) is a modern advancement of mandatory minute ventilation (MMV) with a complex adaptive control taking into account the anatomical dead space. In experienced hands, this procedure allows compliance with pulmonary protection rules, targets minute ventilation, an optimal target breathing pattern (Otis formula), and a safe, patient-based weaning. However, no advantage has yet been shown over other modes for ventilated, tracheotomized patients (Bertram and Brandt 2013).

The intermittent use of CPAP in the late weaning phase may possibly assist with better alveolar recruitment in preventing atelectasis and reducing the work of breathing (Bertram and Brandt 2013). In the case of unsupported spontaneous breathing using a T-piece, automatic tube compensation (ATC) can compensate for an increased work of breathing due to tube resistance (Bertram and Brandt 2013). However, whether the use of these procedures in ventilated patients with neuromuscular weakness and/or respiratory drive disorders shortens the time of weaning or increases the weaning rate has not been adequately studied (Bertram and Brandt 2013). In general, unsupported spontaneous respiratory phases should be performed using a T-piece under close nursing control.

Neurally adjusted ventilatory assist (NAVA) is a "neuronal" controlled ventilation (Moerer et al. 2008; Navalesi and Longhini 2015). The support is synchronous and proportional to the activity of the diaphragm. The diaphragmatic activity is measured by a special electrode applied on a nasogastric tube. This is intended to achieve improved synchronization between the respiration trigger and the patient's breathing demand in order to reduce false triggering and thus an increased work of breathing. In the case of this procedure, it is also unclear as to whether a shortening of the time to successful weaning or an improved outcome can be achieved (Moerer et al. 2008, Navalesi and Longhini 2015).

In principle, the frequency and duration of spontaneous respiration at the T-piece should be successively increased in a fixed step pattern. If successful, the patient can be moved to the next level, and in case of failure they can be moved back to the previous level or the same level re-applied (Bertram and Brandt 2013; Oehmichen et al. 2013). If this step scheme (or weaning protocol) cannot be met, it requires an individual, medically guided weaning plan with close patient surveillance (Bertram and Brandt 2013, Oehmichen et al. 2013).

Classic weaning protocols are aimed at rapid extubation of patients in intensive care units who are ventilated for longer than 24 hours. An important premise of these protocols is the presence of adequate alertness and the ability to assess the patient's neurological status. Weaning and sedation protocols are thus often coupled (Girard et al. 2008). However, for neurological/neurosurgical patients, these conventional weaning parameters can only be used to a very limited extent, if at all

(Ko et al. 2009). This may be due to a lack of consideration of certain aspects of neurological/neurosurgical patients:

- As most prolonged weaning ventilated patients are already tracheotomised— between 91 and 96% (Pohl et al. 2016), there should not be a dichotomous yes/ no decision to extubate but rather a plan involving gradual weaning from the ventilator. This is often achieved by daily extension of time without ventilator support.
- There are often problems with the respiratory pump/respiratory muscles, for example due to CIP/CIM. In contrast, pulmonary insufficiency (as in the case of the classic COPD patient) often plays only a subordinate role or, at most, represents comorbidity.
- The problems of reduced vigilance and neurogenic dysphagia are mostly completely disregarded.

A weaning protocol in neurological patients therefore has fundamentally different requirements compared to a conventional protocol. Examples of a weaning protocol used in the NNER can be found in the literature (Oehmichen et al. 2013).

2.6   Special Features of Prolonged Weaning in Neurological Patients

2.6.1   Definition of Successful Weaning from Mechanical Ventilation

In the respiratory literature, a weaning end point is inconsistently defined. Although non-invasive ventilation is recognized as full-fledged ventilation in the Diagnosis-Related Group (DRG) coding system (Institut für das Entgeltsystem im Krankenhaus (InEK GmbH) 2015), the respiratory literature often suggests that successful weaning is achieved after switching from invasive to non-invasive mechanical ventilation (Schönhofer et al. 2014). Thus, successful withdrawal from ventilation is equated to the removal of invasive ventilation access (endotracheal/tracheostomy tube). In contrast to these patients, the indication for an endotracheal/tracheostomy tube in neurological patients is not only for (invasive) ventilation but also often because of dysphagia and the risk of aspiration (see below). Thus, in principle, there are two indications for an endotracheal/tracheostomy tube.

Patients undergoing early neurological-neurosurgical rehabilitation are considered to have been successfully weaned from respiration if patients manage for at least 48 hours without any mechanical ventilation (Rollnik et al. 2017). Removal of the tracheal cannula occurs when there is no longer a risk of aspiration. This is one of the main differences between respiratory patients who rarely have such dysphagia, and neurological-neurosurgical early rehabilitants (Rollnik et al. 2017). The use of non-invasive ventilation, which plays a fundamental role in early extubation and successful weaning, plays a subordinate role in neurological-neurosurgical early rehabilitation as, in the majority of cases, there are contraindications to this form of ventilation. Examples include lack of cooperation, retention of secretions with impaired/absent coughing, missing protective reflexes, central respiratory drive disorders, and complex dysphagia with risk of aspiration and/or disorders of gastric motility with frequent vomiting (Rollnik et al. 2017). Non-invasive ventilation (NIV) in these patients requires special expertise and close monitoring. It was used as an integral part of the weaning process in only 4.4% of patients according to the NNER study on ventilatory cessation in neurological weaning centres (Oehmichen et al. 2012a). Studies on the use of NIV with pressure support in neurological-neurosurgical patients are lacking. This application remains reserved for experts who are familiar with this type of ventilation and can afford the specific treatment risks and the considerable mechanical and, above all, human resources necessary.

2.6.2 Invasive and Non-Invasive Ventilation

Most patients are invasively ventilated when transferred to a neurological weaning centre—96.7% in one multicentre observational study (Oehmichen et al. 2012a), in whom 99.9% were ventilated via a tracheostomy (Oehmichen et al. 2012a). Comparable data were found in two other multicentre studies (Pohl et al. 2016; Hoffmann et al. 2006). It thus follows that neurological weaning centres need a structured approach to the handling and weaning of the tracheostomy tube.

Non-invasive ventilation (NIV) can be used for hypercapnic respiratory failure or global respiratory insufficiency. This has the advantage that a tracheostomy is avoided, thereby preserving the body's own filtering, moistening and warming of inhaled air. However, NIV with mask ventilation is only possible in cooperative persons without disturbances of consciousness, significant dysphagia and secretion clearance, and with intact swallowing reflexes. Accordingly, their use in neurological weaning centres is severely limited. Non-invasive ventilation should not be used in patients with neurogenic dysphagia or prolonged reduced vigilance and high aspiration risk (Rollnik et al. 2017). In these patients, a blocked-off tracheostomy tube should remain in situ until there is no danger of macro-aspiration (Rollnik et al. 2017). Swallowing status in patients with dysphagia should be determined by a controlled clinical examination (Rollnik et al. 2017).

2.6.3 Accompanying Neurological-Neurosurgical (Early) Rehabilitation

Weaning of neurological patients should always include (early) rehabilitation of various concomitant aspects to achieve the best possible patient participation (Rollnik et al. 2017). Examples include:

• Management of the tracheostomy tube.
• Dysphagia and secretion management.
• Treatment of patients with organic brain syndromes and neurocognitive dysfunction.
• Treatment of patients with spinal cord injury.

- Increasing independence in the activities of daily living.
- Accompanying therapies in neurological-neurosurgical early rehabilitation.
- Nursing techniques and activities.
- Psychological interventions.

3 Clinical Practice Recommendations for Weaning in Stroke Patients (and Other Patients with Neurological Conditions)

3.1 Methodological Explanations

In general, the recommendations given in this book, authorized by the World Federation for NeuroRehabilitation (WFNR), are accompanied by an indication of the level of evidence, e.g. from expert opinion (level 5) to systematic reviews (with homogeneity) of RCTs (level 1a). The overall quality of evidence supporting the recommendations ranges from "very low" when no systematic evidence is available to "high" when there is substantial high-quality evidence and when further evidence is unlikely to change the estimates of therapy effects (and harm). The grading of the recommendations will vary from "*can*" (option), e.g. when based on expert opinion only to "*ought to*" (strong recommendation) when based on high-quality evidence or clinically mandated for ethical reasons.

Levels of evidence for recommendations are indicated below using the "Oxford Centre for Evidence-Based Medicine (CEBM) Levels of Evidence" (version dating from March 2009, http://www.cebm.net/Oxford-centre-evidence-based-medicine). Here, the quality of evidence was rated into four categories according to the "GRADE" ("Grades of Recommendation, Assessment, Development, and Evaluation") system (Owens et al. 2010):

- High quality: further research is unlikely to affect confidence in the estimation of the (therapeutic) effect.
- Medium quality: further research is likely to affect confidence in the estimation of the (therapeutic) effect and may alter the estimate.
- Low quality: further research will most likely influence confidence in the estimation of the (therapeutic) effect and will probably change the estimate.
- Very low quality: any estimation of the (therapy) effect or prognosis is very uncertain.

The GRADE rating of recommendations corresponds to the categories of "*ought to*" (A—strong recommendation) or "*should*" (B—weak recommendation) (Schünemann et al. 2013). As third category "*can*" (0—option) had been introduced (Platz 2017). Recommendation category A is granted for clinically effective interventions with high-quality evidence support; category B for medium-quality evidence, and category 0 for low- or very low-quality evidence. Deviations from this rule could be indicated based on clinical judgement, with individual reasons denoted in [brackets]. A+ and B+ denote a strong or weak recommendation in favour on an intervention, while A− and B− recommend against its use.

3.2 Recommendations

3.2.1 Organizational Setting

Prolonged weaning in stroke patients requires a special setting which can best be provided in neurological weaning and rehabilitation centres. Through the integrated possibilities of an adequate weaning process and a neurologically oriented multi-professional rehabilitation both successful weaning and the goal of the best possible interaction may simultaneously be achieved (CEBM classification: level 2c, GRADE quality: low, recommendation: B+ [clinical reasoning]).

3.2.2 Weaning Strategy

For prolonged weaning of stroke patients, strategies with progressively expanded spontaneous breathing phases can be used, taking into account the underlying pathology and a constant re-evaluation of patient response. In cases of disturbances of neuromuscular transmission, additional pressure support during the spontaneous breathing phases can be useful. Weaning in patients with central respiratory dys-regulation disorders should be individualized, taking into account the underlying injury and also regular adjustments according to patient response (CEBM classification: level 5, GRADE quality: very low, recommendation: 0).

Non-invasive ventilation ought not to be used in patients with neurogenic dys-phagia or prolonged reduced vigilance and a high risk of aspiration; in these patients, a blocked-off tracheostomy tube should remain as a portal for ventilator access until there is no danger of macro-aspiration (CEBM classification: level 5, GRADE quality: very low, recommendation: A− [clinical reasoning]).

Weaning in stroke patients ought to include (early) rehabilitation of various concomitant aspects of care to achieve best possible patient participation (CEBM classification: level 5, GRADE quality: very low, recommendation: A+ [clinical reasoning]).

3.2.3 Weaning Process Characteristics

Weaning protocols can be used during the weaning process of long-term mechanically ventilated stroke patients (CEBM classification: level 5, GRADE quality: very low, recommendation: 0).

The frequency and duration of spontaneous respiration using a T-piece can be increased in a fixed step pattern; if successful, the patient can move to the next level, in case of failure the patient returns to the previous level or the same level is re-applied (CEBM classification: level 2c, GRADE quality: low, recommendation: 0).

Patients undergoing early neurological-neurosurgical rehabilitation are considered to have been successfully weaned if they manage at least 48 h without any mechanical ventilation (CEBM classification: level 5, GRADE quality: very low, recommendation: B+ [clinical reasoning]).

References

Bertram M, Brandt T (2007) Neurologisch-neurochirurgische Frührehabilitation: Eine aktuelle Bestandsaufnahme. Nervenarzt 78:1160–1174

Bertram M, Brandt T (2013) Neurologische Frührehabilitation bei beatmeten Patienten mit ZNS-Störungen. Intensivmedizin Up2date 9:53–71

Boles JM, Bion J, Connors A, Herridge M, Marsh B, Melot C, Pearl R, Silverman H, Stanchina M, Vieillard-Baron A, Welte T (2007) Weaning from mechanical ventilation. Eur Respir J 29:1033–1056

Coplin WM, Pierson DJ, Cooley KD, Newell DW, Rubenfeld GD (2000) Implications of extubation delay in brain-injured patients meeting standard weaning criteria. Am J Respir Crit Care Med 161:1530–1536

Girard TD, Kress JP, Fuchs BD, Thomason JW, Schweickert WD, Pun BT, Taichman DB, Dunn JG, Pohlman AS, Kinniry PA, Jackson JC, Canonico AE, LIGHT RW, Shintani AK, Thompson JL, Gordon SM, Hall JB, Dittus RS, Bernard GR, Ely EW (2008) Efficacy and safety of a paired sedation and ventilator weaning protocol for mechanically ventilated patients in intensive care (awakening and breathing controlled trial): a randomised controlled trial. Lancet 371:126–134

Hoffmann B, Karbe H, Krusch C, Müller B, Pause M, Prosiegel M, Puschendorf W, Schleep J, Spranger M, Steube D, Voss A (2006) Patientencharakteristika in der neurologisch/neurochirurgischen Frührehabilitation (Phase B): Eine multizentrische Erfassung im Jahr 2002 in Deutschland. Akt Neurol 33:287–296

Institut für Das Entgeltsystem im Krankenhaus (Inek GMBH) (2015) Deutsche Kodierrichtlinien—Allgemein und spezielle Kodierrichtlinien für die Verschlüsselung von Krankheiten und Prozeduren. Köln, Deutsche Ärzte-Verlag

Jubran A, Grant BJ, Duffner LA, Collins EG, Lanuza DM, Hoffman LA, Tobin MJ (2013) Effect of pressure support vs unassisted breathing through a tracheostomy collar on weaning duration in patients requiring prolonged mechanical ventilation: a randomized trial. JAMA 309:671–677

Ko R, Ramos L, Chalela JA (2009) Conventional weaning parameters do not predict extubation failure in neurocritical care patients. Neurocrit Care 10:269–273

Ladeira MT, Vital FM, Andriolo RB, Andriolo BN, Atallah AN, Peccin MS (2014) Pressure support versus T-tube for weaning from mechanical ventilation in adults. Cochrane Database Syst Rev 2014:CD006056

Moerer O, Barwing J, Quintel M (2008) Neurally adjusted ventilatory assist: ein neuartiges Beatmungsverfahren. Anästhesist 57:998–1005

Navalesi P, Longhini F (2015) Neurally adjusted ventilatory assist. Curr Opin Crit Care 21:58–64

Neumann A, Schmidt H (2018) SmartCare®/ PS: The automated weaning protocol [online]. https://www.draeger.com/Products/Content/smartcare-bk-9051398-en-gb.pdf. Accessed 18 Dec 2018

Oehmichen F, Ragaller M (2012) Beatmungsentwöhnung bei Chronisch-Kritisch-Kranken. Intensiv- und Notfallbehandlung 37:118–126

Oehmichen F, Ketter G, Mertl-Rotzer M, Platz T, Puschendorf W, Rollnik JD, Schaupp M, Pohl M (2012a) Beatmungsentwöhnung in neurologischen Weaningzentren—Eine Bestandsaufnahme der Arbeitsgemeinschaft Neurologischneurochirurgische Frührehabilitation. Nervenarzt 83:1300–1307

Oehmichen F, Pohl M, Schlosser R, Stogowski D, Toppel D, Mehrholz J (2012b) Critical-illness-Polyneuropathie und -Polymyopathie: Wie sicher ist die klinische Diagnose bei Patienten mit Weaning-Versagen? Nervenarzt 83:220–225

Oehmichen F, Zäumer K, Ragaller M, Mehrholz J, Pohl M (2013) Anwendung eines standardisierten Spontanatmungsprotokolls - Erfahrungen in einem Weaning-Zentrum mit neurologischem Schwerpunkt. Nervenarzt 84:962–972

Owens DK, Lohr KN, Atkins D, Treadwell JR, Reston JT, Bass EB, Chang S, Helfand M (2010) AHRQ series paper 5: grading the strength of a body of evidence when comparing medical interventions—agency for healthcare research and quality and the effective health-care program. J Clin Epidemiol 63:513–523

Platz T (2017) Practice guidelines in neurorehabilitation. Neurol Int Open 1:E148–E152

Pohl M, Mehrholz J (2013) Auf einer Intensivstation erworbenes Schwächesyndrom—Langzeitkomplikationen. Neurorehabil Neural Repair 1:17–20

Pohl M, Bertram M, Bucka C, Hartwich M, Jobges M, Ketter G, Leineweber B, Mertl-Rotzer M, Nowak DA, Platz T, Rollnik JD, Scheidtmann K, Thomas R, Von Rosen F, Wallesch CW, Woldag H, Peschel P, Mehrholz J (2016) Rehabilitationsverlauf von Patienten in der neurologisch-neurochirurgischen Frührehabilitation: Ergebnisse einer multizentrischen Erfassung im Jahr 2014 in Deutschland. Nervenarzt 87:634–644

Ponfick M, Bösl K, Lüdemann-Podubecka J, Neumann G, Pohl M, Nowak DA, Gdynia H-J (2014) Erworbene Muskelschwäche des kritischen Kranken: pathogenese, Behandlung, rehabilitation, outcome. Nervenarzt 85:195–204

Prange H (2004) Akute Schwächesyndrome bei Intensivpatienten (acute weakness syndromes in critically ill patients). In: Prange H, Bitsch A (eds) Neurologische Intensivmedizin. Thieme, Stuttgart

Rollnik JD, Berlinghof K, Lenz O, Bertomeu AM (2010) Beatmung in der neurologischen Frührehabilitation. Akt Neurol 37:316–318

Rollnik JD, Adolphsen J, Bauer J, Bertram M, Brocke J, Dohmen C, Donauer E, Hartwich M, Heidler MD, Huge V, Klarmann S, Lorenzl S, Luck M, Mertl-Rotzer M, Mokrusch T, Nowak DA, Platz T, Riechmann L, Schlachetzki F, Von Helden A, Wallesch CW, Zergiebel D, Pohl M (2017) Prolongiertes Weaning in der neurologisch-neurochirurgischen Frührehabilitation. S2k-Leitlinie herausgegeben von der Weaning-Kommission der Deutschen Gesellschaft für Neurorehabilitation e.V. (DGNR). Nervenarzt 88:652–674

Schönhofer B, Geiseler J, Dellweg D, Moerer O, Barchfeld T, Fuchs H, Karg O, Rosseau S, Sitter H, Weber-Carstens S, Westhoff M, Windisch W (2014) ProlongiertesWeaning - S2k-Leitlinie herausgegeben von der Deutschen Gesellschaft für Pneumologie und Beatmungsmedizin e.V. Pneumologie 68:19–75

Schünemann H, Brożek J, Guyatt G, Oxman A (2013) GRADE handbook for grading quality of evidence and strength of recommendations. The GRADE Working Group. Updated October 2013. www.guidelinedevelopment.org/handbook

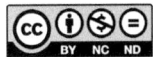

Recovery of Swallowing

Nam-Jong Paik and Won-Seok Kim

1 Introduction

Dysphagia is one of the common impairments after stroke, which ranges widely from 29% to 81% according to the timing of the survey after stroke or the methods used for dysphagia assessment (e.g., questionnaire, clinical examination, instrumental test) (Martino et al. 2005). Pharyngeal phase dysphagia is more prevalent (Han et al. 2001) and brain stem or specific cortical lesions may attribute more for post-stroke dysphagia (Galovic et al. 2013; Martino et al. 2005). Dysphagia is associated with the higher risk of non-silent or silent aspirations and aspiration pneumonia (Ding and Logemann 2000; Falsetti et al. 2009; Perry and Love 2001). In addition, dysphagia is associated with other medical complications such as dehydration, malnutrition, mortality, and recovery after stroke (Perlman 1996). Therefore, detecting and managing dysphagia after stroke could prevent medical complications and reduce the length of hospital stay and socioeconomic burdens (Smithard et al. 1996).

In this chapter, we reviewed the clinical evidence related with dysphagia assessment and management after stroke. The topics selected are: (1) Dysphagia screening; (2) Instrumental assessment of dysphagia; (3) Treatment of dysphagia including behavioral interventions, neuromuscular electrical stimulation, noninvasive brain stimulation, and oral hygiene; and (4) Enteral tube feedings. Five clinical practice guidelines were selected for the review and adaptation (Boddice et al. 2010; Hebert et al. 2016; Smith 2010; Winstein et al. 2016; Kim et al. 2016). Articles published frvom 2014 to 2017 were additionally searched in the PubMed and Cochrane Library using the MeSH keywords "(cerebrovascular disorders OR stroke OR cerebral hemorrhage OR cerebral infarction) AND (Dysphagia OR Deglutition OR oral hygiene)," and in the EMBASE using EMTREE with the keywords, "(cerebrovascular disease)

N.-J. Paik (✉) · W.-S. Kim
Department of Rehabilitation Medicine, Seoul National University College of Medicine,
Seoul National University Bundang Hospital, Seongnam, Republic of Korea
e-mail: njpaik@snu.ac.kr

© The Author(s) 2021
T. Platz (ed.), *Clinical Pathways in Stroke Rehabilitation*,
https://doi.org/10.1007/978-3-030-58505-1_6

AND (Dysphagia OR swallowing disorder OR deglutition)." Total 2118 articles were found by these electronic searches. Titles and abstracts were reviewed for screening and non-English papers, commentaries, case series, narratives, book chapters, editorials, nonsystematic reviews, and conference papers were excluded. Two independent raters screened all 2118 articles and any disagreement was resolved by discussion. In each topic, the systematic review, meta-analyses, and randomized controlled trials (RCTs) were considered for inclusion first, but if no articles were available for the topic, observational studies were additionally selected.

Systematic reviews and meta-analyses ($n = 11$), RCTs ($n = 5$), and observational studies ($n = 10$) relevant to each selected topic in dysphagia (31 articles in total including five clinical practice guidelines) were selected for full-text review for summarizing the currently best available evidence, assessing its overall quality of evidence and for the provision of recommendations. A complete list of selected references is presented online at www.clinical-pathways.org. The recommendations given in this chapter follow the same rules as outlined in chapter "Clinical Pathways in Stroke Rehabilitation: Background, Scope, and Methods" (see Chap. 2).

2 Dysphagia Screening Early after Stroke

One systematic review included 14 studies to detect oropharyngeal dysphagia with bedside screening in patients with neurological disorders. The sensitivity and specificity to detect aspiration ranged from 45% to 100%, and 29% to 86%, respectively (Kertscher et al. 2014). In one systematic review of swallowing screens after acute stroke, four screening protocols that met the quality criteria showed high sensitivities ($\geq 87\%$) and specificities ($\geq 91\%$) (Schepp et al. 2011). A recent prospective, double-blind study in patients with stroke demonstrated that a dysphagia screen protocol has the high sensitivity (96.5%) and acceptable specificity (55.8%) as a screening tool to detect aspiration (Warnecke et al. 2017). Multiple observational multicenter prospective or registry-based studies with large sample size showed that the screening failure of dysphagia after stroke is associated with higher risk of pneumonia or mortality (Hinchey et al. 2005; Joundi et al. 2017a; b; Lakshminarayan et al. 2010). Bedside screening for dysphagia by the trained nurses after acute stroke demonstrated the significant reduction in the time to dysphagia screening and pneumonia rate compared to the screening by speech therapists in the pre- and post-intervention trial (Palli et al. 2017).

Recommendation: Dysphagia screening ought to be administered by the trained healthcare provider early after stroke onset before starting oral feeding to prevent pneumonia and other adverse events such as malnutrition, dehydration, and to reduce the mortality (CEBM classification: level 1, GRADE quality: moderate, recommendation grade: A+).

One of the dysphagia screening tools that showed acceptable reliability, higher sensitivity, and negative predictive value, which consists of items such as alertness assessment, dry swallowing test, and direct swallowing test with water or semisolid and solid foods, should be used (CEBM classification: level 1, Grade quality: moderate, recommendation: B+).

3 Instrumental Assessments to Detect Dysphagia or Aspiration

A bedside screening test alone has a limitation to assess dysphagia after stroke because patients with stroke can aspirate without overt clinical signs or symptoms (silent aspiration), and the assessment for sequential swallowing function (oral, pharyngeal, and esophageal phase) is difficult by a bedside screening tool (Singh and Hamdy 2006). The widely used instrumental assessments for dysphagia are videofluoroscopic swallowing study (VFSS) or fiberoptic endoscopic evaluation of swallowing (FEES), which have advantages to assess the physiological or structural causes of dysphagia necessary for providing the appropriate instruction for dysphagia management (e.g., swallow therapy, compensation maneuver, dietary modification). In a systematic review including 24 observational studies, dysphagia incidence after stroke was higher with the VFSS (64–78%) than those with bedside screening or structured clinical assessments (37–55%) (Martino et al. 2005). High silent aspiration rate (67% of silent aspiration among patients with aspiration) detected by VFSS in one observational study with acute stroke patients indicated that the clinical bedside test alone could not predict the risk of aspiration or pneumonia (Daniels et al. 1998). In a prospective observational study to compare the bedside screening test versus VFSS in patients with acute stroke, 14% of patients who passed the screening test showed aspiration in VFSS and diet recommendations were changed to the more conservative level in 28% of the patients after VFSS (Leigh et al. 2016). One retrospective observational study showed that selective FEES significantly reduced pneumonia (Bax et al. 2014). However, no high-quality study has shown that the instrumental test can reduce the pneumonia rate significantly more than the bedside screening test (Doggett et al. 2001; Kjaersgaard et al. 2014), although one recent study using a decision-analysis model from multiple data sources including meta-analyses and other relevant clinical studies demonstrated that VFSS screening for dysphagia was more cost-effective than a bedside examination alone or a combination of bedside examination with VFSS (Wilson and Howe 2012). The superiority of one method to another between VFSS and FEES was not significant and both can be applied according to the clinical situations (Aviv 2000; Boddice et al. 2010; Hebert et al. 2016; Smith 2010).

Recommendation: Instrumental assessments such as VFSS or FEES ought to be performed to verify the aspiration and to set the appropriate dysphagia management plan in stroke patients who showed the risk for pharyngeal dysphagia or aspiration in the initial or ongoing swallowing screens (CEBM classification: level 1, GRADE quality: moderate, recommendation grade: A+).

4 Treatment of Dysphagia

Early and comprehensive treatment of dysphagia is important, if the dysphagia is detected by the screening or instrumental tests. Conventional dysphagia treatment usually includes the swallowing exercise, compensatory techniques, and appropriate dietary modifications. In this chapter, the evidence for behavioral intervention programs including the conventional dysphagia treatment components were reviewed, because these components are usually provided by rather a program than an isolated component, and the effects of each isolated component cannot be evaluated sufficiently. Based on the current evidence, the evidence for neuromuscular electrical stimulation (NMES), which is commonly used with the behavioral interventions, was reviewed. And since meta-analyses of acupuncture studies were available, the reviews of evidence and recommendation for acupuncture were included. Noninvasive brain stimulations such as repetitive transcranial magnetic stimulation (rTMS) or transcranial direct current stimulation (tDCS) for dysphagia were also reviewed for their evidence because of presence of more recent RCTs and systematic reviews. Lastly, the evidence of oral hygiene to prevent pneumonia in stroke patients with dysphagia was reviewed.

4.1   Behavioral Interventions

One RCT investigated the effect of behavioral interventions on dysphagia in acute stroke with the primary outcome of survival free of an abnormal diet at 6 months (Carnaby et al. 2006). Patients were randomly allocated to usual care ($n = 102$), standard low-intensity intervention ($n = 102$) consisting of compensation strategies (e.g., environmental modification such as the upright positioning for feeding), safe swallowing advice, and appropriate dietary modification, three times per week for a month or standard high-intensity intervention ($n = 102$) comprising direct swallowing exercises and appropriate dietary modification, every working day for a month. A significant reduction in swallowing-related medical complications (RR = 0.73, 95% CI: 0.6 to 0.9), chest infection (RR = 0.56, 95% CI: 0.4 to 0.8), death or institutionalization (RR = 0.73, 95% CI: 0.55 to 0.97), and a significant increased proportion of patients who recovered from swallowing (RR = 1.41, 95% CI: 1.03 to 1.94) were verified in the standard intervention compared to the usual care. Further, a dose–response relation was also apparent with improved recovery of swallowing function and less chest infection in patients receiving intensive standard swallowing therapy compared to less intensive standard therapy and usual care.

One systematic review including 15 RCTs with a broad range of swallowing treatment demonstrated that the general dysphagia treatment programs were related with a less risk of pneumonia in patients with acute stroke (Foley et al. 2008). In a Cochrane systematic review including five studies with behavioral interventions ($n = 423$) consisting of swallowing exercise, environment modifications, and appropriate dietary modification, behavioral interventions reduced the dysphagia at the end of trial ($t = 5$; $n = 423$; OR = 0.52; 95% CI: 0.30 to 0.88); in addition, a nonsignificant reduction in chest infection/pneumonia was noted ($t = 5$; $n = 423$; OR 0.50; 95% CI 0.24 to 1.04; I2 = 34%; $P = 0.06$), but not for case fatality ($t = 2$; $n = 306$; OR 0.83; 95% CI 0.46 to 1.51) or institutionalization ($t = 2$; $n = 306$; OR 0.76; 95% CI 0.39 to 1.48) (Geeganage et al. 2012). Risk of bias assessment indicated a considerable proportion of unclear or high risk of bias of included studies.

Recommendation: Dysphagia treatment program including behavioral interventions should be provided for the dysphagia patients after stroke to prevent dysphagia-related complications and to recover the swallowing (CEBM classification: level 1, GRADE quality: moderate, recommendation grade: B+).

4.2 Neuromuscular Electrical Stimulation (NMES)

One systematic review investigated the effect of NMES on the post-stroke dysphagia (Chen et al. 2016). Six RCTs involving 243 patients with stroke were included for meta-analysis to compare the effect of swallowing treatment with NMES and swallowing treatment without NMES. Swallowing treatment with NMES showed better recovery immediately after the intervention than the swallowing treatment without NMES, with a significant standardized difference of 1.27 (95% CI: 0.51 to 2.02). However, the outcome measures used and the results in included studies were heterogeneous ($I^2 = 85\%$) and long-term effect could not be analyzed. A subgroup analysis suggested that both patients with acute/subacute and with chronic stroke might benefit. Treatment regimens varied with 20- to 60-min sessions applied 3 to 5 days per week for 2 to 4 weeks. A recent randomized controlled trial in subacute stroke patients ($n = 162$) with dysphagia (penetration aspiration score (PAS) in VFSS ≥3) demonstrated no significant effect of NMES for three consecutive days compared to the sham NMES (Bath et al. 2016). The mean treatment current of NMES was 14.8 ± 7.9 mA and duration was 9.9 ± 1.2 min per session, which may be a suboptimal stimulation level. In another recent RCT, 82 patients with dysphagia after acute medullary infarction were allocated to three intervention groups: traditional swallowing treatment, swallowing treatment with NMES of sensory approach, and swallowing treatment with NMES of motor approach. NMES were for 20 min, twice a day, for 5 days/week, over a 4-week period (Zhang et al. 2016). Both sensory and motor NMES with traditional swallowing treatment showed significantly greater improvement than the traditional swallowing treatment alone, and sensory NMES showed better improvement than the motor NMES.

Recommendation: NMES can be used to improve the swallowing function in patients with dysphagia after stroke, combined with a traditional swallowing treatment program including behavioral interventions (CEBM classification: level 1, GRADE quality: low, recommendation grade: 0).

4.3 Acupuncture

Acupuncture has been used as a complementary intervention for stroke recovery in some countries, although its mechanism of action is unclear (Zhang et al. 2014). In a recent Cochrane review, four acupuncture RCTs involving 256 patients were included for the meta-analysis with the outcome of dysphagia at the end of trial, which showed the significant favorable effect (OR = 0.24, 95% CI: 0.13 to 0.46) (Geeganage et al. 2012). In a recent systematic review, efficacy of acupuncture was analyzed with the pooling data from 71 RCTs involving 6010 patients, which showed the superior effect over the control (RR = 1.17, 95% CI: 1.13 to 1.21) (Ye et al. 2017). Although, the pooled effect from these meta-analyses showed the positive effect of acupuncture for the swallowing recovery after stroke, most of the included RCTs in the systematic review by Ye et al. were conducted with small sample sizes and risk of bias (i.e., detection, performance, attrition and reporting bias) was high or unclear for most of the studies included (Ye et al. 2017). In addition, the included RCTs may have been confounded due to the use of routine acupuncture or a different type of acupuncture as control and the variations in the delivery of therapy (Geeganage et al. 2012).

Recommendation: Acupuncture can be considered to treat post-stroke dysphagia. (CEBM classification: level 1, GRADE quality: low, recommendation grade: 0).

4.4 Noninvasive Brain Stimulation (NIBS)

Recovery of swallowing after stroke is associated with the reorganization of the swallowing motor cortex (Hamdy et al. 2000). NIBS, such as repetitive transcranial magnetic stimulation (rTMS) or transcranial direct current stimulation (tDCS), is expected to modulate the swallowing motor cortex reorganization. Traditionally, the concept of interhemispheric rivalry is applied to decide the stimulation site or parameters for NIBS after stroke (Hummel and Cohen 2006) but stimulating either hemisphere can theoretically improve the swallowing because the swallowing musculature is dually innervated by both hemispheres (Hamdy et al. 1996). In recent years, the number of clinical trials investigating the effect of NIBS on post-stroke dysphagia has increased. One recent meta-analysis and systematic review including six RCTs (three rTMS and three tDCS studies) demonstrated that NIBS showed significant improvement of dysphagia compared with the sham stimulation (standardized mean difference = 1.08, 95% CI: 0.29 to 1.88) (Yang et al. 2015). In a subgroup analysis, only rTMS showed significant beneficial effect and no statistically significant difference was found between the stimulation sites (ipsilesional vs. contralesional). No complications of NIBS were reported in these studies. Another systematic review included seven RCTs (four rTMS and three tDCS studies) (Pisegna et al. 2016). A pooled analysis of eight studies showed a significant, moderate pooled effect size (0.55, 95% CI: 0.17 to 0.93). Studies stimulating the contralesional hemisphere showed numerically a somewhat bigger effect size (0.65, 95% CI: 0.14 to 1.16) than that of studies stimulating ipsilesional hemisphere (0.46, 95% CI: 0.17 to 0.93). The long-term effect with pooled analysis of three studies was not statistically significant. A very recent systematic review including only six RCTs with a total of 163 acute and subacute stroke patients with dysphagia investigating rTMS effect showed a significant effect size of 1.24 (95% CI: 0.67 to 1.81) for dysphagia outcome and effect was maintained until 4 weeks after the last session of rTMS (Liao et al. 2017). In a subgroup analysis, both high (SMD = 1.38, 95% CI = 0.47 to 2.29) and low frequency stimulation (SMD = 1.02, 95% CI = 0.51 to 1.53) were significantly effective. Stimulating the contralesional (SMD = 0.91, 95% CI = 0.48 to 1.35) or bilateral hemisphere (SMD = 1.60, 95% CI = 0.57 to 2.63) was effective but ipsilesional stimulation yielded more variable effects and therefore was not significantly effective (SMD = 1.59, 95% CI = −0.14 to 3.31) in a subgroup analysis. Based on these recent systematic reviews and meta-analyses, NIBS in the form of rTMS may be effective on post-stroke dysphagia early after stroke (within 3 months), but the included studies were heterogeneous in terms of stimulation site, mode of stimulation and outcomes, which requires further well-designed clinical trials with larger sample sizes. As a note of caution, international safety standards (Rossi et al. 2009), individual exclusion criteria for rTMS, and medico-legal aspects related to the rTMS device used all need to be taken into consideration.

Recommendation: rTMS can be considered to treat post-stroke dysphagia by the clinical expert in this field as an additional treatment modality to the traditional swallowing treatment, especially within 3 months post-stroke (CEBM classification: level 1, GRADE quality: low, recommendation grade: 0).

4.5   Oral Hygiene

Bacterial species colonized in the oral cavity has been suggested as one of the important sources of pathogens for respiratory infections (Scannapieco et al. 2003). Patients with stroke may have poor oral hygiene due to the limitation of basic activities of daily living. One systematic review included four RCTs to investigate the effect of oral hygiene on pneumonia or respiratory tract infection in elderly people living in the institutions and reported positive preventive effects of oral hygiene on pneumonia and respiratory tract infection with absolute risk reductions from 6.6% to 11.7% (Sjögren et al. 2008). A prospective-controlled trial allocated patients with acute stroke to three groups: intervention (dysphagia screening with Gugging Swallowing Screen and intensified oral hygiene, $n = 58$), internal ($n = 58$), and external control groups (clinical dysphagia screening plus usual care) ($n = 30$) (Sørensen et al. 2013). The incidence of X-ray verified pneumonia was significantly lower in the intervention group (7%), compared with internal (28%) or external control groups (27%). A recent pre- to post-intervention (oral hygiene care) trial with the historical control ($n = 707$ in the historical control, $n = 949$ in the intervention group) in hospitalized patients with acute stroke demonstrated that the oral hygiene care significantly reduced the hospital-acquired pneumonia after adjusting for possible confounders (OR = 0.71, 95% CI: 0.51 to 0.98) (Wagner et al. 2016).

Recommendations: Oral hygiene care should be implemented to reduce the risk of pneumonia after stroke (CEBM classification: level 2, GRADE quality: moderate, recommendation grade: B+).

5   Enteral Tube Feedings

In stroke patients with dysphagia who cannot eat orally safely, enteral tube feeding is often required to provide enough nutrition for short or prolonged periods after stroke. Therefore, the decision on timing and maintenance of enteral feeding and type of enteral feeding (e.g., nasogastric tube or percutaneous gastrostomy) is important. In the well-designed, large sample-sized pragmatic multicenter randomized controlled trial, Feed or Ordinary Diet (FOOD) trials, the effect of timing and method of enteral tube feeding for stroke patients with dysphagia was investigated (Dennis et al. 2005). Dysphagic patients early after stroke who were uncertain when to start enteral tube feeding by the clinician were randomly assigned to early enteral tube feeding ($n = 429$) or avoidance of enteral tube feeding for more than 7 days ($n = 428$). Although it was not statistically significant, early enteral tube feeding showed the trend of reduction in risk of death of 5.8% (95% CI: -0.8 to 12.5), but not for death or poor outcome (modified Rankin scale 4 or 5) of 1.2% (-4.2 to 6.6). In the same trial, 321 dysphagic patients who require enteral feeding by the clinician's decision were randomly allocated to early percutaneous gastrostomy ($n = 162$) or nasogastric tube ($n = 159$). Early percutaneous gastrostomy showed the trend of increase in death or poor outcome of 7.8% (95% CI: 0.0 to 15.5), but not for risk of death alone, i.e., 1.0%, 95% CI: -10.0 to 11.9. Therefore, early gastrostomy cannot be advocated based on this study. In a recent Cochrane systematic review including a small number of studies with small number of total subjects for the pooled analysis, gastrostomy showed better results compared with nasogastric tube feeding, in terms of treatment failure, feed delivery, and albumin concentration (Geeganage et al. 2012). Therefore, if oral intake is not possible after stroke for a prolonged period, it is reasonable to change the nasogastric tube feeding to tube feeding via gastrostomy. Individual factors are also taken into consideration, e.g., a nasogastric tube vs. percutaneous can create a different degree of discomfort for individuals and their family, and some individuals are more prone to risk for accidental nasogastric tube displacement and hence aspiration.

Recommendation: Early enteral tube feeding should be implemented in stroke patients with dysphagia who cannot swallow safely and intake sufficient nutrition orally. (CEBM classification: level 1, GRADE quality: moderate, recommendation grade: B+). Early gastrostomy within 4 weeks after stroke does not have to be prioritized over nasogastric tube feeding, unless there is a mandatory reason for percutaneous gastrostomy (CEBM classification: level 1, GRADE quality: low, recommendation grade: 0). Percutaneous gastrostomy placement should be considered in stroke patients with dysphagia who require enteral tube feeding for a prolonged period (more than 4 weeks) (CEBM classification: level 1, GRADE quality: moderate, recommendation grade: B+).

6 Summary

A decision tree for the rehabilitation of swallowing after acute stroke is suggested in Fig. 1.

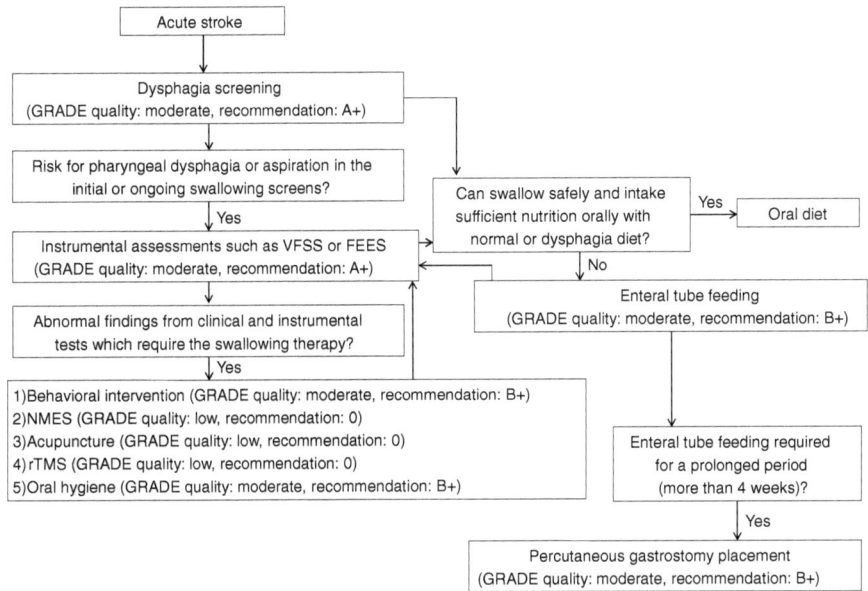

Fig. 1 A decision tree for the rehabilitation of swallowing after acute stroke. *VFSS* videofluoro-scopic swallowing study, *FEES* fiberoptic endoscopic evaluation of swallowing, *NMES* neuromuscular electrical stimulation, *rTMS* repetitive transcranial magnetic stimulation

References

Aviv JE (2000) Prospective, randomized outcome study of endoscopy versus modified barium swallow in patients with dysphagia. Laryngoscope 110:563–574

Bath PM, Scutt P, Love J et al (2016) Pharyngeal electrical stimulation for treatment of dysphagia in subacute stroke. Stroke 47(6):1562–1570

Bax L, McFarlane M, Green E, Miles A (2014) Speech–language pathologist-led fiberoptic endoscopic evaluation of swallowing: functional outcomes for patients after stroke. J Stroke Cerebrovasc Dis 23(3):e195–e200

Boddice G, Brauer S, Gustafsson L, Kenardy J, Hoffmann T (2010) National Stroke Foundation: Clinical Guidelines for Stroke Management 2010. Melbourne, Australia: National Stroke Foundation, ISSBN0-978-0-9805933-3-4

Carnaby G, Hankey GJ, Pizzi J (2006) Behavioural intervention for dysphagia in acute stroke: a randomised controlled trial. Lancet Neurol 5(1):31–37

Chen YW, Chang KH, Chen HC, Liang WM, Wang YH, Lin YN (2016) The effects of surface neuromuscular electrical stimulation on post-stroke dysphagia: a systemic review and meta-analysis. Clin Rehabil 30(1):24–35

Daniels SK, Brailey K, Priestly DH, Herrington LR, Weisberg LA, Foundas AL (1998) Aspiration in patients with acute stroke. Arch Phys Med Rehabil 79:14–19

Dennis MS, Lewis SC, Warlow C, FOOD Trial Collaboration (2005) Effect of timing and method of enteral tube feeding for dysphagic stroke patients (FOOD): a multicentre randomised controlled trial. Lancet 365:764–772

Ding R, Logemann JA (2000) Pneumonia in stroke patients: a retrospective study. Dysphagia 15:51–57

Doggett DL, Tappe KA, Mitchell MD, Chapell R, Coates V, Turkelson CM (2001) Prevention of pneumonia in elderly stroke patients by systematic diagnosis and treatment of dysphagia: an evidence-based comprehensive analysis of the literature. Dysphagia 16:279–295

Falsetti P, Acciai C, Palilla R et al (2009) Oropharyngeal dysphagia after stroke: incidence, diagnosis, and clinical predictors in patients admitted to a neurorehabilitation unit. J Stroke Cerebrovasc Dis 18:329–335

Foley N, Teasell R, Salter K, Kruger E, Martino R (2008) Dysphagia treatment post stroke: a systematic review of randomised controlled trials. Age Ageing 37:258–264

Galovic M, Leisi N, Müller M, Weber J, Abela E, Kägi G, Weder B (2013) Lesion location predicts transient and extended risk of aspiration after supratentorial ischemic stroke. Stroke 44(10):2760–2767

Geeganage C, Beavan J, Ellender S, Bath PM (2012) Interventions for dysphagia and nutritional support in acute and subacute stroke. Cochrane Database Syst Rev 10:CD000323

Hamdy S, Aziz Q, Rothwell JC et al (1996) The cortical topography of human swallowing musculature in health and disease. Nat Med 2:1217–1224

Hamdy S, Rothwell JC, Aziz Q, Thompson DG (2000) Organization and reorganization of human swallowing motor cortex: implications for recovery after stroke. Clin Sci (Lond) 99:151–157

Han TR, Paik N-J, Park JW (2001) Quantifying swallowing function after stroke: a functional dysphagia scale based on videofluoroscopic studies. Arch Phys Med Rehabil 82:677–682

Hebert D, Lindsay MP, McIntyre A et al (2016) Canadian stroke best practice recommendations: stroke rehabilitation practice guidelines, update 2015. Int J Stroke 11:459–484

Hinchey JA, Shephard T, Furie K, Smith D, Wang D, Tonn S (2005) Formal dysphagia screening protocols prevent pneumonia. Stroke 36:1972–1976

Hummel FC, Cohen LG (2006) Non-invasive brain stimulation: a new strategy to improve neurorehabilitation after stroke? Lancet Neurol 5:708–712

Joundi RA, Martino R, Saposnik G, Giannakeas V, Fang J, Kapral MK (2017a) Dysphagia screening after intracerebral hemorrhage. Int J Stroke 1:1747493017729265

Joundi RA, Martino R, Saposnik G, Giannakeas V, Fang J, Kapral MK (2017b) Predictors and outcomes of dysphagia screening after acute ischemic stroke. Stroke 48:900–906

Kertscher B, Speyer R, Palmieri M, Plant C (2014) Bedside screening to detect oropharyngeal dysphagia in patients with neurological disorders: an updated systematic review. Dysphagia 29:204–212

Kim DY, Kim YH, Lee J et al (2016) Clinical practice guideline for stroke rehabilitation in Korea 2016. Brain Neurorehabil 10(Suppl 1)

Kjaersgaard A, Nielsen LH, Sjölund BH (2014) Randomized trial of two swallowing assessment approaches in patients with acquired brain injury: facial-oral tract therapy versus fibreoptic endoscopic evaluation of swallowing. Clin Rehabil 28:243–253

Lakshminarayan K, Tsai AW, Tong X et al (2010) Utility of dysphagia screening results in predicting poststroke pneumonia. Stroke 41:2849–2854

Leigh JH, Lim JY, Han M-K, Bae HJ, Kim WS, Paik NJ (2016) A prospective comparison between bedside swallowing screening test and videofluoroscopic swallowing study in post-stroke dysphagia. Brain Neurorehabil 9:e7

Liao X, Xing G, Guo Z et al (2017) Repetitive transcranial magnetic stimulation as an alternative therapy for dysphagia after stroke: a systematic review and meta-analysis. Clin Rehabil 31:289–298

Martino R, Foley N, Bhogal S, Diamant N, Speechley M, Teasell R (2005) Dysphagia after stroke: incidence, diagnosis, and pulmonary complications. Stroke 36:2756–2763

Palli C, Fandler S, Doppelhofer K et al (2017) Early dysphagia screening by trained nurses reduces pneumonia rate in stroke patients: a clinical intervention study. Stroke 48:2583–2585

Perlman AL (1996) Dysphagia in stroke patients. Semin Neurol 16:341–348

Perry L, Love CP (2001) Screening for dysphagia and aspiration in acute stroke: a systematic review. Dysphagia 16:7–18

Pisegna JM, Kaneoka A, Pearson WG, Kumar S, Langmore SE (2016) Effects of non-invasive brain stimulation on post-stroke dysphagia: a systematic review and meta-analysis of randomized controlled trials. Clin Neurophysiol 127:956–968

Rossi S, Hallett M, Rossini PM, Pascual-Leone A, Safety of TMS Consensus Group (2009) Safety, ethical considerations, and application guidelines for the use of transcranial magnetic stimulation in clinical practice and research. Clin Neurophysiol 120:2008–2039

Scannapieco FA, Bush RB, Paju S (2003) Associations between periodontal disease and risk for nosocomial bacterial pneumonia and chronic obstructive pulmonary disease. A systematic review. Ann Periodontol 8:54–69

Schepp SK, Tirschwell DL, Miller RM, Longstreth W (2011) Swallowing screens after acute stroke. Stroke 43(3):869–871

Singh S, Hamdy S (2006) Dysphagia in stroke patients. Postgrad Med J 82:383–391

Sjögren P, Nilsson E, Forsell M, Johansson O, Hoogstraate J (2008) A systematic review of the preventive effect of oral hygiene on pneumonia and respiratory tract infection in elderly people in hospitals and nursing homes: effect estimates and methodological quality of randomized controlled trials. J Am Geriatr Soc 56:2124–2130

Smith L (2010) Management of Patients with Stroke: rehabilitation, prevention and Management of Complications, and discharge planning: a National Clinical Guideline. SIGN

Smithard D, O'Neill P, Park C, Morris J, Wyatt R, England R, Martin D (1996) Complications and outcome after acute stroke. Stroke 27:1200–1204

Sørensen RT, Rasmussen RS, Overgaard K, Lerche A, Johansen AM, Lindhardt T (2013) Dysphagia screening and intensified oral hygiene reduce pneumonia after stroke. J Neurosci Nurs 45:139–146

Wagner C, Marchina S, Deveau JA, Frayne C, Sulmonte K, Kumar S (2016) Risk of stroke-associated pneumonia and oral hygiene. Cerebrovasc Dis 41:35–39

Warnecke T, Im S, Kaiser C, Hamacher C, Oelenberg S, Dziewas R (2017) Aspiration and dysphagia screening in acute stroke—the Gugging swallowing screen revisited. Eur J Neurol 24:594–601

Wilson RD, Howe EC (2012) A cost-effectiveness analysis of screening methods for dysphagia after stroke. PM&R 4:273–282

Winstein CJ, Stein J, Arena R et al (2016) Guidelines for adult stroke rehabilitation and recovery. Stroke 47:e98–e169

Yang SN, Pyun S-B, Kim HJ, Ahn HS, Rhyu BJ (2015) Effectiveness of non-invasive brain stimulation in dysphagia subsequent to stroke: a systemic review and meta-analysis. Dysphagia 30:383–391

Ye Q, Xie Y, Shi J, Xu Z, Ou A, Xu N (2017) Systematic review on acupuncture for treatment of dysphagia after stroke. Evid Based Complement Alternat Med 2017:6421852

Zhang JH, Wang D, Liu M (2014) Overview of systematic reviews and meta-analyses of acupuncture for stroke. Neuroepidemiology 42:50–58

Zhang M, Tao T, Zhang Z-B et al (2016) Effectiveness of neuromuscular electrical stimulation on patients with dysphagia with medullary infarction. Arch Phys Med Rehabil 97:355–362

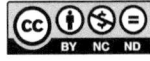

Arm Rehabilitation

Thomas Platz, Linda Schmuck, Sybille Roschka,
and Jane Burridge

1   Introduction

Stroke is the leading cause of long-term disability among adults. Even with appropriate acute care and neurorehabilitation, recovery of motor function after stroke is usually incomplete (Ward and Cohen 2004). More than 60% of stroke survivors suffer from persistent neurological deficits with impaired motor function compromising their independence with activities of daily living (Feigin et al. 2003; Levin et al. 2009). Motor function of the affected arm can explain up to 50% of the variance in functional autonomy in stroke patients (Mercier et al. 2001). Further, both arm impairment (i.e. the ability to move the arm and its segments selectively) and arm activities (i.e. the ability to handle objects successfully) as assessed at discharge

T. Platz (✉)
Institute for Neurorehabilitation and Evidence-based Practice ("An-Institute", University of Greifswald), BDH-Klinik Greifswald, Greifswald, Germany

Neurorehabilitation Research Group, University Medical Centre Greifswald (UMG), Greifswald, Germany

Special Interest Group Clinical Pathways, World Federation Neurorehabilitation (WFNR), North Shields, UK
e-mail: T.Platz@bdh-klinik-greifswald.de

L. Schmuck
Department of Psychiatry and Psychotherapy, University Medical Centre (UMG), Greifswald, Germany
e-mail: linda.schmuck@med.uni-greifswald.de

S. Roschka
Institute for Community Medicine, University Medical Centre Greifswald (UMG), Greifswald, Germany

J. Burridge
Health Sciences, University of Southampton, Southampton, UK
e-mail: J.H.Burridge@soton.ac.uk

© The Author(s) 2021   97
T. Platz (ed.), *Clinical Pathways in Stroke Rehabilitation*,
https://doi.org/10.1007/978-3-030-58505-1_7

from rehabilitation are associated with the level of activity and participation 6 months later, that is, the degree of difficulty and help needed in daily life and instrumental activities, and in social roles (Desrosiers et al. 2003).

Thus, arm paresis after stroke and its therapeutic management is a key element of stroke rehabilitation. Treatment of arm paresis has been ranked among the top ten research priorities relating to life after stroke by stroke survivors, caregivers, and health professionals (Pollock et al. 2014a). A wide variety of therapeutic interventions exist that aim to improve arm impairment, activity limitations, and the amount of actual use of the affected arm in daily life (Pollock et al. 2014b). Therapeutic decisions need to be individualized based on factors such as individual therapeutic goals, time post-stroke, and severity of paresis. Indeed, arm paresis after stroke shows a bimodal distribution: there are many people with either mild or severe arm activity limitations, but fewer with moderate activity limitations (Nakayama et al. 1994). And the course and expected level of recovery are different for patients with more or less profound arm paresis initially after stroke (Kwah and Herbert 2016). Therefore, subgroups with different severity of arm paresis do have different therapeutic needs.

Based on a systematic search of the best evidence available, i.e. randomized controlled trials (RCTs) and systematic reviews (SRs), with or without meta-analysis, and their critical appraisal, a best evidence synthesis was performed for treatment of arm paresis post-stroke, and clinical practice recommendations are given based on this synthesis.

2 Methods for the Best Evidence Synthesis

Within the framework of stroke rehabilitation guideline development of the German neurorehabilitation society (DGNR) (Platz 2017), systematic PubMed searches for RCTs and SRs addressing rehabilitative therapy for arm paresis after stroke had been performed in 2006, 2013, 2016, and on 23.07.2017 (PubMed and Cochrane Library). Search terms had been ((((Cerebrovascular Accident OR Stroke OR cerebrovascular disorders)) AND (Upper Extremity OR arm)) AND (Rehabilitation OR Physical Therapy Modalities OR Biofeedback OR Durable Medical Equipment OR Occupational therapy OR exercise therapy OR physiotherapy OR therapy); few additional reports (3 SRs, 1 RCT) were included based on hand search. Retrieved abstracts and, if necessary, full-text references were checked for defined eligibility criteria by two independent raters and any disagreement was resolved by a third author. Overall, a total of 411 RCT and 114 SR reports were eligible and selected for the best evidence synthesis provided below. The following steps were taken from critical appraisal of evidence to the provision of recommendations (Chap. 2):

I. For each included source (original paper, systematic review), the following was performed:
    1. Standardized evaluation of the methodology (internal validity with regard to study design issues and risk of bias).
    2. Classification of evidence level (1a to 5 according to the "Oxford Center for Evidence-Based Medicine—Levels of Evidence", last version from March

2009, http://www.cebm.net/Oxford-centre-evidence-based-medicine):levels-evidence, March-2009 /).

3. summarizing the results, conclusions, and deriving recommendations as applicable to the individual source,

II. Based on data from all sources on a specific therapy method (across original papers, systematic reviews, and meta-analyses), the following steps were taken:

4. rating the overall quality of evidence of the sources included and thereby the confidence in the estimation of the effect strength (of a therapy) and,

5. provision of graded recommendations.

The quality of evidence is grouped into four categories according to the "GRADE" system ("Grades of Recommendation, Assessment, Development and Evaluation, GRADE", www.gradeworkinggroup.org) (Schünemann et al. 2013):

- High quality: further research is unlikely to affect our confidence in the estimation of the (therapeutic) effect or prognosis.
- Medium quality: further research is likely to affect our confidence in the estimation of the (therapeutic) effect or prognosis and may alter the estimate.
- Low quality: further research will most likely influence our confidence in the estimation of the (therapeutic) effect or prognosis and will probably change the estimate.
- Very low quality: any estimation of the (therapy) effect or prognosis is very uncertain.

The grading of the recommendations according to GRADE (Schünemann et al. 2013) corresponds to the categories "ought to" (A) (strong recommendation) and "should" (B) (weak recommendation); for the purpose of this practice recommendation project, we added the category "can" (0) (option) (Platz 2017; Chap. 2). Recommendation category A is granted for clinically effective interventions with high-quality evidence support; with medium-quality evidence category B; and with low- or very low-quality evidence category 0 can be appropriate. Grading of recommendations is based on both quality of evidence including risk of bias, imprecision or heterogeneity of results, publication bias and other relevant factors for clinical decision-making such as clinical relevance of the approach, effect sizes reported, the benefit-risk ratio, scientific plausibility, and ease to transfer an approach to routine clinical practice.

3 Assessment

A systematic Cochrane overview performed a data synthesis across all Cochrane reviews for interventions targeting upper limb function after stroke. It describes a large variety of assessment tools for arm/hand impairment and function (activity limitations) (Pollock et al. 2014b). Some of the more frequently used measures that can be considered as valid, reliable, and with a clinically important focus are presented below. An indication is given whether the tests can be used for patients with mild, moderate, or severe arm paresis. These measures can be recommended for clinical use when the construct measured is of importance for clinical assessment, monitoring, or decision-making. It should be noted that no single measure is right or wrong, but has its role depending on the specific intention for assessment.

3.1   Measures of Impairment

3.1.1   Active Motor Control

- Fugl-Meyer Assessment of Sensorimotor Recovery after Stroke (upper limb section) (FM Arm) (Fugl-Meyer et al. 1975) (mild-to-severe paresis).
- Wolf Motor Function Test (WMFT) (Wolf et al. 2001) (mild-to-moderate paresis).
- Rivermead Motor Assessment, arm section (RMA arm) (Lincoln and Leadbetter 1979) (mild-to-severe paresis).
- Motricity Index (MI) (Demeurisse et al. 1980) (mild-to-severe paresis).
- Dynamometer scores (including Jamar) (Bohannon 1997) (mild-to-moderate paresis).

The arm section of the Fugl-Meyer test is among the most widely used assessments in post-stroke rehabilitation research; it measures selective motion capacity with its motor subscale (range 0–66), somatosensory function (range 0–24), and passive joint motion/pain (range 0–44). Individual items are ordinally scaled (0–2). The Wolf Motor function test includes selective movement tasks and handling object tasks, each item ordinally scaled (0–5). In addition, time to complete tasks is measured. The Rivermead Motor Assessment arm section has 15 movement tasks with dichotomous evaluation. It is a hierarchical test (range 0–38). The Motricity Index is a simple three-item measure of degree of arm paresis (range 1–100); it is based on a weighted grading of MRC strength grades (Medical Research Council 1975). Dynamometer measure strength for a given movement, e.g. grip, numerically.

3.1.2   Spasticity/Resistance to Passive Movement

Ashworth Scale (AS) (Ashworth 1964), or Modified Ashworth Scale (MAS) (Bohannon and Smith 1987) or Resistance to Passive movement Scale (REPAS) (Platz et al. 2008).

Spasticity as clinically assessed with resistance to passive joint movements has most frequently been measured with the ordinally scaled Ashworth or Modified Ashworth Scale (range 0–4). The REPAS is a summary rating scale across joints based on the Ashworth scale and provides detailed instructions for performance and scoring to support reliability.

3.2   Measures of Arm, Hand, and/or Finger Function

- Action Research Arm Test (ARAT) (Lyle 1981) (mild-to-moderate paresis).
- Box and Block Test (BBT) (Desrosiers et al. 1994) (mild-to-moderate paresis).
- Nine-Hole Peg Test (NHPT) (Kellor et al. 1971) (mild paresis).
- Wolf Motor Function Test (WMFT) (Wolf et al. 2001) (mild-to-moderate paresis).

The ARAT is a hierarchical assessment of the ability to grasp, handle, and transport larger and smaller objects with different grips, which consists of four subtests and a total of 19 tasks (score ranges from 0 to 57). It has widely been used in stroke rehabilitation research. The BBT is a measure of manual dexterity. The number of one-inch cubes grasped and transported from one compartment of a box to the adjacent compartment within 1 min is measured. The NHPT measures finger dexterity by the time needed to grasp and place nine pegs in their holes.

3.3 Measure of Self-Perceived Usefulness of the Affected Arm in Daily Life

- Motor Activity Log, MAL (Taub et al. 1993) (mild-to-moderate paresis).

The MAL is a structured interview intended to examine how much and how well people use their more-affected arm outside of the laboratory setting. Participants are asked standardized questions about the amount of use of their more-affected arm (amount of use, AOU) and the quality of their movement (QOM) during the 30 different functional activities indicated. Each item and subscale are rated between 0 (not used) and 5 (as before stroke) with half scores when indicated, i.e. 0.5, 4.5.

4 Therapy

The best evidence synthesis was grouped in the following sections: training, technology-supported training, and medication. Only a selection of relevant references has been cited. The complete list of references is presented online (www.clinical-pathways.org) for further information.

4.1 Training

A large variety of training strategies without the need for specific technical support is available for stroke survivors with arm paresis.

4.1.1 Dosage of the Therapeutic Time Prescribed and Organizational Forms of Therapy

A simple dose–response relationship does not exist for arm rehabilitation. In addition, it seems that a dedicated *active* arm motor training is a prerequisite to achieve further improvements when dosages are increased. Such a training provided for 2.5 h (Kwakkel et al. 1999) to 4–5 h (Winstein et al. 2004) per week over 4–20 weeks can accelerate arm motor recovery in the acute and subacute phase post-stroke. Two hours of training per week (Sehatzadeh 2015) or a total of more than 15 h of training seem to be necessary to achieve measurable effects on arm motor recovery (Pollock et al. 2014). Increasing therapy time up to 2 or 3 h per day has been shown to generate an additional benefit in the subacute phase post-stroke (Han et al. 2013). Improvement in the chronic phase was demonstrated after prolonged specific active motor training of ≥3 h per week (Cauraugh et al. 2011; Corti et al. 2012), while that was not the case for more passive "mobilization and tactile stimulation" therapy (Hunter et al. 2011). Of note, there was no significant effect for additional time spent in exercise therapy for very high intensity (6 h per day) vs. moderately high intensity (up to 3 h per day) constraint-induced movement therapy (Kwakkel et al. 2015).

Aside from one-to-one therapy, treatment can be organized as arm rehabilitation circuit training (Blennerhassett and Dite 2004; Pang et al. 2006) or as supervised home training (e.g. Harris et al. 2009; Almhdawi et al. 2016). For the latter, dedicated manuals for patients with mild, moderate, or severe paresis with repetitive impairment- and activity-oriented training seem to support therapeutic success in the subacute phase and client-centred individualized functional goal-oriented practice in the chronic phase.

An alternative form of organizing rehabilitation service is telerehabilitation that with limited evidence has been shown to be feasible (Wolf et al. 2015) and equally effective as institution-based arm therapy (Laver et al. 2013). Caregiver-mediated exercises have not been shown to be beneficial for arm rehabilitation post-stroke (Vloothuis et al. 2016).

In case an individual has very poor predicted recovery (complete arm paralysis with diagnosed severe corticospinal tract damage; i.e. loss of motor evoked potentials (MEP) with transcranial magnetic stimulation (TMS), posterior limb of internal capsule damage on MRI diffusion tensor imaging (DTI)), a therapeutic focus on prevention of secondary complications (only) for the plegic arm and teaching compensatory strategies already early after stroke can be effective and show little risk to miss out a recovery potential (Stinear et al. 2017).

4.1.2 "Schools" of Therapy
Bobath therapy (neurodevelopmental therapy, NDT) and other "schools" of therapy have not been shown to specifically support arm motor recovery post-stroke (Langhorne et al. 2009).

4.1.3 Type of Feedback Given
Extrinsic feedback has its role in clinical practice. Proof of clinical effectiveness is, however, rather limited (e.g. Israely and Carmeli 2016).

4.1.4 Bilateral Training
Quite a few RCTs compared bilateral to unilateral training approaches. Overall, equivocal or inferior benefits after bilateral training were reported. Among mildly affected chronic stroke survivors, activities and actual amount of use were better promoted with unilateral training: a Cochrane review (Pollock et al. 2014) indicated better arm function (6 trials, 375 participants; standardized mean difference, SMD 0.20, 95% confidence interval, 95% CI 0.00 to 0.41) and ADL improvement (3 trials, $n = 146$) after unilateral compared to bilateral training. Effects at impairment level had been comparable (4 trials, $n = 228$).

When repetitive bilateral symmetrical active–passive movements were, however, used as priming before active rehabilitation of the affected limb, recovery could be accelerated in subacute stroke patients (Stinear et al. 2014).

4.1.5 Impairment-Oriented Training
One single-centre ($n = 60$) and two multicentre RCTs ($n = 60$ and $n = 148$, resp.) demonstrated a superior effect of the impairment-oriented arm training, i.e. the arm basis training for severe arm paresis and the arm ability training for mild arm

paresis. The arm basis training had a bigger effect on selective motion capacity (FM Arm) with incomplete severe arm paresis compared to therapeutic time equivalent control therapies, i.e. Bobath therapy or "best conventional" therapy (Platz et al. 2005; Platz et al. 2009). The graded training enhances selective motion capacities by a systematic repetitive training of individual joint motions without gravity influence to start with, with gravity influence next, and finally multi-joint movements in a progressive training scheme. The arm ability training improved sensorimotor efficiency with arm activities (TEMPA; Desrosiers et al. 1993) with a long-term effect (Platz et al. 2001) and superiority compared to therapeutic time-equivalent "best conventional" therapy (Platz et al. 2009). It specifically trains speed and accuracy of abilities such as fast finger movements, aiming, visuomotor tracking, steadiness, and dexterity as well as endurance. Taken together, the training techniques provide a comprehensive modular approach for arm paresis after stroke with a moderate differential beneficial effect compared to an active control arm therapy of the same therapeutic time (SMD 0.47, 95% CI 0.12 to 0.81; two studies, number of participants analyzed by individual patient data meta-analysis = 135) (Platz et al. 2015/in preparation).

4.1.6 Task-Specific Training

Task-specific training where training tasks resemble an activity received substantial attention in RCTs with variable results, mostly indicating no or a comparable effect to control therapies both for subacute and chronic patients and a lack of dose–response relationship. A Cochrane review summarized that there is low-quality evidence that repetitive task training (RTT) improves arm function (SMD 0.25, 95% CI 0.01 to 0.49; 11 studies, number of participants analyzed = 749), hand function (SMD 0.25, 95% CI 0.00 to 0.51; eight studies, number of participants analyzed = 619) with significant differences between groups up to 6 months post-treatment (SMD 0.92, 95% CI 0.58 to 1.26; three studies, number of participants analyzed = 153), but not after 6 months; effects were not modified by intervention type, dosage of task practice, or time post-stroke and were no longer significant when studies with high or unclear risk of bias were removed from the meta-analysis (French et al. 2016).

A stronger benefit had been substantiated in one RCT included in the meta-analysis where patients received training tasks that resemble a meaningful activity while the therapist nevertheless focused on motor control issues (impairment level) as therapeutic target (Arya et al. 2012). This was similarly demonstrated for task-oriented mirror therapy (Arya et al. 2015).

4.1.7 Constraint-Induced Movement Therapy (CIMT)

The constraint-induced movement therapy (CIMT) is a response to the observed behaviour that some stroke survivors who suffer from arm paresis learn to cope with their non-affected arm. Even when their affected arm recovers, the learnt non-use behaviour persists. The psychologist Edward Taub, Ph.D. provided a therapeutic approach that reverses the learnt non-use behaviour by restraint of the non-affected arm and massed practice of the affected arm with gradual increase of motor challenges, i.e. "shaping" (Taub et al. 1993). The original CIMT includes 6 h of "shaping" as one-to-one therapy and 90% of waking hours restraint of the non-affected arm. Modified versions, i.e. mCIMT, use up to 3 h therapy sessions with massed practice and less than 90% of waking hours restraint (if any), e.g. a couple of hours per day. The approach (CIMT and mCIMT) is suitable for individuals with learnt non-use and only moderate arm paresis with some preserved hand function and no severe pain or spasticity problem in their affected arm.

CIMT is the arm rehabilitation technique with the broadest evidence base including >50 RCTs and many systematic reviews.

A Cochrane review (Corbetta et al. 2015) (systematic search up to January 2015) with 42 RCTs (1453 participants) and 40 RCTs being used for meta-analysis assessed effects of CIMT and mCIMT or "Forced Use, FU" (restraint only) compared to different control interventions. A high risk for bias by small trials was noted.

Immediate post-training effects were non-significant for ADL activities (Functional Independence Measure, FIM or Barthel Index, BI; 11 studies, 344 participants; SMD 0.24, 95% CI −0.05 to 0.52). A small significant effect on arm motor function (ARAT, WMFT, Emory Motor Function Test, Manual Function Test, RMA; 28 studies, 858 participants; SMD 0.34, 95% CI 0.12 to 0.55) was documented. A moderate significant effect was found for dexterity (Peg Tests, BBT; 4 studies, 113 participants; SMD 0.42, 95% CI 0.04 to 0.79), a significant effect on perceived arm motor function (MAL quality of movement, 24 studies, 891 participants; +0.68 points, 95% CI 0.47 to 0.88; MAL amount of use, 23 studies, 851 participants; +0.79 points, 95% CI 0.50 to 1.08), a moderate to large statistically significant effect on arm motor impairment (FM arm, Chedoke McMaster Impairment Inventory, grip strength, isometric strength; 16 studies, 372 participants; SMD 0.82, 95% CI 0.31 to 1.34), and a non-significant effect on quality of life, QoL (SIS, 3 studies, 96 participants; mean difference, MD +6,54 points, 95% CI −1.2 to 14.28). Three studies involving 125 participants explored disability after a few months of follow-up and found no significant difference (FIM or BI; SMD −0.20, 95% CI −0.57 to 0.16), yet numerically in favour of conventional treatment.

Overall, small effects on arm motor function and perceived arm motor function, moderate effects on dexterity, and larger effects on arm motor impairment could be substantiated after training, while effects on disability and QoL remained non-significant; evidence for long-term effects is rather limited.

Time post-stroke and type of CIMT (mCIMT vs. CIMT) seem not to be critical factors for its effectiveness (Kwakkel et al. 2015) with the exception that early after stroke mCIMT seems preferable over CIMT (Nijland et al. 2011).

A restraint outside therapeutic sessions promotes actual amount of use (only) when combined with a "transfer package", i.e. an individualized critical reflection of "obstacles" to use the affected arm in daily life and how to overcome them individually (Taub et al. 2013).

4.1.8 Strength Training

Strengthening exercises, at least when offered as one component of training, were shown to have a positive effect on grip strength (SMD 0.97, 95% CI 0.05 to 1.85; 6 studies, 306 participants) and arm function (SMD 0.21, 95% CI 0.03 to 0.39; 11

studies, 465 participants), but not on disability (ADL) for patients with (mild to) moderate arm paresis (subacute and chronic phase) as indicated by a systematic review (Harris and Eng 2010).

In a large multicentre RCT recruiting acute/subacute stroke patients with significant, yet incomplete arm paresis (288 participants, 2 to 60 days post-stroke) received up to 1.5 h daily training for 6 weeks either as functional strength training (FST) or movement performance therapy (MPT), each combined with conventional therapy. FST consisted of progressive resistive exercise during functional tasks and MPT of "hands on" guidance for smooth and accurate movements. No significant intergroup differences were observed at the end of intervention (ARAT, WMFT, hand and pinch grip force) (Pomeroy et al. 2018).

4.1.9   Mirror Therapy

During mirror therapy a patient performs certain movements with their non-affected arm while looking into a mirror. The mirror is placed in the patient's midsagittal plane and therefore reflects the non-paretic side as if it were the affected side that moves. It is assumed that by the virtual visual image of the normally moving affected arm, the brain network subserving its control is activated. If this therapy is performed for about 30 min every day for several weeks, motor function has improved and disability reduced in both subacute and chronic phases.

A Cochrane review (Thieme et al. 2018) included 62 studies (ten studies addressing the lower limb) with a total of 1982 participants that compared mirror therapy with other interventions. When compared with all other interventions, mirror therapy for the arm had a significant effect on motor function (activity level) (post-intervention data: SMD 0.46, 95% CI 0.23 to 0.69; 31 studies, 1048 participants). In addition, mirror therapy improved the capability for selective movements (post-intervention data: FM, arm motor score MD 4.32, 95% CI 2.46 to 6.19; 28 studies, 898 participants). The authors found a significant positive effect on pain (SMD -1.10; 95% CI -2.10 to -0.09) which is influenced by patient population and a non-significant positive effect on visuospatial neglect (SMD 1.06; 95% CI -0.10 to 2.23). The effects on motor function could not be substantiated at follow-up assessment after 6 months. The therapeutic effects on motor function were statistically significant when mirror therapy was compared with a sham intervention where the affected arm was invisible, but not when it could be seen.

Therefore, mirror therapy could be applied as an additional intervention in the rehabilitation of patients after stroke. This includes supervised training, including home training for selected patients with a high degree of compliance (Tyson et al. 2015). It is still unclear whether mirror therapy can replace other interventions for improving motor function of the arm. It might especially be suitable as additional training for patients with more severe arm paresis who could not train their affected arm actively by themselves.

4.1.10   Mental Practice

During mental practice (MP) a subject repeatedly mentally rehearses an action or task without physically performing it. In rehabilitation trials, MP was typically used after an actual training session with the paretic arm, ranging from twice a week to daily sessions, each lasting 10 to 60 min for 3–10 weeks.

According to two Cochrane reviews, MP in combination with other treatment appeared more effective in improving upper extremity (impairment and) activity than the other treatment alone (5 studies, 105 participants; SMD 1.37, 95% CI 0.60 to 2.15; Barclay-Goddard et al. 2011; 7 studies, 197 participants; SMD 0.62, 95% CI 0.05 to 1.19; Pollock et al. 2014b). Effects on disability (ADL) were not substantiated. Due to small numbers in each group, subgroup analyses based on time since stroke and dosage of MP were not feasible.

4.1.11 Action Observation

The evidence reviewed is too weak and inconsistent to serve as a basis for clinical practice recommendations.

4.1.12 Music Therapy and Rhythmic Auditory Stimulation

A Cochrane review (Magee et al. 2017) examined the effects of music interventions on upper extremity function. The review included nine studies with a total of 308 participants and found no evidence of effect for music interventions for general upper extremity function, range of motion (shoulder flexion), hand function, upper limb strength, and manual dexterity; two studies indicated that music therapy improved timed performance somewhat.

Further, the addition of rhythmic auditory stimulation or rhythmic auditory cueing with repetitive training of reaching movements might generate some benefit (Yoo and Kim 2016).

4.2   Technology-Supported Training

4.2.1   Passive Devices for Repetitive Arm and Hand Training

A variety of passive devices have been developed for repetitive practice in arm and hand rehabilitation. They include a "reha-slide" the "Bilateral Arm Training with Rhythmic Auditory Cueing, BATRAC", an "Upper Limbs' Encircling Motion, ULEM" apparatus, an arm ergometer (bidirectional hand cycle commonly used for upper body aerobic exercise), and hand orthoses that passively assist finger extension. The devices have been tested in a few RCTs with subacute and chronic stroke patients with moderate-to-severe arm paresis without big effects or superiority; they are an option, e.g. when integrated in a circuit class approach.

4.2.2   Trunk Restraint

Trunk restraint has been used when reaching movements are trained and accompanied by excess trunk movements as compensation for limited shoulder flexion. It has a moderate effect on reduction of upper extremity impairment (improvement of FM Arm score) and increase of active shoulder flexion during reaching as shown for chronic stroke patients with (mild to) moderate upper extremity impairment (FM Arm: SMD 0.54, 95% CI 0.06 to 1.01; 3 trials with 71 participants; active shoulder flexion: SMD 0.45, 95% CI 0.11 to 0.79; 5 trials with 138 patients) (Wee et al. 2014).

4.2.3 Splints and Strapping

Using splints and other orthoses to immobilize joints, e.g. the wrist of the severely affected arm, or shoulder strapping (glenohumeral, sacapulo-thoracal) does not facilitate motor recovery (Veerbeek et al. 2014). It can have a positive therapeutic and prophylactic effect on pain of the joint treated (wrist orthosis and shoulder strapping) (Appel et al. 2014; Bürge et al. 2008).

4.2.4 Arm Rehabilitation Using Virtual Reality (VR) Applications

Both VR games using a commercially available gaming consoles and purpose-built VR-based rehabilitation systems have been used clinically and in clinical trials for arm rehabilitation post-stroke.

Laver et al. (2017) presented in an updated Cochrane review a meta-analysis, which indicated no differential effect on arm function and activities when comparing virtual reality to conventional therapy (SMD 0.07, 95% CI −0.05 to 0.20; 22 studies, 1038 participants, low-quality evidence). However, when virtual reality was used in addition to usual care (providing a higher dose of therapy for those in the intervention group), there was a statistically significant difference between groups in favour of VR (SMD 0.49, 95% CI 0.21 to 0.77; 10 studies, 210 participants, low-quality evidence). These results were mainly based on FM Arm scores (16 trials with 599 participants; MD 2.85, 95% CI 1.06 to 4.65). In subgroup analyses, beneficial effects were corroborated for trials providing more than 15 h of intervention (trend) and when using a specialized rehabilitation training system rather than a commercially available gaming console; comparisons between subgroups were, however, not significant. Time after stroke and severity of arm paresis did not modify the effects significantly.

In one of these non-robot purpose-built VR intervention systems, the therapist's arm movement with an object as shown in the VR ("end effector"-based training) has to be mimicked by a patient. The system provides both "knowledge of performance" (quality of the arm movement) and "knowledge of result" (precision of the movement) based on movement tracking with an electromagnetic system. It has been tested in subacute to chronic stroke patients with mild-to-moderate arm paresis with 1 h VR training plus 1 h traditional arm training five times a week for 4 weeks compared to 2 h per day traditional training. This consistently showed some differential beneficial effect on selective motion capacity and disability (e.g. Kiper et al. 2014). For subjects with more severe arm paresis, a system that integrates arm weight support can be used; the therapy is equally effective as time-equivalent conventional therapy (e.g. Prange et al. 2015).

4.2.5 EMG- and Neuro-Biofeedback

Only low-quality evidence comparing EMG biofeedback with physiotherapy is available with some suggestion that biofeedback may have some beneficial impact (Pollock et al. 2014).

Neurofeedback therapy activation of cerebral motor areas can either be used for direct feedback training, e.g. as target domain during motor imagery or as signal to induce electrical stimulation or robot-assisted movements of the paretic limb. Data from first clinical trials suggest that neurofeedback can have a therapeutic effect (e.g. Mihara et al. 2013; Ramos-Murguialday et al. 2013). Currently, the technology is seen as investigational.

4.2.6 Neuromuscular Electrical Stimulation (NMES)

NMES either can stimulate nerves and muscles cyclically independent of a person's volition to move (cNMES) or triggered by an EMG signal induced by voluntary muscle activity (EMG-triggered NMES, EMG-NMES), controlled by voluntary movements of the non-affected side ("contralaterally controlled FES, CCFES") or can be used within a functional task as functional electrical stimulation, FES, e.g. when single- or multi-channel NMES is used for grasp and release activities.

License and restrictions for use need to be considered for each device used as provided by its manufacturer.

Veerbeek et al. 2014 have carried out a series of meta-analyses of RCT data related to electrical stimulation (49 RCTs, $n = 1521$).

Their meta-analyses indicated that cNMES of wrist and finger flexors and extensors (22 trials, 894 participants) (but not cNMES of wrist and finger extensors) improved selective movement capacity (modified FM Arm: SMD 0.91, 95% CI 0.29 to 1.53; 41 participants) and hand function (Jebsen-Taylor hand function test, JTHFT: SMD 0.88, 95% CI 0.05 to 1.71; 23 participants), but not arm-hand activities. EMG-NMES of wrist and finger extensors (25 trials, 492 participants) improved active range of motion (SMD 1.16, 95% CI 0.28 to 2.03; 61 participants), selective movements (FM Arm, Chedoke-McMaster stroke assessment, CMMSA: SMD 0.58, 95% CI 0.04 to 1.12; 49 participants), arm-hand activities (ARAT, BBT, JTHFT, 10CMT (10-cup moving test), and FTHUE (Functional test for the hemiplegic upper extremity: SMD 0.72, 95% CI 0.41 to 1.03; 162 participants), but had no significant effect on muscle strength and muscle tone. Subgroup analyses revealed no significant differences between post-stroke phases. No evidence revealed a beneficial effect of transcutaneous electrical nerve stimulation (TENS) (four trials, 484 participants).

cNMES of shoulder muscles decreased shoulder subluxation (x-ray: SMD 0.58, 95% CI 0.15 to 1.01; 190 participants) while it did not significantly affect motor function, ROM, or pain; the effect might be restricted to the subacute phase (Vafadar et al. 2015).

For a selection of patients, FES can be used to facilitate high-intensity self-training, e.g. when hand opening is induced by EMG-NMES integrated in an FES orthosis for patients with severe finger extension paresis, and thereby motor function improved (effect size for intergroup differences of change scores: FM Arm-distal d = 1.16, 95% CI 0.21 to 2.10; 24 participants) (Shindo et al. 2011).

4.2.7 Arm Robot Therapy

Arm robots have been developed to repetitively train shoulder and elbow movements (e.g. MIT-manus, MIME, NeReBot, InMotion Linear Robot, UL-EX07, ReoGo), forearm and wrist movements (e.g. NeReBot, Bi-Manu-Track, Hand Mentor, UL-EX07), or finger movements (e.g. Reha-Digit, Amadeo, Hand Mentor, Gloreha). They have the advantage that with assistance by the robot (as needed) stroke survivors can repetitively train active movements even when they have severe arm paresis. High repetition rates for selective movements can thus be achieved during training sessions.

Mehrholz et al. (2018) included 45 trials (involving 1615 participants) in their updated Cochrane review. In these trials, therapy has usually been applied five times a week for 20–105 min, mostly for 2–6 weeks.

Electromechanical and robot-assisted arm training improved activities of daily living scores (SMD 0.31, 95% CI 0.09 to 0.52; 24 studies, 957 participants, high quality of evidence), arm function (SMD 0.32, 95% CI 0.18 to 0.46; 41 studies, 1452 participants, high quality of evidence), and arm muscle strength (SMD 0.46, 95% CI 0.16 to 0.77; 23 studies, 826 participants, high quality of evidence). Electromechanical and robot-assisted arm training did not increase the risk of participant drop-out (RD 0.00, 95% CI −0.02 to 0.02; 45 studies, 1615 participants, high quality of evidence), and adverse events were rare. The test for subgroup differences between a subgroup of participants who received mainly training for the distal arm and the hand (finger, hand, and radioulnar joints) and a subgroup of participants who received training mainly of the proximal arm (shoulder and elbow joints) revealed no significant difference for either arm function or activities of daily living scores at the end of intervention. Effects on ADL could be substantiated for the subgroup treated during the acute and subacute phase, but not for the subgroup with participants in the chronic phase (i.e. more than 3 months after stroke).

Taken together, people who receive electromechanical and robot-assisted arm and/or hand training during the acute/subacute phase after stroke improve their activities of daily living, arm and hand function, and muscle strength while effects in the chronic phase are uncertain.

Another systematic review with meta-analyses excluding RCTs of "insufficient quality" corroborated a small effect of robot therapy on motor function (FM Arm: MD 2.23, 95% CI 0.87 to 3.59; 28 RCTs, 884 participants) and (only) at trend level for activities of daily living (SMD 0.27, 95% CI −0.05 to 0.59; 14 studies with 427 participants) (Veerbeek et al. 2017). In dose-matched trials (i.e. equal therapeutic time allocated), a differential benefit of robot-assisted therapy on motor recovery was still observed (FM Arm: MD 2.28, 95% CI 0.89 to 3.68; 26 RCTs, 808 participants).

The high number of selective repetitive movements generated during robot therapy is probably the main reason for its therapeutic effect.

A specifically task-oriented robot therapy used by high functioning stroke survivors did not achieve a superior benefit at the activity level compared to task-oriented training without robot (Timmermans et al. 2014).

4.2.8 Repetitive Transcranial Magnetic Stimulation (rTMS)

rTMS has been applied during the acute, post-acute, and chronic post-stroke phases to improve motor recovery in stroke patients having upper and/or lower limb paresis. The rationale has been that priming the arm motor cortex by an excitatory stimulation of the lesioned hemisphere or by an inhibitory stimulation of the non-lesioned hemisphere (that itself might inhibit the ipsilesional motor cortex) can promote arm motor recovery.

The following "inhibitory" (I) or "excitatory" (E) types of rTMS have been used in arm motor rehabilitation:

Low-frequency (LF) rTMS (I) of the contralesional primary motor cortex (M1),
Continuous theta burst stimulation (cTBS) (I) of the contralesional M1,
High-frequency (HF) rTMS (E) of the ipsilesional M1, and,
Intermittent theta burst stimulation (iTBS) (E) of the ipsilesional M1.

Thirty-four studies with 904 participants were included in the systematic review by Zhang et al. (2017). Upper limb function was measured by grip force, movement accuracy, keyboard, tapping, pinch and lift force, or complex hand movements. Pooled estimates show that rTMS significantly improved short-term (SMD 0.43, 95% CI 0.30 to 0.56) and long-term (SMD 0.49, 95% CI 0.29 to 0.68) manual dexterity. The mean effect size for the acute subgroup was 0.69 (95% CI 0.41 to 0.97), for subacute stroke 0.43 (95% CI 0.16 to 0.70), and for chronic stroke 0.34 (95% CI 0.00 to 0.69; $P = 0.048$), respectively. The mean effect size for the high-frequency rTMS subgroup was 0.45 (95% CI 0.22 to 0.69) versus 0.42 (95% CI 0.26 to 0.58) for the low-frequency rTMS subgroup. The mean effect size was significant for intermittent theta burst stimulation (iTBS) subgroup at 0.60 (95% CI 0.10 to 1.10), but was only at a trend level for continuous theta burst stimulation (cTBS) at 0.35 (95% CI −0.11 to 0.81; n.s.). The pooled effect size for the subcortical subgroup was 0.66 (95% CI 0.36 to 0.95); the mean effect size for non-specified subgroup was 0.39 (95% CI 0.24 to 0.54). In addition, 25 studies were divided into four subgroups based on the numbers of sessions of the treatment: 1 session, 5 sessions, 10 sessions, and 15 to 16 sessions, with the mean effect sizes as follows: 0.55 (95% CI 0.29 to 0.81) for 1 session; 0.67 (95% CI 0.41 to 0.92) for 5 sessions; 0.20 (95% CI −0.06 to 0.41; n.s.) for 10 sessions; and 0.08 (95% CI −0.36 to 0.51; n.s.) for 15–16 sessions. Only three studies reported mild adverse events such as headache and increased anxiety.

In summary, the data showed a moderate short- and long-term benefit and only rarely reported mild adverse events, i.e. harm. Contralesional LF rTMS and ipsilesional HF rTMS or iTBS were effective with a maximum effect for trials applying 5 sessions; the situation is less clear for contralesional cTBS. The modifiers of treatment effect are to be taken into account with bigger benefits earlier after stroke and with patients suffering from subcortical stroke. Trials frequently included patients with mild-to-moderate arm paresis.

The systematic review by Xiang et al. 2019 including 42 RCTs with a total of 1168 participants reported qualitatively similar results.

Evidence for combined treatments (bilateral HF and LF rTMS within sessions or across series of sessions) also showed benefits. E.g., 2 weeks contralesional LF rTMS, followed by ipsilesional iTBS, had superior effects to the reverse order and sham stimulation in subacute stroke survivors with moderate-to-severe arm paresis (Wang et al. 2014). The database for such combinations is, however, still limited.

Although rTMS appears generally safe for stroke patients, it is necessary to follow the safety guidelines to prevent or minimize the risk of side effects (Rossi et al. 2009). In addition, characteristics of the medical product used for rTMS (including licensing) need to be taken into consideration.

4.2.9   Repetitive Peripheral Magnetic Stimulation (rPMS)

A Cochrane review documented one RCT (63 participants with spastic paresis) with no effect of rPMS in addition to rehabilitation treatment on arm function (FM Arm), while there was some effect on elbow spasticity (Momosaki et al. 2017).

4.2.10   Transcranial Direct Current Stimulation (tDCS)

Compared to rTMS, tDCS is a less focal non-invasive method. tDCS is used to modulate cortical excitability by applying a direct current to the brain; tDCS using anodal stimulation (a-tDCS) might lead to increased cortical excitability (e.g. of the lesioned hemisphere), whereas cathodal stimulation (c-tDCS) might lead to decreased excitability (e.g. of the non-lesioned hemisphere); in addition, anodal stimulation and cathodal stimulation may be applied simultaneously (dual-tDCS).

A systematic Cochrane review including 12 trials with a total of 431 participants measured upper extremity function at the end of a tDCS intervention period and revealed no evidence of an effect in favour of tDCS (a-tDCS, c-tDCS, dual-tDCS) compared to any type of placebo or passive control intervention (SMD 0.01, 95% CI −0.48 to 0.50 for studies presenting absolute values (low-quality evidence) and SMD 0.32, 95% CI −0.51 to 1.15 (low-quality evidence) for studies presenting change values) (Elsner et al. 2016). Regarding the effects of tDCS on upper extremity function at the end of follow-up, four studies with a total of 187 participants (absolute values) showed no evidence of an effect (SMD 0.01, 95% CI −0.48 to 0.50; low-quality evidence). Similarly, a network meta-analysis failed to substantiate an effect of tDCS on arm function among stroke survivors (16 RCTs, 302 participants) (Elsner et al. 2017).

4.2.11   Somatosensory Stimulation

Somatosensory stimulation that can be provided as tactile, thermal, vibratory, pneumatic, or electrical stimulation might have a potential to enhance recovery not only in the somatosensory but also in the motor domain. Overall, the efficacy data from clinical trials is not yet convincing regarding its effects on motor recovery (Veerbeek et al. 2014). Moderate-quality evidence, arising from a small RCT (29 participants), showed that sensory stimulation (alternating cold and "hot" thermal stimulation) combined with active movement efforts had a beneficial effect on arm activities and impairment, when compared to no treatment in acute and subacute stroke patients with moderate-to-severe arm paresis (Modified Motor Assessment Scale: MD 1.58, 95% CI 0.98 to 2.18; Brunnstrom Score: MD 0.19, 95% CI 0.09 to 0.29; 29 participants) (Chen et al. 2005). Similar results (Stroke Rehabilitation Assessment of Movement, ARAT) of thermal stimulation were reported for mostly chronic patients (23 participants; Wu et al. 2010).

4.2.12 Acupuncture

The evidence for acupuncture in arm rehabilitation post-stroke—more frequently assessed for the subacute phase—is considered of low quality due to design issues, heterogeneity, or lack of differential effects in clinical trials. A systematic review highlights the big issues of risk of bias in the published data (Cai et al. 2017). A bigger RCT randomizing 295 subacute stroke patients with moderate-to-severe arm paresis documented acupuncture for 30 min six times a week for 4 weeks to be equally effective as physiotherapy (60 min neurodevelopmental therapy) and occupational therapy (45 min) or the combination of both acupuncture and physiotherapy as well as occupational therapy (Zhuang et al. 2012).

4.2.13 Investigational Devices

Clinical evidence for post-stroke arm rehabilitation with other investigational devices such as the brain–machine interface-supported therapy, vagal nerve stimulation, or epidural electrical motor cortex stimulation is too limited for a recommendation for their use outside study protocols.

4.3 Medication

4.3.1 Botulinum Neurotoxin A (BoNT A)

Treatment of spasticity is covered in the corresponding chapter of this book. There is considerable evidence that BoNT A reduces spasticity, pain associated with spasticity, and consequently difficulties to integrate a plegic severely spastic arm in daily activities (Andringa et al. 2019); there is, however, less evidence to suggest that BoNT A improves active arm function even though this can be the case individually (e.g. Foley et al. 2013).

4.3.2 Drugs to Enhance Recovery

Medication thought to modify neuroplasticity and motor recovery post-stroke has not been investigated extensively. Any data regarding arm rehabilitation is regarded preliminary, e.g. for L-dopa, donepezil, D-amphetamine, fluoxetine, or cerebrolysin and not yet sufficient to recommend its routine clinical use. Individualized treatment decisions (e.g. for L-dopa, fluoxetine, or cerebrolysin) are at the discretion of the physician in charge, mostly as "off-label" treatment.

5   Clinical Pathway and Practice Recommendations

5.1   General Comments

As presented in the paragraph "therapy", there is ample evidence for benefits gained by dedicated arm rehabilitation therapy in terms of improvement of active motor control (impairment) and activities. Self-perceived usefulness of the affected arm as well as disability has been shown to improve with some interventions. Overall, the immediate benefits from various interventions are moderate, long-term effects were less systematically assessed. If applied appropriately, the interventions show little risk to harm and are by and large very acceptable for patients. The question of feasibility to apply these clinically effective therapies rests largely on access to and the availability of skilled human therapeutic resources. The use of technical devices such as arm rehabilitation "robots" ($$), NMES ($), or rTMS ($$) (), NMES ($) requires additional investment (high $$, moderate $) and therapeutic skills. Our knowledge of cost-effectiveness, i.e. the change in costs to the change in therapeutic effects, is limited.

Arm rehabilitation therapy is always embedded in the overall goal-oriented rehabilitation plan. As such, there is no tight link between an individual arm impairment or activity limitations and a certain therapeutic intervention and strategy. Rather, arm rehabilitation needs individually to be tailored and therapeutic decisions need to be weighed with a reflection of the overall rehabilitation goals and their priority.

In addition, therapeutic decisions in arm rehabilitation rest on underlying therapeutic principles, e.g. what are the next steps of motor control improvement to be taken. They might well be achievable by alternative therapeutic options as locally available. Teams might want to use the recommendations given below to structure their service and local "arm rehabilitation pathway" in such a way that the diverse patients' needs can effectively be addressed. As stated above, this is not primarily a matter of technical devices: Evidence-based smart and skilled therapeutic approaches do not have to imply huge "costs" for equipment. Conversely, technical devices can reduce the workload for human resources and can be cost-effective.

This chapter gives insight into the currently best available evidence when improvement of (sensori)motor control, i.e. body functions, or activities performed with the affected arm and hand is a therapeutic goal. Therapeutic affordances will tentatively differ early after stroke, when functional restauration might be a prevailing goal, while in the chronic stage therapeutic goals might more frequently focus on activities primarily. Further, therapeutic steps to be taken by patients with severe arm paresis are quite different from those with mild-to-moderate arm paresis and therapeutic interventions need to be chosen accordingly. Hence, the evidence-based recommendations provided below will be given for the acute, subacute, and the chronic phase and for patients with severe or mild-to-moderate paresis separately. On an individual basis, there might be good reasons to take different decisions based on a patient's values and preferences and a healthcare professional's expertise.

5.2   Dosage and Organization of Treatment

5.2.1   Acute and Subacute Phase After Stroke

A dedicated active arm motor control training of at least 2 h per week over several weeks ought to be provided when acceleration of arm motor recovery is intended post-stroke (level of evidence 1a, quality of evidence high, A+). Increasing the therapy time up to 3 h per day can create a benefit in the subacute stage and can be considered individually (level of evidence 1b, quality of evidence moderate, 0).

Depending on individual circumstances (patient and service) (I) one-to-one therapy, (II) circuit class training that can integrate the use of passive training apparatuses, and (III) intermittently supervised home training, the latter ideally with dedicated training manuals for patients with mild, moderate, or severe paresis, resp., with a focus on repetitive impairment- and activity-oriented training, and documentation of the training should be entertained as therapeutic options (level of evidence 1b, quality of evidence moderate, B+).

In cases with an individually very poor prediction (complete paralysis with diagnosed severe corticospinal tract damage (loss of motor evoked potentials (MEP) with transcranial magnetic stimulation (TMS), posterior limb of internal capsule damage on MRI diffusion tensor imaging (DTI)), a therapeutic focus on prevention of secondary complications (only) for the plegic arm and teaching compensatory strategies with the non-paretic arm can be considered already early after stroke (level of evidence 2b, quality of evidence low [imprecision], 0).

5.2.2   Chronic Phase After Stroke

At least 3 h per week of dedicated active arm motor rehabilitation (including circuit class approaches and the use of training apparatuses or home practice with intermittent supervision) with regular evaluation of therapeutic progress are recommended for prolonged therapy in the chronic stage when improvements at impairment or activity level are intended and can be observed (level of evidence 1b, quality of evidence moderate, B+).

When improved performance of the affected arm in individually valued functional tasks is the therapeutic goal, intensified home practice with intermittent supervision for a couple of weeks is recommended; the training should then focus on client-centred individualized functional goal-oriented practice (level of evidence 1b, quality of evidence moderate, B+).

5.3   Therapeutic Options (Table 1)

5.3.1   Therapeutic Options for Stroke Survivors with Severe Paresis

Daily arm basis training should be considered in the acute and subacute phase when improvement of selective motion capacity is the therapeutic goal for patients with incomplete severe arm paresis (level of evidence 1b, quality of evidence moderate, B+); it is an option in the chronic phase (0).

Table 1 Clinical pathway—therapeutic options in arm rehabilitation post-stroke

Severity	Basic vs. optional	Type of therapy	Acute/ subacute	Chronic
Severe paresis	Basic	Arm basis training	B+	0
		Arm robot therapy	B+	0
		Mirror therapy (additional)	B+	B+
		Bilateral training	0	0
		cNMES, EMG-NMES	0	0
		Therapy with VR and arm weight support	0	
	Optional	Somatosensory stimulation	0	0
		Acupuncture	0	
Mild-to-moderate paresis	Basic	Arm ability training	B+	0
		Repetitive task training	0	0
		Strengthening exercises	0	0
		Therapy with VR	0	0
		Mirror therapy (additional)	B+	B+
		mCIMT/CIMT (learnt non-use)	B+	B+
	Optional	Trunk restraint (reaching)	0	0
		Mental practice	0	0
		rTMS	0	0
		Transfer package	B+	B+
Mild to severe	Discouraged	tDCS	B−	B−

The grading of the recommendations according to GRADE corresponds to the categories "ought to" (A) and "should" (B); the category (0) implies "can". Abbreviations: *cNMES* cyclical neuromuscular electrical stimulation; *EMG* electromyographically triggered; *CIMT* constraint-induced movement therapy; *rTMS* repetitive transcranial magnetic stimulation; *tDCS* transcranial direct current stimulation; *VR* virtual reality.

If available, arm robot therapy should be offered on a daily base especially to increase dosage/intensity of repetitive selective movements in the acute/subacute phase when selective movement capacity recovery is therapeutic goal (level of evidence 1a, quality of evidence high, B+ [unclear long-term effects]); it is also an option in the chronic phase (level of evidence 1a, quality of evidence low [uncertain effects], 0).

Daily mirror therapy as additional training for several weeks, e.g. as supervised self-training, should be considered when motor improvement at impairment and/or activity level is intended (and likely to be achieved) (level of evidence 1a, quality of evidence moderate, B+); patients with neuropathic pain or neglect might have an additional benefit.

Bilateral training is a therapeutic option (level of evidence 1a, quality of evidence moderate, 0).

cNMES of wrist and finger flexors and extensors, or when EMG-triggering is voluntarily possible, EMG-NMES of wrist and finger extensors, in selected cases as FES can be used to enhance selective motion capacity and arm activities (level of evidence 1a, quality of evidence low, 0). cNMES of shoulder muscles can be applied to treat subluxation (level of evidence 1a, quality of evidence low, 0).

Purpose-built virtual reality therapy systems with arm weight support can be used to improve selective motion capacity and arm activities with severe incomplete arm paresis (level of evidence 1b, quality of evidence low, 0).

Somatosensory (especially thermal) stimulation is an option as adjunct therapy (level of evidence 1b, quality of evidence moderate, 0), in the subacute phase also acupuncture (level of evidence 1b, quality of evidence low, 0).

Using splints and other orthoses to intermittently immobilize joints, e.g. the wrist of the severely affected arm or shoulder strapping (glenohumeral, scapulo-thoracal), does not facilitate motor recovery and should not be used for this therapeutic goal (level of evidence 1a, quality of evidence moderate, B−). It can be used to prevent or treat pain associated with severe paresis at these joints (level of evidence 1a, quality of evidence low, 0).

Substantial difficulties to integrate a plegic and severely spastic arm in daily activities and spasticity-associated pain should trigger the evaluation of a botulinum neurotoxin A treatment of the affected muscle groups (level of evidence 1a, quality of evidence moderate, B+).

5.3.2   Therapeutic Options for Stroke Survivors with Moderate and Mild Paresis

A three-week course of daily arm ability training should be considered when improvement of sensorimotor skilfulness (e.g. dexterity) is the therapeutic goal for patients with mild-to-moderate arm paresis (level of evidence 1b, quality of evidence moderate, B+).

Repetitive task training is a therapeutic option when improvement of arm activities is the therapeutic goal (level of evidence 1a, quality of evidence moderate, 0).

Strengthening exercises can be an element of individualized therapy (level of evidence 1a, quality of evidence moderate, 0).

Purpose-built virtual reality therapy systems (and gaming consoles) can be used to improve selective motion capacity (level of evidence 1a, quality of evidence low, 0).

For patients with moderate arm paresis showing compensatory trunk displacement during reaching, using a trunk restraint while training reaching movements can be considered (level of evidence 1a, quality of evidence low, 0).

Daily mirror therapy as additional training for several weeks, e.g. as supervised self-training, should be considered when motor improvement at impairment and/or activity level is intended (level of evidence 1a, quality of evidence moderate, B+); patients with neuropathic pain or neglect might have an additional benefit.

Mental practice is an alternative option after actual motor training sessions with the paretic arm (level of evidence 1a, quality of evidence moderate, 0).

Contralesional LF rTMS or ipsilesional HF rTMS or iTBS of the primary hand motor cortex (e.g. five sessions) can be considered as adjunct therapy by experienced personnel when available and when used within safety guidelines, preferably early after stroke (level of evidence 1a, quality of evidence moderate, 0 [resource implications]).

Patients showing learnt non-use while having only mild-to-moderate paresis with some preserved hand function and no major problems with pain or spasticity in their affected arm should be offered mCIMT or CIMT (the latter when beyond the acute phase) when the actual amount of use of the affected arm is the therapeutic target, i.e. to reverse learnt non-use (level of evidence 1a, quality of evidence high, B+); wearing a restraint of the non-affected arm outside therapeutic sessions is recommended when a "transfer package" is offered during therapy (level of evidence 1b, quality of evidence moderate, B+).

5.3.3 Therapeutic Options Independent of Stage of Disease or Severity of Paresis

For Bobath therapy (neurodevelopmental therapy, NDT), no recommendation can be given (level of evidence 1a, quality of evidence moderate).

The use of tDCS (a-tDCS, c-tDCS, dual-tDCS) to improve upper limb motor function is discouraged outside study protocols (level of evidence 1a, quality of evidence low, B−). The same holds true for rPMS (level of evidence 1a, quality of evidence low, B−).

References

Almhdawi KA, Mathiowetz VG, White M, delMas RC (2016) Efficacy of occupational therapy task-oriented approach in upper extremity post-stroke rehabilitation. Occup Ther Int 23:444–456

Andringa A, van de Port I, van Wegen E, Ket J, Meskers C, Kwakkel G (2019) Effectiveness of Botulinum toxin treatment for upper limb spasticity Poststroke over different ICF domains: a systematic review and meta-analysis. Arch Phys Med Rehabil 100:1703–1725

Appel C, Perry L, Jones F (2014) Shoulder strapping for stroke-related upper limb dysfunction and shoulder impairments: systematic review. NeuroRehabilitation 35:191–204

Arya KN, Verma R, Garg RK, Sharma VP, Agarwal M, Aggarwal GG (2012) Meaningful task-specific training (MTST) for stroke rehabilitation: a randomized controlled trial. Top Stroke Rehabil 19:193–211

Arya KN, Pandian S, Kumar D, Puri V (2015) Task-based Mirror therapy augmenting motor recovery in poststroke hemiparesis: a randomized controlled trial. J Stroke Cerebrovasc Dis 24:1738

Ashworth B (1964) Preliminary trial of carisoprodol in multiple sclerosis. Practitioner 192:540–542

Barclay-Goddard RE, Stevenson TJ, Poluha W, Thalman L (2011) Mental practice for treating upper extremity deficits in individuals with hemiparesis after stroke. Cochrane Database Syst Rev (5):CD005950

Blennerhassett J, Dite W (2004) Additional task-related practice improves mobility and upper limb function early after stroke: a randomised controlled trial. Aust J Physiother 50(4):219–224

Bohannon RW (1997) Reference values for extremity muscle strength obtained by hand-held dynamometry from adults aged 20 to 79 years. Arch Phys Med Rehabil 78(1):26–32. https://doi.org/10.1016/s0003-9993(97)90005-8

Bohannon RW, Smith MB (1987) Inter-rater reliability of a modified Ashworth scale of muscle spasticity. Phys Ther 67:206–207

Bürge E, Kupper D, Finckh A, Ryerson S, Schnider A, Leemann B (2008) Neutral functional realignment orthosis prevents hand pain in patients with subacute stroke: a randomized trial. Arch Phys Med Rehabil 89:1857–1862

Cai Y, Zhang CS, Liu S, Wen Z, Zhang AL, Guo X, Lu C, Xue CC (2017) Electroacupuncture for poststroke spasticity: a systematic review and meta-analysis. Arch Phys Med Rehabil 98:2578–2589

Cauraugh JH, Naik SK, Lodha N, Coombes SA, Summers JJ (2011) Long-term rehabilitation for chronic stroke arm movements: a randomized controlled trial. Clin Rehabil 25:1086–1096

Chen JC, Liang CC, Shaw FZ (2005) Facilitation of sensory and motor recovery by thermal intervention for the hemiplegic upper limb in acute stroke patients: a single-blind randomized clinical trial. Stroke 36:2665–2669

Corbetta D, Sirtori V, Castellini G, Moja L, Gatti R (2015) Constraint-induced movement therapy for upper extremities in people with stroke. Cochrane Database Syst Rev (10):CD004433

Corti M, McGuirk TE, Wu SS, Patten C (2012) Differential effects of power training versus functional task practice on compensation and restoration of arm function after stroke. Neurorehabil Neural Repair 26:842–854

Demeurisse G, Demol O, Robaye E (1980) Motor evaluation in vascular hemiplegia. Eur Neurol 19:382–389

Desrosiers J, Hebert R, Dutil E, Bravo G (1993) Development and reliability of an upper extremity function test for the elderly: the TEMPA. Can J Occup Ther 60:9–16

Desrosiers J, Bravo G, Herbert R, Dutil E, Mercier L (1994) Validation of the box and block test as a measure of dexterity of elderly people: reliability, validity, and norms studies. Arch Phys Med Rehabil 75:751–755

Desrosiers J, Malouin F, Bourbonnais D, Richards CL, Rochette A, Bravo G (2003) Arm and leg impairments and disabilities after stroke rehabilitation: relation to handicap. Clin Rehabil 17:666–673

Elsner B, Kugler J, Pohl M, Mehrholz J (2016) Transcranial direct current stimulation (tDCS) for improving activities of daily living, and physical and cognitive functioning, in people after stroke. Cochrane Database Syst Rev (3):CD009645

Elsner B, Kwakkel G, Kugler J, Mehrholz J (2017) Transcranial direct current stimulation (tDCS) for improving capacity in activities and arm function after stroke: a network meta-analysis of randomised controlled trials. J Neuroeng Rehabil 14:95

Feigin VL, Lawes CM, Bennett DA, Anderson CS (2003) Stroke epidemiology: a review of population-based studies of incidence, prevalence, and case-fatality in the late 20th century. Lancet Neurol 2:43–53

Foley N, Pereira S, Salter K, Fernandez MM, Speechley M, Sequeira K, Miller T, Teasell R (2013) Treatment with Botulinum toxin improves upper-extremity function post stroke: a systematic review and meta-analysis. Arch Phys Med Rehabil 94:977–989

French B, Thomas LH, Coupe J, McMahon NE, Connell L, Harrison J, Sutton CJ, Tishkovskaya S, Watkins CL (2016) Repetitive task training for improving functional ability after stroke. Cochrane Database Syst Rev (11):CD006073

Fugl-Meyer AR, Jaasko L, Leyman IL, Olsson S, Steglind S (1975) The post-stroke hemiplegic patient. I A method for evaluation of physical performance. Scand J Rehabil Med 7:13–31

Han C, Wang Q, Pp M, Mz Q (2013) Effects of intensity of arm training on hemiplegic upper extremity motor recovery in stroke patients: a randomized controlled trial. Clin Rehabil 27:75–81

Harris JE, Eng JJ, Miller WC, Dawson AS (2009) A self-administered Graded Repetitive Arm Supplementary Program (GRASP) improves arm function during inpatient stroke rehabilitation: a multi-site randomized controlled trial. Stroke 40(6):2123–2128

Harris JEH, Eng JJ (2010) Strength training improves upper-limb function in individuals with stroke. a meta-analysis. Stroke 41:136–140

Hunter SM, Hammett L, Ball S, Smith N, Anderson C, Clark A et al (2011) Dose-response study of mobilisation and tactile stimulation therapy for the upper extremity early after stroke: a phase I trial. Neurorehabil Neural Repair 25(4):314–322

Israely S, Carmeli E (2016) Error augmentation as a possible technique for improving upper extremity motor performance after a stroke—a systematic review. Top Stroke Rehabil 23:116–125

Kellor M, Frost J, Silberberg N (1971) Hand strength and dexterity. Am J Occup Ther 25:77–83

Kiper P, Agostini M, Luque-Moreno C, Tonin P, Turolla A (2014) Reinforced feedback in virtual environment for rehabilitation of upper extremity dysfunction after stroke: preliminary data from a randomized controlled trial. Biomed Res Int 2014:752128

Kwah LK, Herbert RD (2016) Prediction of walking and arm recovery after stroke: a critical review. Brain Sci 6:4

Kwakkel G, Veerbeek JM, van Wegen EEH, Wolf SL (2015) Constraint-induced movement therapy after stroke. Lancet Neurol 14:224–234

Kwakkel G, Wagenaar RC, Twisk JW, Lankhorst GJ, Koetsier JC (1999) Intensity of leg and arm training after primary middle-cerebral-artery stroke: a randomised trial. Lancet 354:191–196

Langhorne P, Coupar F, Pollock A (2009) Motor recovery after stroke: a systematic review. Lancet Neurol 8:741–754

Laver KE, Schoene D, Crotty M, George S, Lannin NA, Sherrington C (2013) Telerehabilitation services for stroke. Cochrane Database Syst Rev (12):CD010255

Laver KE, Lange B, George S, Deutsch JE, Saposnik G, Crotty M (2017) Virtual reality for stroke rehabilitation. Cochrane Database Syst Rev 11:CD008349

Levin MF, Kleim JA, Wolf SL (2009) What do motor "recovery" and "compensation" mean in patients following stroke? Neurorehabil Neural Repair 23:313–319

Lincoln NB, Leadbetter D (1979) Assessment of motor function in stroke function. Physiotherapy 65:48–51

Lyle RC (1981) A performance test for assessment of upper limb function in physical rehabilitation treatment and research. Int J Rehabil Res 4:483–492

Magee WL, Clark I, Tamplin J, Bradt J (2017) Music interventions for acquired brain injury. Cochrane Database Syst Rev 1(1):CD006787

Medical Research Council (1975) Aids to the investigation of peripheral nerve injuries. Medical Research Council, HMSO, London

Mehrholz J, Pohl M, Platz T, Kugler J, Elsner B (2018) Electromechanical and robot-assisted arm training for improving activities of daily living, arm function, and arm muscle strength after stroke. Cochrane Database Syst Rev 9(9):CD006876

Mercier L, Audet T, Herbert R, Rochette A, Dubois MF (2001) Impact of motor, cognitive, and perceptual disorders on the ability to perform activities of daily living after stroke. Stroke 32:2602–2608

Mihara M, Hattori N, Hatakenaka M, Yagura H, Kawano T, Hino T, Miyai I (2013) Near-infrared spectroscopy-mediated Neurofeedback enhances efficacy of motor imagery-based training in Poststroke victims: a pilot study. Stroke 44:1091–1098

Momosaki R, Yamada M, Ota E, Abo M (2017) Repetitive peripheral magnetic stimulation for activities of daily living and functional ability in people after stroke. Cochrane Database Syst Rev 6(6):CD011968

Nakayama H, Jorgensen HS, Raaschou HO, Olsen TS (1994) Recovery of upper extremity function in stroke patients: the Copenhagen study. Arch Phys Med Rehabil 75:394–398

Nijland R, Kwakkel G, Bakers J, van Wegen E (2011) Constraint-induced movement therapy for the upper paretic limb in acute or sub-acute stroke: a systematic review. Int J Stroke 6:425–433

Pang MY, Harris JE, Eng JJ (2006) A community-based upper-extremity group exercise program improves motor function and performance of functional activities in chronic stroke: a randomized controlled trial. Arch Phys Med Rehabil 87(1):1–9

Platz T (2017) Practice guidelines in neurorehabilitation. Neurol Int Open 1:E148–E152

Platz T, Winter T, Müller N, Pinkowski C, Eickhof C, Mauritz K-H (2001) Arm ability training for stroke and traumatic brain injury patients with mild arm paresis. A single-blind, randomized, controlled trial. Arch Phys Med Rehabil 82:961–968

Platz T, Eickhof C, van Kaick S, Engel U, Pinkowski C, Kalok S, Pause M (2005) Impairment-oriented training or Bobath therapy for arm paresis after stroke: a single blind, multi-centre randomized controlled trial. Clin Rehabil 19:714–724

Platz T, Vuadens P, Eickhof C, Arnold P, Van Kaick S, Heise K (2008) REPAS, a summary rating scale for resistance to passive movement: item selection, reliability and validity. Disabil Rehabil 30:44–53

Platz T, van Kaick S, Mehrholz J, Leidner O, Eickhof C, Pohl M (2009) Best conventional therapy versus modular impairment-oriented training (IOT) for arm paresis after stroke: a single blind, multi-Centre randomized controlled trial. Neurorehabil Neural Repair 23:706–716

Platz T, Elsner B, Mehrholz J (2015) Arm basis training and arm ability training: two impairment-oriented exercise training techniques for improving arm function after stroke (protocol). Cochrane Database Syst Rev (9):CD011854

Pollock A, Farmer SE, Brady MC, Langhorne P, Mead GE, Mehrholz J et al (2014) Interventions for improving upper limb function after stroke. Cochrane Database Syst Rev Issue 11. Art.No.: CD010820

Pollock A, St George B, Fenton M, Firkins L (2014a) Top 10 research priorities relating to life after stroke—consensus from stroke survivors, caregivers, and health professionals. Int J Stroke 9:313–320

Pollock A, Farmer SE, Brady MC, Langhorne P, Mead GE, Mehrholz J, van Wijck F (2014b) Interventions for improving upper limb function after stroke. Cochrane Database Syst Rev 2014(11):CD010820

Pomeroy VM, Hunter SM, Johansen-Berg H, Ward NS, Kennedy N, Chandler E, Weir CJ, Rothwell J, Wing A, Grey M, Barton G, Leavey N (2018) Functional strength training versus movement performance therapy for upper limb motor recovery early after stroke: a RCT. NIHR Journals Library, Southampton

Prange GB, Kottink AI, Buurke JH, Eckhardt MM, van Keulen-Rouweler BJ, Ribbers GM, Rietman JS (2015) The effect of arm support combined with rehabilitation games on upper-extremity function in subacute stroke: a randomized controlled trial. Neurorehabil Neural Repair 29:174–182

Ramos-Murguialday A, Broetz D, Rea M, Läer L, Yilmaz Ö, Brasil FL, Liberati G, Curado MR, Garcia-Cossio E, Vyziotis A, Cho W, Agostini M, Soares E, Soekadar S, Caria A, Cohen LG, Birbaumer N (2013) Brain-machine Interface in chronic stroke rehabilitation: a controlled study. Ann Neurol 74:100–108

Rossi S, Hallett M, Rossini PM, Pascual-Leone A (2009) Safety, ethical considerations, and application guidelines for the use of transcranial magnetic stimulation in clinical practice and research. Clin Neurophysiol 120:2008–2039

Schünemann H, Brożek J, Guyatt G, Oxman A, editors (2013) GRADE handbook for grading quality of evidence and strength of recommendations. Updated October 2013. The GRADE Working Group. Available from http://www.guidelinedevelopment.org/handbook

Sehatzadeh S (2015) Effect of Increased Intensity of Physiotherapy on Patient Outcomes After Stroke: An Evidence-Based Analysis. Ont Health Technol Assess Ser 15(6):1–42

Shindo K, Fujiwara T, Hara J, Oba H, Hotta F, Tsuji T, Hase K, Liu M (2011) Effectiveness of hybrid assistive neuromuscular dynamic stimulation therapy in patients with subacute stroke: a randomized controlled pilot trial. Neurorehabil Neural Repair 25:830–837

Stinear CM, Petoe MA, Anwar S, Barber PA, Byblow WD (2014) Bilateral priming accelerates recovery of upper limb function after stroke: a randomized controlled trial. Stroke 45:205–210

Stinear CM, Byblow WD, Ackerley SJ, Barber PA, Smith MC (2017) Predicting recovery potential for individual stroke patients increases rehabilitation efficiency. Stroke 48:1011–1019

Taub E, Miller NE, Novack TA, Cook EW, Fleming WC, Nepomuceno CS et al (1993) Technique to improve chronic motor deficit after stroke. Arch Phys Med Rehabil 74:347–354

Taub E, Uswatte G, Mark VW, Morris DM, Barman J, Bowman MH, Bryson C, Delgado A, Bishop-McKary S (2013) Method for enhancing real-world use of a more affected arm in chronic stroke: transfer package of constraint-induced movement therapy. Stroke 44:1383–1388

Thieme H, Morkisch N, Mehrholz J, Pohl M, Behrens J, Borgetto B, Dohle C (2018) Mirror therapy for improving motor function after stroke. Cochrane Database Syst Rev 7(7):CD008449

Timmermans AA, Lemmens RJ, Monfrance M, Geers RP, Bakx W, Smeets RJ et al (2014) Effects of task-oriented robot training on arm function, activity, and quality of life in chronic stroke patients: a randomized controlled trial. J Neuroeng Rehabil 11:45

Tyson S, Wilkinson J, Thomas N, Selles R, McCabe C, Tyrrell P et al (2015) Phase II pragmatic randomized controlled trial of patient-led therapies (mirror therapy and lower-limb exercises) during inpatient stroke rehabilitation. Neurorehabil Neural Repair 29:818–826

Vafadar AK, Côté JN, Archambault PS (2015) Effectiveness of functional electrical stimulation in improving clinical outcomes in the upper arm following stroke: a systematic review and meta-analysis. Biomed Res Int 2015:729768

Veerbeek JM, van Wegen E, van Peppen R, van der Wees PJ, Hendriks E et al (2014) What is the evidence for physical therapy poststroke? A systematic review and meta-analysis. PLoS One 9(2):e87987

Veerbeek JM, Langbroek-Amersfoort AC, van Wegen EE, Meskers CG, Kwakkel G (2017) Effects of robot-assisted therapy for the upper limb after stroke. Neurorehabil Neural Repair 31:107–121

Vloothuis JD, Mulder M, Veerbeek JM, Konijnenbelt M, Visser-Meily JM, Ket JC, Kwakkel G, van Wegen EE (2016) Caregiver-mediated exercises for improving outcomes after stroke. Cochrane Database Syst Rev 12(12):CD011058

Wang CP, Tsai PY, Yang TF, Yang KY, Wang CC (2014) Differential effect of conditioning sequences in coupling inhibitory/facilitatory repetitive transcranial magnetic stimulation for poststroke motor recovery. CNS. Neurosci Ther 20:355–363

Ward NS, Cohen LG (2004) Mechanisms underlying recovery of motor function after stroke. Arch Neurol 61:1844–1848

Wee SK, Hughes AM, Warner M, Burridge JH (2014) Trunk restraint to promote upper extremity recovery in stroke patients: a systematic review and meta-analysis. Neurorehabil Neural Repair 28:660–677

Winstein CJ, Rose DK, Tan SM, Lewthwaite R, Chui HC, Azen SP (2004) A randomized controlled comparison of upper-extremity rehabilitation strategies in acute stroke: A pilot study of immediate and long-term outcomes. Arch Phys Med Rehabil 85(4):620–628

Wolf SL, Catlin PA, Ellis M, Archer AL, Morgan B, Piacentino A (2001) Assessing Wolf Motor function test as outcome measure for research in patients after stroke. Stroke 32:1635–1639

Wolf SL, Sahu K, Bay RC, Buchanan S, Reiss A, Linder S et al (2015) The HAAPI (home arm assistance progression initiative) trial: a novel robotics delivery approach in stroke rehabilitation. Neurorehabil Neural Repair 29:958–968

Wu HC, Lin YC, Hsu MJ, Liu SH, Hsieh CL, Lin JH (2010) Effect of thermal stimulation on upper extremity motor recovery 3 months after stroke. Stroke 41:2378–2380

Xiang H, Sun J, Tang X, Zeng K, Wu X (2019) The effect and optimal parameters of repetitive transcranial magnetic stimulation on motor recovery in stroke patients: a systematic review and meta-analysis of randomized controlled trials. Clin Rehabil 33:847–864

Yoo GE, Kim SJ (2016) Rhythmic auditory cueing in motor rehabilitation for stroke patients: systematic review and meta-analysis. J Music Ther 53:149–177

Zhang L, Xing G, Fan Y, Guo Z, Chen H, Mu Q (2017) Short- and long-term effects of repetitive transcranial magnetic stimulation on upper limb motor function after stroke: a systematic review and meta-analysis. Clin Rehabil 31:1137–1153

Zhuang LX, Xu SF, D'Adamo CR, Jia C, He J, Han DX, Lao LX (2012) An effectiveness study comparing acupuncture, physiotherapy, and their combination in poststroke rehabilitation: a multicentered, randomized, controlled clinical trial. Altern Ther Health Med 18:8–14

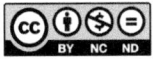

Mobility After Stroke: Relearning to Walk

Klaus Martin Stephan and Dominic Pérennou

1 Introduction

Stroke is one of the leading causes for disability in adults. Approximately two-thirds of stroke patients suffer initially from disturbed mobility (Jorgensen et al. 1995). The scope for functional recovery is greatest during the first few months (Kwakkel et al. 2006). Therefore, early and effective rehabilitation training is an important denominator for the final functional outcome of the patients and subsequently for their quality of life.

In the last years, more and more evidence has been accumulated for well-defined rehabilitative interventions including good-quality multicenter studies (e.g., Duncan et al. 2011) and Cochrane reviews (e.g., Saunders et al. 2009). In the German guideline about rehabilitation of mobility after stroke (ReMoS), this evidence has been structured according to clinical meaningful outcome variables separately for the acute/subacute and the chronic phase after stroke (ReMoS Working Group 2015). A similar approach has been chosen by most of the other guidelines the present results were compared with.

Practical therapy recommendations were given for restoration or improvement of gait separately in patients who are initially not able to walk without help and for those who are able to walk, for the improvement of gait velocity, of walking distance and of balance (Flowchart 1).

Unfortunately, there are hardly any high-quality studies of walking as part of everyday activities: e.g., getting up from a low, unstable chair, maneuvering a

K. M. Stephan (✉)
Department of Neurology, SRH Gesundheitszentrum Waldbronn, Waldbronn, Germany
e-mail: KlausMartin.Stephan@gns.srh.de

D. Pérennou
Grenoble University Hospital, Grenoble, France Grenoble-Alpes University, Grenoble, France
e-mail: DPerennou@chu-grenoble.fr

© The Author(s) 2021
T. Platz (ed.), *Clinical Pathways in Stroke Rehabilitation*,
https://doi.org/10.1007/978-3-030-58505-1_8

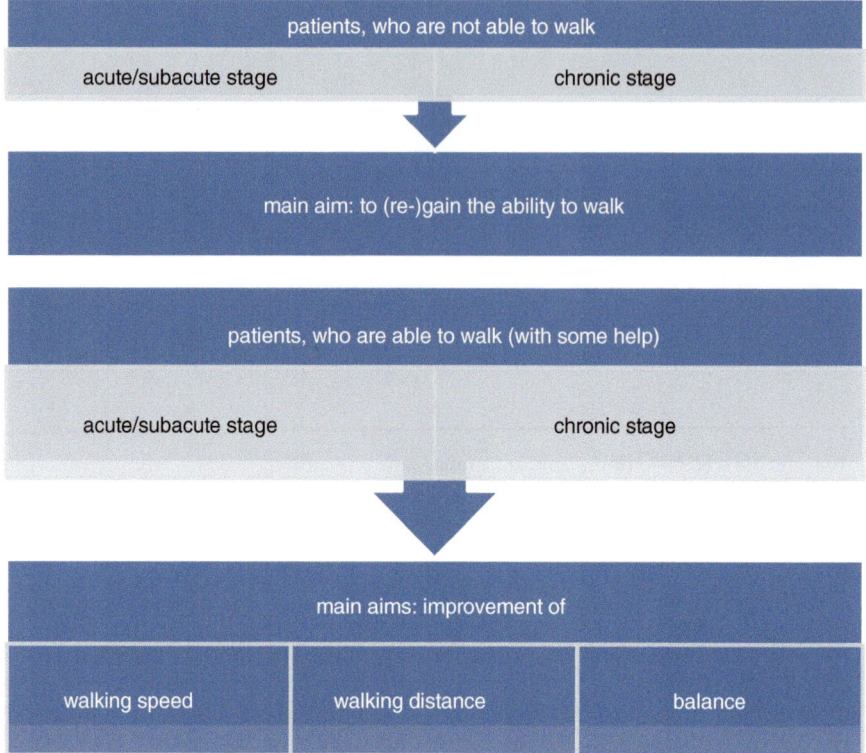

Flowchart 1 Practical therapy recommendations according to clinical status and recovery phase after stroke

slippery surface, and carrying fragile dishes or hot meals from the kitchen to the living room.

As it is very difficult to establish a meaningful, reliable, and standardized test for these basic activities, it might be more promising to search for the underlying elementary requirements for such movements. One of the most important requirements is the ability to balance oneself in many different positions and situations. These requirements and strategies to cope with these challenges have been studied in detail by Pérennou and coworkers in the last decades.

2   Best Evidence for Rehabilitations of Gait: Methodology

A German guideline about rehabilitation of gait after stroke (ReMoS Working Group 2015, Dohle et al. 2016) forms the basis for this chapter. As part of their systematic guideline development program, the German Society for Neurorehabilitation (DGNR) joined forces with "Physio Deutschland," the German Society for Physiotherapy (Deutscher Verband für Physiotherapie), to develop **a**

guideline for rehabilitation of gait after stroke (ReMoS). As an S2e-guideline, a systematic review of the literature has been performed using Medline (PubMed), Pedro und the Cochrane Library (2012), and performing additional hand search (in 2012, 2014, and again in 2015). Eleven systematic reviews and 188 RCTs were identified. Forty-one different principles of interventions have been identified.

Many RCTs present the effect of an intervention for several of the outcome parameters: restoration or improvement of gait, improvement of gait velocity and walking distance, and improvement of balance. Functional Ambulation Categories (FAC) were the predominant assessment for the ability to walk, and the 10-m walking test and 6-min walking test were most commonly used to measure the walking speed and walking distance/walking capacity and the Berg Balance Scale and the Timed Up and Go (TUG) test are most often used to assess functional aspects of balance. In addition, we distinguished whether the intervention took place within the first 6 months in the acute or subacute phase after stroke, or after 6 months in the chronic phase after stroke.

For each intervention, a coherent evaluation was performed, separately for each outcome criteria and clinical phase. The evaluation was based on the evidence of all the available literature and performed according to the principles of the GRADE scheme. The resulting quality of evidence category (high, medium, low, or very low) served as a basis for our recommendations taking into account possible side effects: (A—"ought to," B—"should," 0—"can," "therapeutic option"). The recommendations given in this chapter follow the same rules as outlined in chapter "Clinical Pathways in Stroke Rehabilitation: Background, Scope, and Methods" (see Chap. 2).

The specific ReMoS guideline methodology has been described in detail in German (ReMoS Working Group). The present version has been updated to include recent literature and developments. The German version of the guideline can be obtained in print by the Hippocampus Verlag, Bad Honnef, Germany (www.hippocampus.de) or downloaded from the website of the German Society for Neurorehabilitation (https://www.dgnr.de/images/pdf/leitlinien/S2e_Leitlinie_Rehabilitation_der_Mobilitaet_nach_Schlaganfall.pdf). Tables 1, 2, 3, 4 and 5 of the present publication are modified translations from the original German version of the ReMoS guideline.

The original evidence and the resulting recommendations were compared with the evidence and the resulting recommendations presented in four other international guidelines, which also studied sensorimotor interventions after stroke in detail:

- Practice Guideline for Physical Therapy in patients with stroke (**Royal Dutch Society for Physical Therapy** 2014); (KNGF guideline).
- Guideline for adult stroke rehabilitation and recovery (**American Heart Association/American Stroke Association** 2016) (AHA/ASA guideline).
- Canadian Stroke Best Practice Recommendations, **Canadian Heart and Stroke Foundation**, 6th Edition, 2019 (Canadian guideline)
- Clinical Practice Guideline to improve locomotor function following chronic stroke, incomplete spinal cord injury, and brain injury; **American Physical Therapy Association**, 2020. (APTA guideline).

Similarities and differences between the main recommendations of the different guidelines are discussed. The structure of the ReMoS guideline was used as the structural basis for the comparison. An additional paragraph has been added about early intensive training in the acute phase after stroke (paragraph 3).

3   Early Intensive Training in the Acute Phase (24 H) After Stroke

Early intensive training in the acute phase directly after stroke may be counterproductive: a steady, but less intensive training scheme leads to a less positive effect directly after the training session, but a more positive outcome 3 months later (e.g., Avert Trial Collaboration Group 2015). This result is in line with results in some animal studies, which show that early intensive training leads to additional damage of tissue at risk close to the lesion site (e.g., Humm et al. 1998). Marzolini et al. (2019) have studied this question in more detail and argue that initial therapy sessions should be brief, and cerebral hypotension should be avoided. Furthermore, as stroke can also affect the function of the heart, possible cardiac manifestations should be kept in mind (Marzolini et al. 2019).

Thus, during the first 24 h, mobilization should be performed cautiously even in seemingly fit patients and exercise intensity should be light in the first days, slowly increasing to moderate. Specific clinical guidelines based on recovery stages from neurological and cardiovascular perspectives are provided by Marzolini et al. (2019).

4   Restoration of Gait in Severely Affected Patients Who cannot Walk Without Help

In patients who cannot walk without help, rehabilitation training with a high number of walking cycles early after stroke improves the chances of patients to walk independently at 6 months considerably (Pohl et al. 2007). The present literature suggests that several hundred walking cycles should be achieved in each training session during the first weeks after stroke (e.g., Pohl et al. 2007). This aim can be achieved by the dedicated personal effort of two or more therapists who help the patient to keep in an upright position and continue to move the feet of the patients continuously early after stroke (Peurala et al. 2009). This approach is dependent on a considerable physical effort by the therapists. Machine supported training regimes have also been used for the neurologically severely affected patients based on either exoskeletons or end-effector devices (e.g., Mehrholz and Pohl 2012). A recent Cochrane analysis showed comparable evidence for both technical approaches: Patients who received physiotherapy in combination with electromechanical-assisted gait training after stroke were more likely to achieve independent walking than people who receive gait training without these devices (Mehrholz et al. 2017). This justifies now an equal recommendation for both end-effector devices and exoskeletons, (B—recommendation; different to the original ReMoS recommendation (2015)).

Table 1 Restoration of gait in patients who cannot walk without help *(modified from the original German version of the ReMoS guideline)*

	Subacute phase after stroke	Chronic phase after stroke
A (ought to)		
B (should)	• Intensive, progressive gait training, combining conventional physiotherapy and gait training with—If available and appropriate—End-effector or exoskeleton–based training	
0 (can)	• Intensive gait training with motor imagery as one component • Intensive gait training, also using a treadmill if available and appropriate • Cyclic multichannel stimulation to generate movements similar to a walking pattern • For patients with neglect: Specific neglect training	

An improvement of gait categories from non-ambulatory (FAC 0–1) to independent ambulatory (FAC 4 + 5) was only seen in patients in their acute or early subacute phases. It was not achieved, when intensive training of gait was commenced in non-ambulatory patients in their late subacute or chronic phases after stroke.

In the subacute stage after stroke, intensive gait training should be performed, in order to reestablish the ability to walk (low-to-moderate level of evidence). If available and appropriate, intensive physiotherapy should be combined with the use of an end-effector–based device or an exoskeleton (high quality of evidence; B—recommendation, see also Table 1).

For patients, who are still bedridden, there is low quality of evidence that cyclic multichannel stimulation to generate movements similar to a walking pattern can facilitate the ability to walk later on (Yan et al. 2005); 0—recommendation, Table 1). Interestingly, an adjoining neglect training also facilitates the ability to learn to walk again (Paolucci et al. 1996); (low quality of evidence; 0—recommendation, Table 1). The same is true for motor imagery as a component of gait training (low quality of evidence, 0—recommendation, Table 1).

4.1   Discussion: Restoration of Gait in Non-Ambulatory Patients

"Intensive, repetitive mobility-task training" is recommended by the AHA/ASA guideline for all individuals with gait limitations after stroke (2016) based on a high quality of evidence. Intensive training of mobility is also advocated by the Dutch and Canadian guidelines with similarly high evidence levels. Even though there is only limited direct evidence for intensive conventional gait training in non-ambulatory patients (FAC 1–2; see for example, Peurala et al. 2009), there is strong evidence for the benefit of higher number of steps during training sessions using mechanical devices in this patient group (Table 1, see discussion above).

Similar to the present recommendations for the use of an end-effector–based device or an exoskeleton in combination with conventional physiotherapy and gait training (Table 1, see above), the Dutch KNGF guideline (2014) stated that "it has been demonstrated that robot-assisted gait training for stroke patients who are unable to walk independently improves their … walking ability and performance of basic activities of daily living, compared to conventional therapy (including overground walking)." The two North American guidelines (AHA/ASA Guideline 2016; Canadian Guideline 2019) base their recommendations on basically the same evidence as the two European guidelines of 2014 and 2015 and especially on the Cochrane reviews by Mehrholz et al. (2013, 2017). However, their recommendations are more cautious: "mechanically assisted walking *may be considered* in patients who are non-ambulatory or have low ambulatory ability early after stroke" (AHA/ASA Guideline 2016); "Electromechanical (robotic) assisted gait training devices *could be considered* for patients who would not otherwise practice walking. They should not be used in place of conventional gait therapy." (Canadian Guideline 2019).

Three of the guidelines (ReMoS; KNGF; and AHA/ASA) advocate to consider the use of these mechanical devices mainly in the early subacute phase (up to 3 months) after stroke. The guideline of the American physiotherapists (APTA Guideline 2020) does not address the ability to walk directly. However, with regard to walking speed und duration it states explicitly that "clinicians should not perform walking interventions with exoskeletal robotics on a treadmill or elliptical devices to improve walking speed and distance in individuals greater than 6 months following acute-onset CNS injury as compared with alternative interventions (APTA Guideline 2020)."

4.2 Summary

*For non-ambulatory patients after stroke, all the guidelines advocate <u>intensive, progressive, and task-related mobility training</u>, with direct and indirect evidence for <u>intensive gait training especially during the (early) subacute phase after stroke</u>. A Cochrane review (*Mehrholz et al. 2017*) showed that patients who received physiotherapy in combination with electromechanical-assisted gait training after stroke were more likely to achieve independent walking than people who receive gait training without these devices. However, the strength of recommendations for the use of these devices in the first months after stroke varies between guidelines.*

5 Improvement of Gait in Patients Who Walk Independently or With Little Help

The high number of steps is again the key to improvement in this patient group. However, support by devices such as an exoskeleton or an end-effector device does not improve patient's performance further (Dias et al. 2007). In rehabilitative

Table 2 Restoration of gait in patients who can walk independently with or without an aid or with little help *(modified from the original German version of the ReMoS guideline)*

	Subacute phase after stroke	Chronic phase after stroke
A (ought to)		
B (should)	• Intensive and progressive gait training: Conventional or using a treadmill	• For patients with spastic Equinovarus-deformity: Injections of Botulinum toxin to reduce the need of supportive devices
0 (can)	• Task-specific training combined with motor imagery • Functional electrical stimulation • Additional electroacupuncture • Usage of walking devices (e.g., crane, stick)	• Intensive and progressive task-specific training • Intensive and progressive training in the chronic phase after stroke combined with VR

practice, intensive training of walking on the ground and/or walking on treadmills are often used (e.g., Duncan et al. 2011). Regardless of the exact mode of training (with or without a treadmill), intensity of therapy should be progressive, e.g., with an increase of speed, difficulties or complexity over time (Pohl et al. 2002). Such training can also be performed as "circuit training."

Progressive high-intensity training is especially effective in the subacute phase after stroke (B—recommendations, Table 2). In chronic stroke, it also led to an improvement of gait in these patients, although with a lower quality of evidence for this patient group (0—recommendation, Table 2).

The effect of botulinum toxin injections was evaluated in chronic patients with a spastic equinovarus deformity. A reduction of the use of supportive devices was achieved. There was however no improvement of the abovementioned clinical outcome parameters (Pittock et al. 2003) (B—recommendation for chronic patients with spastic equinovarus deformity).

> **In patients who can walk independently with or without an aid or with little help an intensive and progressive gait training should be performed in the subacute stage after stroke (moderate quality of evidence; B–recommendation, see also** Table 2 **) and can be performed (intermittently) in the chronic phase after stroke (low quality of evidence, 0–recommendation).**

Task-specific training combined with motor imagery, usage of walking devices (e.g., crane, stick), the use of functional electrical stimulation, and additional electroacupuncture all had lower levels of evidence and may be used during training (0—recommendations for the subacute phase, Table 2). The same was true for intensive and progressive training in the chronic phase after stroke (0—recommendation for the chronic phase, Table 2).

5.1   Discussion: Improving Walking Ability in Ambulatory and Nearly Ambulatory Patients

The AHA/ASA guidelines (2016) recommend an intensive, repetitive, and task-related training also for this group of patients—similar to the recommendation above. The KGNF and the Canadian guidelines support this recommendation: e.g., "task and goal-oriented training that is repetitive and progressively adapted should be used to improve performance of selected lower-extremity tasks such as sit to stand, walking distance and walking speed" (Canadian Guideline 2019). There are however open questions: Where should such training be performed: on the ground or on a treadmill? What is the advantage of circle training, which is advocated by several of the guidelines? And do the level of evidence and the class of recommendation differ between the guidelines, especially for some of "our" low-level recommendations?

Training on the ground is the most natural place and does not need any additional technical equipment. And at least for chronic stroke patients, it has been demonstrated that "overground gait training by stroke patients who are able to walk without physical support is more effective in increasing walking distance and reducing anxiety than walking on a treadmill" (KGNF Guideline 2014).

"Group therapy with circuit training is a reasonable approach to improve walking." (AHA/ASA guideline) "It has been demonstrated that circuit class training (CCT) for walking and other mobility-related functions and activities improves walking distance/speed, sitting and standing balance and walking ability, and reduces inactivity in patients with a stroke" (KNGF Guideline 2014; evidence for patients in the subacute and chronic phases after stroke). Circuit class training allows therapists to combine advantages of group and individual treatments: if a reasonable ratio between patients and therapists is guaranteed (e.g., 2:1), therapists can use the positive aspects of group dynamics and also concentrate during individual time slots on those aspects of gait, which are especially important for individual patients. Thus, circle training tries to combine the advantages of the traditional one therapist–one patient relationship with the economically more effective therapist-patient ratio in group settings.

Overground walking exercises can be combined with treadmill training with or without body support to improve walking ability (AHA/ASA guideline). Treadmill-based training "should be used … as an adjunct to over-ground training or when over-ground training is not available or appropriate" (Canadian guideline, evidence for subacute and chronic stroke patients). Treadmill training can be especially useful for patients, which are more severely affected and may profit from body weight support to train more effectively. It has even been demonstrated "that overground gait training for patients with a stroke who are unable to walk independently at the start of therapy has an adverse effect on their aerobic endurance compared to body-weight supported walking exercises" (KNGF Guideline 2014).

Treadmill-based gait training (with or without body weight support) can also been used to enhance specific aspects of gait: walking speed and distance walked (*see paragraphs 7 and 8*). Thus, treadmill-based training can be used twofold: either for specifically defined patient groups (e.g., with body weight support) or for the training and optimization of specific tasks (e.g., maximal speed training (see 7) or training of endurance (see 8)). And sometimes it will just provide an alternative to a training session within a cold and rainy or snowy environment outside the building!

When we prepared the ReMoS guideline, we saw cognitive training (e.g., motor imagery in the subacute phase), external stimulation instead of usage of walking aids (e.g., FES in the subacute phase after stroke), and virtual reality in the chronic phase after stroke as treatment options, which might rapidly develop and become standard treatment methods (see Table 2).

According to the Canadian guidelines (2019), "mental practice should be considered as an adjunct to lower extremity motor retraining." The role of cognitive training in daily routine seems to increase slowly over time. Mental imagery, movement observation, and dual-task paradigms become more and more popular (see also Table 4, paragraph 7). Cognitive training allows patients to concentrate on specific details of the tasks (motor imagery, motor observation) during a learning phase before trying to automatize the task, e.g., with the help of dual-task paradigms. It is important that the learning phase does always include not only imagined or observed but also "real practice." Physiologically this may correspond to changing functional connections between different sensorimotor areas (e.g., Stephan et al. 1995; Hardwick et al. 2018). Only then will cognitive training develop its full potential during the learning process.

In patients with remedial foot paresis (foot drop) ankle foot orthoses (AFO) remain the standard (e.g. AHA/ASA Guideline 2016). Similarly, the Canadian Guidelines (2019) advise that "ankle-foot orthoses should be used on selected patients with foot drop following proper assessment and with follow-up to verify its effectiveness" (evidence for the subacute and chronic stages after stroke). Neuromuscular electrical stimulation remains a valid alternative to an AFO (AHA/ASA Guideline 2016).

Functional electrical stimulation (FES) is often used to improve strength and function (gait). According to the Canadian guideline, "FES should be used in selected patients, but the effects may not be sustained" (Canadian Guideline 2019, evidence for subacute and chronic stages after stroke). There was no substantial change of the quality of evidence in the last years.

Finally, VR combined with progressive training may be used in the chronic phase after stroke (Table 2). The Dutch guideline (2014) is uncertain about the advantages of VR in combination with conventional therapy. The North American guidelines consider VR as possibly beneficial (AHA/ASA Guideline 2016) or as a possible adjunct (Canadian Guideline 2019). The APTA Guideline (2020) is the only guideline which gives a strong recommendation for the use of VR in conjunction with gait training in chronic patients.

These diverging classes of recommendations even in the two guidelines which were published within the last 2 months (Canadian Guideline Dec. 2019 and APTA Guideline Jan. 2020) indicate that for the lower extremities there is still uncertainty about the exact role of VR in routine clinical therapy. Thus, a strong recommendation cannot (yet) be given.

5.2   Summary

In ambulatory patients and patients who need a little help to walk after stroke all guidelines advocate intensive, progressive, and task-related gait training in order to further improve walking ability. Recommendations are given for overground walking and additional treadmill-based therapy. Treadmill-based therapies have different advantages: a) they may be especially useful for more severely affected patients and b) they support the training of specific aspects of walking, walking speed, and distance walked (paragraphs 7 and 8).

Cognitive training, external stimulation, and virtual reality are specific methods of training, which have become more popular over the last years. However, until now, the quality of evidence is not yet very high and therefore recommendations for their therapeutic use are not yet very strong.

6   Improvement of Balance, Reduction of Falls

Isolated balance training does not lead to an improvement of balance during walking or to a reduction of falls in stroke patients. An integration of balance training into the context of standing and walking seems to be the key aspect for clinical meaningful improvements. (Duncan et al. 2003). It is therefore not surprising that a "motor relearning program" with a focus on activities of daily living shows a clear improvement of functionally relevant balance parameters (Chan et al. 2006). This evidence exists mainly for the subacute phase (moderate quality of evidence, B—recommendations for the subacute phase, Table 3) and with a lower quality of evidence also for the chronic phase (0—recommendation). Such an integration of balance exercises into gait-related training may also lead to a reduction of the number of falls (Duncan 2011).

> **In order to improve balance in the subacute stage after stroke and reduce the number of falls in patients who can walk independently with or without an aid or with little help dynamic balance training should be performed as an integral part of an intensive gait training (moderate quality of evidence, B—recommendation, see also** Table 3). **An intensive supervised home training program with progression and a motor relearning program have the same quality of evidence for the subacute stage after stroke (moderate quality of evidence, B—recommendations).**

There is low quality of evidence that an increase in gait speed without accompanying balance training may lead to a higher number of falls (Duncan et al. 2011). Therefore, context dependent balance training should be part of any mobility training after stroke.

Conventional gait training combined with training using mechanical devices (treadmill, end-effector device, or exoskeleton), and strength and endurance

Table 3 Improvement of balance (static, dynamic, reduction of falls) *(modified from the original German version of the ReMoS guideline)*

	Subacute phase after stroke	Chronic phase after stroke
A (ought to)		
B (should)	• Intensive gait training including balance training without treadmill **or** • Intensive gait training including balance training with the use of a treadmill **or** • Intensive supervised home training program (strength, endurance and balance training) with progression • Motor relearning program	
0 (can)	• Conventional gait training including balance training combined with training using an exoskeleton (e.g., Lokomat) or an end-effector–based device • Strength–endurance training • Training to stand on an unstable support base • Acoustic feedback during walking • Orthopedic shoe when indicated	• Conventional gait training including balance training combined with training of a treadmill or other mechanical training devices • Exercises on an unstable support base • Exercises on a progressively smaller support base • Progressive increase of perturbations of the support base • Additional VR-based training

training may also improve balance, especially in the subacute and chronic stages after stroke (low quality of evidence, 0—recommendation, Table 3). If balance training is performed as a specific training session, training with an unstable support base (Saeys et al. 2012) or with a systematic reduction of the size of the support base (McClellan and Ada 2004) is recommended. Ai Chi (Tai Chi in the water) seems also be beneficial (Noh et al. 2008) (low quality of evidence and 0—recommendations for those interventions in the subacute and/or chronic phases after stroke; see Table 3).

6.1 Discussion: Improvement of Balance, Reduction of Falls

Balance training programs are encouraged for those stroke patients who fall or who have fear of falling (e.g., AHA/ASA Guidelines 2016). The Dutch KNGF Guideline (2014) and the ReMoS guideline also encourage the use of such programs (see Table 3).

At first sight, however, the other recommendations of the different guidelines vary widely regarding the best therapies to improve balance: e.g., training on a force platform is advocated (Canadian guideline and to a lesser extent KNGF guideline) or dismissed (ReMoS Guideline, APTA guideline); similarly treadmill training may lead to an improvement of balance (Canadian guideline) or may increase the number of falls (Duncan 2011; ReMoS Guideline, paragraph 7).

A second look however reveals that the goals of the different recommendations differ; taking these different goals into account, the full picture becomes more unified again.

(A) Exercising postural control with visual feedback while standing on a force platform improves the postural sway in stance (KNGF Guideline 2014), such exercises are also advocated by the Canadian guidelines (2019) to train standing. These exercises do, however, not improve dynamic balance e.g., while walking (ReMoS guideline) and are therefore discouraged, if patients want to improve their balance during walking (see also (APTA guideline for the chronic phase, 2020)).

(B) Balance training on an unstable support base and balance boards (ReMoS guideline, subacute, and chronic phase (Table 3); Canadian Guideline 2019, chronic phase), and balance training with virtual reality while standing in the chronic phase (ReMoS guideline (Table 3) and Canadian Guideline 2019), but not in the subacute phase after stroke (Canadian Guideline 2019) may improve dynamic balance and especially balance while walking.

(C) Treadmill training with partial body weight support in the subacute phase (Canadian Guideline 2019) and training with other mechanical devices (see Table 3, especially in severely affected patients) may improve dynamic balance. However, intensive gait training on a treadmill to improve gait speed may also lead to a higher number of falls compared to intensive home-based training (Duncan 2011; for discussion see also Nave et al. 2019). Duncan et al. (2011) argue that presumably the intensity of balance training was too low compared to the intensity of gait speed training on the treadmill. Thus, it may depend on the context whether treadmill training is facilitating or inhibiting the rehabilitation of dynamic balance during walking.

(D) Exercising balance may not only improve walking abilities. It has also been demonstrated that exercising balance during various activities results in improved performance of basic activities of daily living in the subacute and chronic phases after stroke (KNGF guideline).

(E) Balance may also be stabilized using assistive devices or an orthosis if appropriate (AHA/ASA Guideline 2016;).

Thus, balance training while performing functional relevant tasks will lead to an improvement of balance within the context of these tasks. As far as we know, there is not much carryover of "balance abilities" from one functional task to another. In clinical practice, patients may show different degrees of balance control between slow and fast walking, between walking in an open space, and while navigating obstacles between walking with and without carrying objects in their hands. It is important to identify those differences and address them during the rehabilitative process if necessary.

6.2   Summary

In stroke patients, environmentally adapted balance training improves those aspects of balance which are specifically trained: (a) exercising postural control on a force platform improves postural sway in stance, (b) training of walking abilities by over-ground gait training, circle training, or with the help of walking devices (e.g., treadmill, end-effector devices, exoskeletons) improves standing balance, walking ability, and walking distance and speed, and (c) exercising balance during various basic activities results in improved performance of those basic activities in daily living. According to the clinical data, there seems to be very limited carryover between different aspects of balance control. Therefore, balance should be trained within the context of walking, and while performing, ADL tasks in order to reduce the risk of falls and resulting injuries.

7   Improvement of Walking Speed

Once walking ability including basic balance control has been achieved, other outcome variables become important such as walking speed or walking distance. To improve walking speed, a progressive increase of training requirements is the dominant therapeutic principle. Progressive circuit training (Outermans et al. 2010) and progressive treadmill training (Pohl et al. 2002; Eich et al. 2004) have the highest quality of evidence (A—recommendations for the subacute phase, Table 4). Treadmill training without monitoring of heart frequency or perceived exertion or an intensive home exercise programs also have a positive effect (Duncan et al. 2011), but at a lower quality of evidence (B—recommendations for the subacute phase, Table 4). Progressive anaerobic training without direct functional relevance, however, does not lead to a further improvement of maximal gait speed, even when compared to "relaxation" (Nave et al. 2019). In this study (PHYS-stroke), both subacute patient groups showed a comparable increase in gait speed when the interventions were added to a standard rehabilitation program. This result demonstrates the importance of task- and goal-directed training, when patients, who have already learned the basic walking skills, try to achieve maximal walking speed.

An increase of walking velocity can also be achieved by intensive training in the chronic phase after stroke (see, for example, (Duncan et al. 2011)), however, the overall quality of evidence is lower than for patients in the subacute phase (0—recommendation, Table 4).

Stimulation of flexor-reflex afferents synchronous to the steps (Spaich et al. 2014) leads to an increase of velocity in the subacute phase (moderate quality of evidence, B—recommendation). In patients with a leg paresis, gait training with an orthosis (Thijssen et al. 2007; Erel et al. 2011) may also increase gait velocity (moderate quality of evidence, B—recommendation for the chronic phase, Table 4). Until today, there is however no evidence for a differential effectiveness of static or dynamic devices (de Seze et al. 2011).

Table 4 Improvement of walking speed in patients who can walk independently, with supervision or with a little help *(modified from the original German version of the ReMoS guideline)*

	Subacute phase after stroke	Chronic phase after stroke
A (ought to)	• Intensive task-specific progressive gait training (using a treadmill or performing a task specific circuit training)	
B (should)	• Intensive gait training without treadmill **or** • Intensive gait training with the use of a treadmill **or** • Intensive supervised home training program (strength, endurance, and balance training) with progression • Gait training with stimulation of flexor-reflex afferences	• Orthosis with or without electrical stimulation (indirect effect)
0 (can)	• Task-specific strength–endurance training • Gait training with acoustic rhythmic stimulation • Task-specific training using additional cognitive elements e.g., motor imagery • Acoustic (e.g., musical) feedback, knowledge of results	• Intensive, task-specific gait training • Task-specific endurance training (e.g., aerobic treadmill training combined with gait training on the floor) • Task-specific strength training • Task-specific cognitive training, e.g., motor observation, dual-task paradigms • Functional electrical stimulation

- **In order to increase walking velocity in patients who can walk independently with or without an aid or with little help, goal-directed progressive training of gait velocity ought to be performed (high quality of evidence, A—recommendation for the subacute phase after stroke, see also** Table 4).
- **If this is not possible, an intensive gait training with or without a use of a treadmill, an intensive supervised home training program or training with stimulation of flexor-reflex afferents should be performed in the subacute stage (moderate quality of evidence, B—recommendation).**
- **In the chronic stage, an orthosis with or without electrical stimulation should be applied in appropriate patients if available (moderate quality of evidence, B—recommendation).**
- **Intensive task specific gait, strength, endurance, and cognitive training can also be performed in the chronic stage (0—recommendation).**

The effectiveness of the different intervention may be further improved by the combination of gait training with other techniques in the subacute and chronic stages. There are encouraging results for the combination of gait training with cognitive training (e.g., movement observation, movement imagery (Verma et al. 2011), training under dual-task conditions), with additional stimulations and/or feedback (electrical stimulation, acupuncture, rhythmic acoustic stimulation (Thaut et al. 1997), and acoustic feedback (Schauer and Mauritz 2003)) as well as with additional strength and endurance training (low quality of evidence and 0—recommendations for all interventions; for some interventions only for the subacute or for the chronic phase, see also Table 4). An isolated use of these techniques out of a functional context does, however, not lead to the desired improvements.

7.1 Discussion: Improvement of Walking Speed

Again repetitive, progressive, and task-related training forms, the basis for any training-related improvement of gait speed in the subacute phase (Table 4; AHA/ASA Guideline 2016; Canadian Guideline 2019).

Training on the ground, possibly also in the form of circuit training and treadmill training are the two main modes of training which are often combined. Treadmill training with or without body weight support should (Canadian guideline) or could (Dutch guideline) be used to improve walking speed after stroke. Especially with regard to maximum walking speed, it has been demonstrated that treadmill training without body weight support is more effective than conventional gait training (Dutch guideline). Mehrholz et al. (2017) have shown that the quality of evidence for the use of treadmills is highest for ambulatory patients in the first 3 months. However, although the improvement of maximum walking speed was statistically significant at the end of treatment, even these patients had no persisting beneficial effects.

Thus, whenever possible, the achieved improvements in walking speed should be transferred into meaningful and relevant tasks of daily routine (see Table 4).

Strength and endurance training and balance training are further components of such an intensive training program. Strength and aerobic endurance training are advocated by all guidelines in this context (e.g., Canadian guideline (2019) and Dutch Guideline 2014). The role of aerobic endurance training in stroke rehabilitation will be discussed in more detail in the next paragraph chapter (paragraph 8). The importance of balance training was already shown in the previous paragraph (paragraph 6).

Rhythmic acoustic stimulation (RAS) is a further technique to facilitate the speed of repetitive movements and furthermore to influence the gait dynamics. While the Dutch (2014), the ReMoS and the AHA/ASA guideline (2016) identified a low quality of evidence and gave weak recommendations (e.g., Table 4), the Canadian guideline (2019) advised that "rhythmic auditory stimulation should be considered for improving gait parameters in stroke patients, including gait velocity ...." Evidence for RAS in stroke is building up, although there is still a need for long-term evaluations and for a deeper understanding of its (patho-)physiology in healthy subjects (Stephan et al. 2002) and patients. As a reduced effect over time is known, it might be advisable to try to preserve the gain in walking speed by including such tasks in daily routine similar to the strategy after treadmill training (see above). As RAS is much easier to administer than treadmill training, shorter RAS sessions can easily be included in daily or weekly routines.

7.2   Summary

Task- and goal-oriented training that is repetitive and progressively adapted should be used to improve walking speed. Overground training and treadmill training are the most common forms of training.

In order to improve comfortable walking speed, strength and aerobic endurance training, balance training, rhythmic acoustic stimulation and mental observation, and motor imagery help to train further aspects of mobility. In order to improve specifically maximal walking speed, structured treadmill training may be most promising as it allows the patients to concentrate on this specific aspect of mobility. Thus, similar to training in sports, basic skills are the basis for advanced training with specific goals.

Unfortunately, the training at the rehabilitation center does not lead to a permanent improvement of function on a stable level. Therefore, whenever possible, the achieved improvements in walking speed should be transferred into meaningful and relevant tasks of daily routine.

8   Improvement of Walking Distance

Walking longer distances (e.g., for 6 min as in the 6-min walking test) does not only require a sufficient quality of gait parameters but also cardiovascular fitness. The American Heart Association (AHA) has developed criteria for effective endurance training such as a minimal training duration, optimal heart frequency, and perceived levels of exertion (Gordon et al. 2004). In order to improve walking distance, the cardiovascular fitness training has to be embedded into a specific functional context, e.g., treadmill training (16) or task-specific circuit training (Outermans et al. 2010) (high quality of evidence and A—recommendations for the subacute phase; moderate quality of evidence and B—recommendation for the chronic phase, Table 5). Isolated aerobic endurance training on a cycling ergometer does not improve walking distance (Katz-Leurer et al. 2003). This result stresses the importance of task- and goal-directed training also for the improvement of walking distance.

Other progressive forms of training without monitoring of heart frequency or perceived exertion such as supervised home training (Duncan et al. 2011) or progressive treadmill training (Pohl et al. 2002) have a lower quality of evidence (moderate quality of evidence and B—recommendations for the subacute phase; low quality of evidence and 0—recommendations for the chronic phase, Table 5).

Improvement can be achieved both in the subacute and in the chronic phases after stroke, once basic walking ability has been achieved (e.g., (Duncan et al.

Table 5 Improvement of walking distance in patients who can walk with supervision or little help *(modified from the original German version of the ReMoS guideline)*

	Subacute phase after stroke	Chronic phase after stroke
A (ought to)	• Task- and goal-specific endurance training	
B (should)	• Intensive supervised home training program (strength, endurance, and balance training) with progression • Intensive gait training with the use of a treadmill, especially progressive aerobic treadmill training	• Task-specific endurance training, e.g., progressive aerobic treadmill training • Orthosis with electrical peroneal stimulation (indirect effect)
0 (can)	• Strength and endurance with or without feedback • Cognitive training (motor imagery) • Functional electrical stimulation during gait training	• Intensive progressive training • Treadmill training and variable training on the floor • Feedback, motor observation

2011)). However, the overall quality of evidence is higher for patients in the subacute phase than for patients in the chronic phase leading to different levels of recommendation (see above).

In chronic stroke, patients with paresis may benefit from the use of assistive devices such as an orthosis. Continuous use of an orthosis with electrical stimulation also leads to an improvement of walking distance (Kottink et al. 2007) (moderate quality of evidence, B—recommendation).

- **In the chronic stage, task-specific endurance training, e.g., progressive aerobic treadmill training should be performed or an orthosis with electrical peroneal stimulation should be applied if indicated and available (moderate quality of evidence, B—recommendation).**
- **In order to increase walking distance in patients who can walk independently with or without an aid or with little help task- and goal-specific endurance training ought to be performed, especially in the subacute phase after stroke (high quality of evidence, A—recommendation, see also Table 5).**
- **If this is not possible, an intensive gait training with or without a use of a treadmill, an intensive supervised home training program should be performed in the subacute stage (moderate quality of evidence, B—recommendation).**

Elements of cognitive training (motor imagery, motor observation), additional stimulation techniques (peroneal stimulation, functional electrical stimulation), and especially task-specific endurance and strength training with or without feedback can also enhance walking distance (low quality of evidence and 0—recommendations for all interventions in the subacute and/or chronic phases after stroke, Table 5).

8.1   Discussion: Increasing Walking Distance

<u>Strength and aerobic endurance training</u> within a task- and goal-related training program is the key to build up walking capacity after stroke. Strength and endurance training should be repetitive and progressively adapted (e.g., Canadian Guideline 2019).

Again, a <u>combination of overground training with treadmill training</u> seems to be most useful to combine the strength of both training forms (see the Dutch Guideline 2014, for the advantages of overground training, the Canadian Guideline 2019 for the advantages of treadmill training).

Such a setting also allows to include <u>strength training in a functional context</u>. It has been shown to be less effective: for persons with mild-to-moderate impairment in lower extremity function when performed on its own (Canadian Guideline 2019). The Canadian Guideline (2019) suggests that "individually-tailored <u>aerobic training</u> involving large muscle groups should be incorporated into a comprehensive stroke rehabilitation program to enhance cardiovascular endurance and cognitive function." Such training can be easily performed as part of a comprehensive training regime to further walking capacity.

The Canadian Guideline (2019) gives recommendations, which investigations should be performed and which precautions should be taken to avoid harm to the patients. They further recommend "patients should participate in aerobic exercise at least 3 times weekly for a minimum of 8 weeks, progressing as tolerated to 20 minutes or more per session, exclusive of warm-up and cooldown" and "heart rate and blood pressure should be monitored during training to ensure safety and attainment of target exercise intensity." More detailed recommendations for patient safety are given by Marzolini et al. (2019).

Training walking distance provides implicitly some <u>feedback</u> about the distance walked to every patient. Different forms of structured feedback have been used to provide the patients with information about their progress and details of their performance: verbal feedback (Dutch Guideline 2014), biofeedback, in the form of visual and/or auditory signals to indicate unequal weight bearing and timing (Canadian Guideline 2019), and EMG feedback (AHA/ASA Guideline 2016; Dutch Guideline 2014). However, none of the technical feedback signals have led to a substantial enhancement of functional recovery and were strongly recommended in the guidelines. Verbal feedback seems to be the most promising form of feedback, possibly associated with a caring and supportive attitude of the therapist.

<u>Continuous training after discharge</u> is a problem for most patients after stroke. For aerobic exercise, the Canadian Guideline (2019) suggest: "to ensure long-term maintenance of health benefits, a planned transition from structured aerobic exercise to more self-directed physical activity at home or in the community should be implemented." Furthermore, strategies to address specific barriers to physical activity related to patients, healthcare providers, family, and/or the

environment should be employed. These recommendations are important for the transition of most learned skills on discharge from the rehabilitation hospital or center.

8.2   Summary

Task- and goal-specific strength and aerobic endurance training should be the focus of training to enhance walking distance after stroke. It should incorporate both overground training and treadmill training, if available. Pre-participation screening and monitoring during aerobic training should be performed to ensure patient safety.

Treadmill training has the advantage that it allows easy monitoring during training and attainment of target exercise intensity. However, it is difficult to maintain such a structure outside a rehabilitative setting. Therefore, a planned transition from a structured therapy setting to more self-directed physical activity at home or in the community should be implemented.

9   General Discussion and Conclusions

Five different guidelines with recommendations for rehabilitative therapies were compared. All of them were published by scientific societies. Their description of the timeline of rehabilitation was similar: the acute stage or phase lasted for about a week after stroke, the subacute stage until the end of the sixth month with a subdivision between an early subacute phase (up to 3 months) and a late subacute phase (after 3 months up to 6 months). Thereafter began the chronic phase after stroke.

Most of the evidence for specific interventions and the recommendations based on the evidence were similar between the guidelines. This is not surprising, as more or less the same literature formed the basis for the guideline, and the process of writing a guideline is now standardized internationally.

Nevertheless, the classification of the literature and the critical appraisal process also led to some different recommendations in different regions of the world.

First, the critical appraisal of a study may lead to different results regarding the level and/or quality of evidence. Second, synthesis of the evidence of individual studies may lead to different categories of quality of evidence for specific interventions. Furthermore, the quality of evidence for a specific intervention may change over time: there are up to 5 years difference between the years of publication of the different guidelines. And during this time, further studies have been published, which may change the overall quality of evidence or the estimate of therapeutic effect itself.

More often, however, the writers of the guideline will disagree about the level of recommendation. The GRADE system does explicitly require the guideline writers to include not only the quality of evidence but also relevant context factors and the degree of certainty of the recommendation. Therefore, it is not surprising when two or more writers disagree about the class of recommendation, especially when they have a different methodological, cultural, economic, and/or geographic background. From this perspective, the more or less unified view on the process of rehabilitation of walking after stroke is more surprising than the discrepancies between the guidelines.

The evidence underlying the recommendations suggests <u>elementary rules for recovery and rehabilitation of gait</u> according to the different stages of recovery after stroke. These elementary rules are valid for patients regardless of the country or region they live in and form a basis to shape local and regional clinical pathways.

- In the acute phase, directly after stroke (first 24 h), very intensive training may impair the degree of recovery 3 months later.
- In **patients who cannot walk,** intensive task-specific training (e.g., a high number of repetitions of the full gait cycle) supports recovery of basic walking abilities in patients who cannot walk in the subacute stage after stroke. There is no evidence that such an intensive training is still effective to regain basic walking abilities in the chronic stage after stroke in this patient group. Thus, the training of compensatory modes of mobility (e.g., wheelchair handling) may be a major therapeutic aim in these patients (see Flowchart 2).
- In **patients who can walk independently or with some help,** intensive task-specific training supports improvement or even restoration of gait. Often balance, walking speed, and walking distance are the main therapeutic goals in

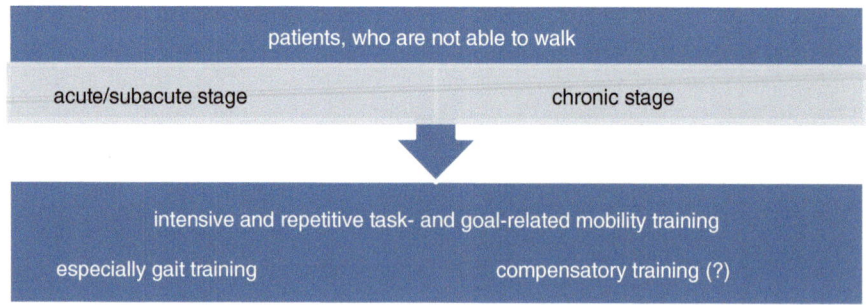

Flowchart 2 Main therapeutic goals and interventions in the different phases of recovery in patients who are not able to walk

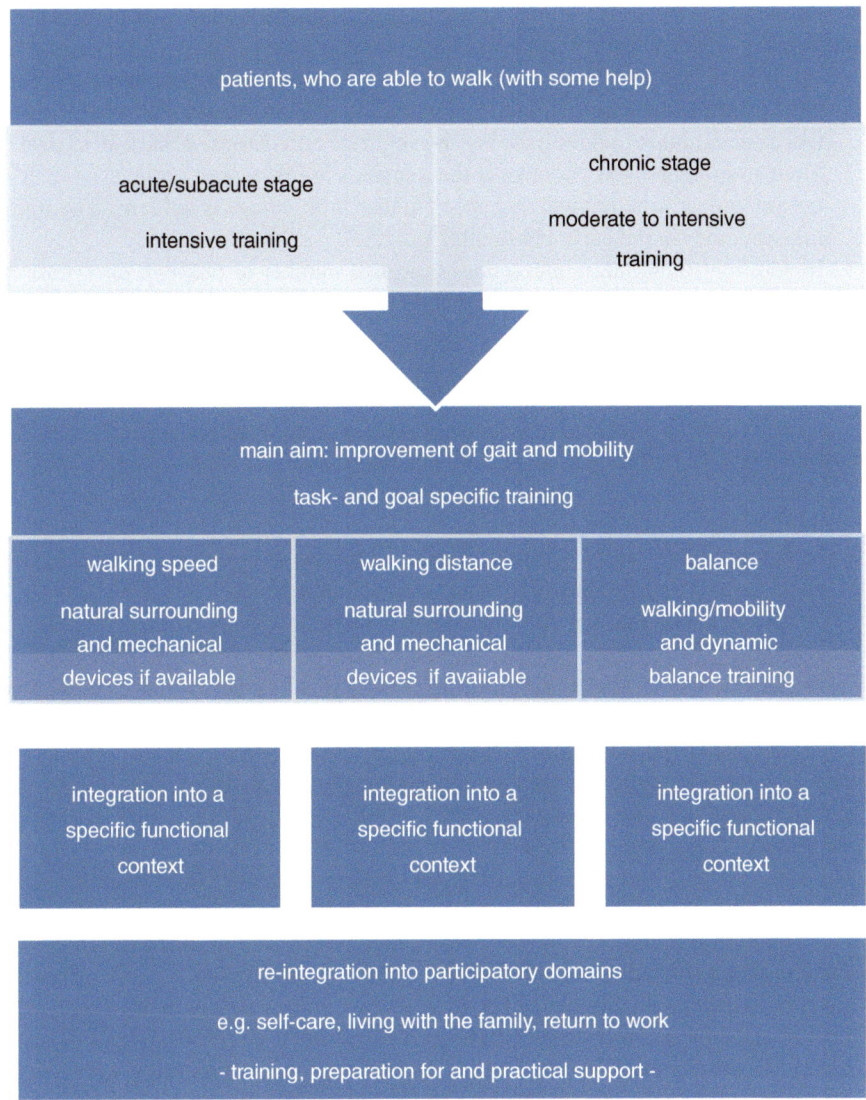

Flowchart 3 Main therapeutic goals and therapeutic principles depending on different rehabilitative priorities in patients who are able to walk (with some help)

these patients (see Flowchart 3). There is higher quality of evidence for such training in the subacute than in the chronic stage after stroke.

• Clinically meaningful improvements of balance are best achieved when dynamic balance training is performed as an integral part of stance and gait training and/ or during relevant ADL sessions. Such training may also lead to a reduction of the number of falls after stroke. Again, there is higher quality of evidence for training in the subacute than in the chronic stage after stroke.

- While basic walking abilities and balance seem to be basic elements of mobility which have to be relearned early after stroke, walking speed and walking distance can be improved both during the subacute and chronic phases after stroke. Their training is most effective if the demands are increased progressively. It is not yet known, whether walking speed in the chronic stage is influenced by training schedules in the early phase after stroke.
- In addition to the main interventions, a great number of possible interventions are available, which have also been shown to be effective. These may be chosen according to the specificity of the clinical deficits and the individual preferences of the patients.
- In contrast to other tasks and activities after stroke (e.g., hand motor control, speech), gait and balance training seems to be more effective when the relevant functions are trained task and goal-specific with regard to the relevant activity. There is not much carryover from one task to another. This is even true for the training of strength and endurance.
- In the same line, additional stimulation techniques in order to further plasticity (e.g., central and peripheral stimulation) seem to be only effective when performed in combination with functionally relevant aspects of gait training.

In the last years, goal setting during neurological rehabilitation concentrated more and more on activities, which are often more meaningful to patients than basic functions, which were mainly trained earlier in the twentieth century. Not surprisingly, the main outcome parameters of scientific studies are today mostly activities and participation including quality of life—but not functions any longer. Therefore, we learned a lot about how to help patients to regain predefined activities and skills—but less on how to change basic networks in the brain and train basic sensorimotor abilities outside the labs.

The aim of our work was not only to evaluate the different forms of rehabilitative interventions but also to distill the principles of effective treatment for the different aspects of mobility. This is especially important as worldwide most strokes happen in low- and middle-income countries (Norrving and Kissela 2013) and thus not in Western Europe, North America, or Australia, where most of the guideline development takes place. Local and regional culture and traditions in Africa, the Middle East, or South America may stress the importance of other aspects of mobility, e.g., "standing and walking without a visible aid" and of therapeutic settings, e.g., "therapeutic sessions with individual therapists instead of sessions in a group setting." Regional and local traditions and the cultural background will influence goal setting and the choice of therapeutic interventions. Regardless of regional and local traditions, the above described elementary rules should be part of these clinical pathways to further the recovery of walking ability after stroke.

Acknowledgments K. M. Stephan is member of the ReMoS working group (Dohle C, Quintern J, Saal S, Stephan KM, Tholen R, Wittenberg H; in alphabetical order) that developed the evidence-based guideline on "Rehabilitation of Mobility after Stroke (ReMoS)" for the German Society of Neurorehabilitation (DGNR). As the systematic search, critical appraisal and best evidence synthesis of that guideline development has been a major information source for this chapter the work of the ReMoS working group is gratefully acknowledged.

References

AHA/ASA Guideline (2016) Guidelines for adult stroke rehabilitation and recovery. A guideline for healthcare professionals from the American Heart Association/American Stroke Association. Stroke 47:e98–e169. https://doi.org/10.1161/STR.0000000000000098

APTA Guideline (2020) Clinical practice guideline to improve locomotor function following chronic stroke, incomplete spinal cord injury, and brain injury. Academy of Neurologic Physical Therapy. JNPT 44:49–100

AVERT Trial Collaboration Group, Bernhardt J, Langhorne P, Lindley RI, Thrift AG, Ellery F, Collier J, Churilov L, Moodie M, Dewey H, Donnan G (2015) Efficacy and safety of very early mobilisation within 24 h of stroke onset (AVERT): a randomised controlled trial. Lancet 386:46–55

Canadian Guideline (2019) Rehabilitation and recovery following stroke module 2019. Canadian stroke best practice reecommendations, 2019. Heart and Stroke Foundation, Ottawa, ON

Chan DY, Chan CC, Au DK (2006) Motor relearning programme for stroke patients: a randomized controlled trial. Clin Rehabil 20(3):191–200

de Seze MP, Bonhomme C, Daviet JC, Burguete E, Machat H, Rousseaux M, Mazaux JM (2011) Effect of early compensation of distal motor deficiency by the chignon ankle-foot orthosis on gait in hemiplegic patients: a randomized pilot study. Clin Rehabil 25(11):989–998

Dias D, Lains J, Pereira A, Nunes R, Caldas J, Amaral C et al (2007) Can we improve gait skills in chronic hemiplegics? A randomised control trial with gait trainer. Eura Medicophys 43(4):499–504

Dohle C, Tholen R, Wittenberg H, Quintern J, Saal S, Stephan KM (2016) Evidence-based rehabilitation of mobility after stroke. [Article in German]. Nervenarzt 87(10):1062–1067. https://doi.org/10.1007/s00115-016-0188-8

Duncan P, Studenski S, Richards L, Gollub S, Lai SM, Reker D et al (2003) Randomized clinical trial of therapeutic exercise in subacute stroke. Stroke 34(9):2173–2180

Duncan PW, Sullivan KJ, Behrman AL, Azen SP, Wu SS, Nadeau SE et al (2011) Body-weight-supported treadmill rehabilitation after stroke. N Engl J Med 364(21):2026–2036. https://doi.org/10.1056/NEJMoa1010790

Eich HJ, Mach H, Werner C, Hesse S (2004) Aerobic treadmill plus Bobath walking training improves walking in subacute stroke: a randomized controlled trial. Clin Rehabil 18(6):640–651

Erel S, Uygur F, Engin SI, Yakut Y (2011) The effects of dynamic ankle-foot orthoses in chronic stroke patients at three-month follow-up: a randomized controlled trial. Clin Rehabil 25(6):515–523

Gordon NF, Gulanick M, Costa F, Fletcher G, Franklin BA, Roth EJ, Shephard T (2004) Physical activity and exercise recommendations for stroke survivors: an American Heart Association scientific statement from the council on clinical cardiology, subcommittee on exercise, cardiac rehabilitation, and prevention; the council on cardiovascular nursing; the council on nutrition, physical activity, and metabolism; and the stroke council. Circulation 109(16):2031–2041

Hardwick RM, Caspers S, Eickhoff SB, Swinnen SP (2018) Neural correlates of action: comparing meta-analyses of imagery, observation, and execution. Neurosci Biobehav Rev 94:31–44

Humm JL, Kozlowski DA, James DC, Gotts JE, Schallert T (1998) Use-dependent exacerbation of brain damage occurs during an early post-lesion vulnerable period. Brain Res 783:286–292

Jorgensen HS, Nakayama H, Raaschou HO, Vive-Larsen J, Stoier M, Olsen TS (1995) Outcome and time course of recovery in stroke. Part I: outcome. The Copenhagen Stroke Study. Arch Phys Med Rehabil 76(5):399–405

Katz-Leurer M, Shochina M, Carmeli E, Friedlander Y (2003) The influence of early aerobic training on the functional capacity in patients with cerebrovascular accident at the subacute stage. Arch Phys Med Rehabil 84(11):1609–1614

KNGF Guideline (2014) Royal Dutch Society for physical therapy (Koninklijk Nederlands Genootschap voor Fysiotherapie, KNGF)

Kottink AI, Hermens HJ, Nene AV, Tenniglo MJ, van der Aa HE, Buschman HP, Ijzerman MJ (2007) A randomized controlled trial of an implantable 2-channel peroneal nerve stimulator on walking speed and activity in poststroke hemiplegia. Arch Phys Med Rehabil 88(8):971–978

Kwakkel G, Kollen B, Twisk J (2006) Impact of time on improvement of outcome after stroke. Stroke 37(9):2348–2353

Marzolini S, Robertson AD, Oh P, Goodman JM, Corbett D, Du X, MacIntosh BJ (2019) Aerobic training and mobilization early post-stroke: cautions and consideration. Front Neurol 10:article 1187

McClellan R, Ada L (2004) A six-week, resource-efficient mobility program after discharge from rehabilitation improves standing in people affected by stroke: placebo-controlled, randomised trial. Aust J Physiother 50(3):163–167

Mehrholz J, Pohl M (2012) Electromechanical-assisted gait training after stroke: a systematic review comparing end-effector and exoskeleton devices. J Rehabil Med 44(3):193–199

Mehrholz J, Elsner B, Werner C, Kugler J, Pohl M (2013) Electromechanical-assisted training for walking after stroke: updated evidence. Stroke 44(10):e127–e128

Mehrholz J, Thomas S, Werner C, Kugler J, Pohl M, Elsner B (2017) Electromechanical-assisted training for walking after stroke. Cochrane Database Syst Rev 5:CD006185. https://doi.org/10.1002/14651858.CD006185

Nave AH, Rackoll T, Grittner U et al (2019) Physical fitness training in patients with subacute stroke (PHYS-STROKE): multicentre, randomised controlled, endpoint blinded trial. BMJ 366:l5101

Noh DK, Lim JY, Shin HI, Paik NJ (2008) The effect of aquatic therapy on postural balance and muscle strength in stroke survivors--a randomized controlled pilot trial. Clin Rehabil 22(10–11):966–976

Norrving B, Kissela B (2013) The global burden of stroke and need for a continuum of care. Neurol 80(Suppl 2):S5–S12. https://doi.org/10.1212/WNL.0b013e3182762397

Outermans JC, Van Peppen RP, Wittink H, Takken T, Kwakkel G (2010) Effects of a high-intensity task-oriented training on gait performance early after stroke: a pilot study. Clin Rehabil 24(11):979–987

Paolucci S, Antonucci G, Guariglia C, Magnotti L, Pizzamiglio L, Zoccolotti P (1996) Facilitatory effect of neglect rehabilitation on the recovery of left hemiplegic stroke patients: a cross-over study. J Neurol 243(4):308–314

Peurala SH, Airaksinen O, Huuskonen P, Jakala P, Juhakoski M, Sandell K et al (2009) Effects of intensive therapy using gait trainer or floor walking exercises early after stroke. J Rehabil Med 41(3):166–173

Pittock SJ, Moore AP, Hardiman O, Ehler E, Kovac M, Bojakowski J et al (2003) A double-blind randomised placebo-controlled evaluation of three doses of botulinum toxin type a (Dysport) in the treatment of spastic equinovarus deformity after stroke. Cerebrovasc Dis 15(4):289–300

Pohl M, Mehrholz J, Ritschel C, Ruckriem S (2002) Speed-dependent treadmill training in ambulatory hemiparetic stroke patients: a randomized controlled trial. Stroke 33(2):553–558

Pohl M, Werner C, Holzgraefe M, Kroczek G, Mehrholz J, Wingendorf I, Hoölig G, Koch R, Hesse S (2007) Repetitive locomotor training and physiotherapy improve walking and basic activities of daily living after stroke: a single-blind, randomized multicentre trial (DEutsche GAngtrainerStudie, DEGAS). Clin Rehabil 21:17–27

ReMoS Arbeitsgruppe, Dohle C, Quintern J, Saal S, Stephan KM, Tholen R, Wittenberg H (2015) S2e-Leitlinie Rehabilitation der Mobilität nach Schlaganfall (ReMoS). Neurol Rehabil 21(7):355–494

Saeys W, Vereeck L, Truijen S, Lafosse C, Wuyts FP, Heyning PV (2012) Randomized controlled trial of truncal exercises early after stroke to improve balance and mobility. Neurorehabil Neural Repair 26(3):231–238

Saunders DH, Greig CA, Mead GE, Young A (2009) Physical fitness training for stroke patients. Cochrane Database Syst Rev (4):CD003316

Schauer M, Mauritz KH (2003) Musical motor feedback (MMF) in walking hemiparetic stroke patients: randomized trials of gait improvement. Clin Rehabil 17(7):713–722

Spaich EG, Svaneborg N, Jorgensen HR, Andersen OK (2014) Rehabilitation of the hemiparetic gait by nociceptive withdrawal reflex-based functional electrical therapy: a randomized, single-blinded study. J Neuroeng Rehabil 11(81)

Stephan KM, Fink GR, Passingham RE, Silbersweig D, Ceballos-Baumann AO, Frith CD, Frackowiak RS (1995) Functional anatomy of the mental representation of upper extremity movements in healthy subjects. J Neurophysiol 73(1):373–386

Stephan KM, Thaut MH, Wunderlich G, Schicks W, Tian B, Tellmann L, Schmitz T, Herzog H, McIntosh GC, Seitz RJ, Hömberg V (2002) Conscious and subconscious sensorimotor synchronization—prefrontal cortex and the influence of awareness. Neuroimage 15(2):345–352

Thaut MH, McIntosh GC, Rice RR (1997) Rhythmic facilitation of gait training in hemiparetic stroke rehabilitation. J Neurol Sci 151(2):207–212

Thijssen DH, Paulus R, van Uden CJ, Kooloos JG, Hopman MT (2007) Decreased energy cost and improved gait pattern using a new orthosis in persons with long-term stroke. Arch Phys Med Rehabil 88(2):181–186

Verma R, Arya KN, Garg RK, Singh T (2011) Task-oriented circuit class training program with motor imagery for gait rehabilitation in poststroke patients: a randomized controlled trial. Top Stroke Rehabil 18(Suppl 1):620–632

Yan T, Hui-Chan CW, Li LS (2005) Functional electrical stimulation improves motor recovery of the lower extremity and walking ability of subjects with first acute stroke: a randomized placebo-controlled trial. Stroke 36(1):80–85

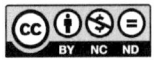

Post-Stroke Spasticity

Gerard E. Francisco, Jörg Wissel, Thomas Platz, and Sheng Li

1 Introduction

Post-stroke spasticity (PSS) is a complication that contributes to limitations in performance of activities and community participation. It occurs in anywhere from 19% (Sommerfeld et al. 2004) to 92% (Malhotra et al. 2011) of stroke survivors. Its prevalence may be as high as 38% in the first year following a stroke (Watkins et al. 2002). Estimates of incidence and prevalence vary widely perhaps due differences in the definition and clinical measurement of spasticity in varying severity and chronicity of stroke. As well, based on a prospective, observational study, Wissel et al. (2010) found a prevalence of spasticity in 24.5% at 6 days, 26.7% 6 weeks, and 21.7% (18 of 83 survivors at 16 weeks). The same group also found that in 98% of

G. E. Francisco (✉) · S. Li
Department of Physical Medicine and Rehabilitation, The University of Texas
Health Science Center at Houston McGovern Medical School
and TIRR Memorial Hermann Hospital, Houston, TX, USA
e-mail: gerard.e.francisco@uth.tmc.edu; Sheng.Li@uth.tmc.edu

J. Wissel
Department of Neurology, Neurorehabilitation and Physical Therapy,
VIVANTES Hospital Spandau, Berlin, Germany

University of Potsdam, Health Science, Health Campus Brandenburg, Potsdam, Germany
e-mail: Joerg.Wissel@vivantes.de

T. Platz
Institute for Neurorehabilitation and Evidence-based Practice ("An-Institute", University of Greifswald), BDH-Klinik Greifswald, Greifswald, Germany

Neurorehabilitation Research Group, University Medical Centre Greifswald (UMG), Greifswald, Germany

Special Interest Group Clinical Pathways, World Federation Neurorehabilitation (WFNR), North Shields, UK
e-mail: T.Platz@bdh-klinik-greifswald.de

© The Author(s) 2021
T. Platz (ed.), *Clinical Pathways in Stroke Rehabilitation*,
https://doi.org/10.1007/978-3-030-58505-1_9

subjects with PSS, velocity-dependent increase in muscle tone in one joint was evident at about 6 weeks post-stroke.

Beside identified early clinical signs that predict PSS (velocity-dependent increase in muscle tone in two or more joints, severe paresis and loss of function resulting in severe disability/loss of ADL), recent studies showed that brain lesions involving the basal ganglia, thalamus, insula, and white matter tracts especially the internal capsule, corona radiata, external capsule, and superior longitudinal fasciculus are also predictive for PSS when lesion load is compromising the corticospinal tract (Wissel et al. 2015; Lee et al. 2019).

There is a heightened awareness of the need to manage spasticity because not only can it limit limb movement and overall mobility but also can predispose to other complications, such as joint contractures and pain, which further magnify motor weakness and functional limitations. In this chapter, current evidence will be assessed in the following key clinical areas:

- Problem identification and clinical assessment.
- Treatment goal setting.
- Pharmacological and surgical treatment.

2   Methods Used for Evidence Synthesis and Practice Recommendations

A comprehensive literature search was performed on 30 July, 2017 on PubMed (MEDLINE database) for guidelines, systematic reviews and meta-analyses (SR), and randomized controlled studies (RCT) published in the last 5 years on the topic of spasticity treatment across etiologies. This was performed in conjunction with preparations for the German Neurology Society S2k (consensus) guideline on the "Treatment of spasticity" (Platz et al. 2019). Search terms for SR and RCT were: (1) (Search (meta analysis [Publication Type] OR meta analysis [Title/Abstract] OR meta analysis [MeSH Terms] OR review[Publication Type] OR search*[Title/Abstract]) AND (spast*)); (2) (Search ((clinical[Title/Abstract] AND trial[Title/Abstract]) OR clinical trials as topic[MeSH Terms] OR clinical trial[Publication Type] OR random*[Title/Abstract] OR random allocation[MeSH Terms] OR therapeutic use[MeSH Subheading]) AND (spast* OR ton*)) AND ("last 5 years"[PDat]). The search initially yielded 297 references, and after eliminating duplicates, 215 references remained, of which 28 were directly relevant for the preparation of said guideline. The vast majority of the 28 manuscripts were systematic reviews.

Additionally, the S2e (evidence-based) German Society for Neurorehabilitation (DGNR) guideline on "Treatment of Spasticity after Stroke" (Winter and Wissel 2013) was referenced and all essential information included. For the DGNR guideline (Winter and Wissel 2013), 172 references (164 original papers, 8 reviews) were evaluated, of which 111 served as a basis for the guideline, which included non-experimental studies (e.g., case series and cohort studies). In addition, further studies and reviews that were known to the authors and relevant for the healthcare question addressed were included.

The recommendations given below are based on the evidence as presented below. We categorized the level of evidence used for recommendations according to the

Oxford Centre for Evidence-Based Medicine Levels of Evidence (CEBM 2009). Further, the quality of this evidence has been grouped into four categories according to "GRADE" ("Grades of Recommendation, Assessment, Development and Evaluation") (Owens et al. 2010):

- High quality: further research is unlikely to affect our confidence in the estimation of the (therapeutic) effect.
- Medium quality: further research is likely to affect our confidence in the estimation of the (therapeutic) effect and may alter the estimate.
- Low quality: further research will most likely influence our confidence in the estimation of the (therapeutic) effect and will probably change the estimate.
- Very low quality: any estimation of the (therapy) effect or prognosis is very uncertain.

The grading of the recommendations according to GRADE (Schünemann et al. 2013) corresponds to the categories "ought to" (A) (strong recommendation), "should" (B) (weak recommendation). As a third category had been introduced "can" (0) (option) (Platz 2017). Recommendation category A is granted for clinically effective interventions with high-quality evidence support (and when mandatory, e.g., for ethical reasons); with medium-quality evidence category B, and with low- or very low-quality evidence category 0 can be appropriate. Reasons to upgrade or downgrade are given: A+ or B+ denote a strong or weak recommendation in favor on an intervention and A− or B− against its use.

3   Problem Identification and Clinical Assessment

When assessing clinical problems associate with post-stroke spasticity, it is very important to keep in mind that spasticity defined as muscle overactivity as a positive sign of the upper motor neuron syndrome (UMNS) is only one component. The problems may be caused by other motor impairments, such as weakness, and/or disordered motor control. For example, patients may complain of abnormal joint positions, or that a limb could not be moved, or the resultant functional limitations, such as the inability to release a grasped object or difficulty with walking due to an inverted foot. In the majority of post-stroke patients, these problems are a combination of the above motor impairments. Thus, it is important to obtain a thorough, yet focused, history to identify clinical problems, to guide the examination, and to formulate treatment goals and plans. A systematic approach to history-taking and clinical assessment of spasticity that can be modified to suit different clinical scenarios is proposed in Tables 1 and 2.

With respect to the distribution of the positive signs of the UMNS identified as involuntary muscle overactivity (velocity-depended increase in muscle tone, spasms, clonus, spastic dystonia, and co-contracting muscle activation) spasticity could be classified as focal (one joint/functional region, e.g., the wrist and fingers), multifocal (minimal two or more joints, e.g., wrist, fingers, and ankle), segmental (adjacent joints in one or more limbs, e.g., toes, ankle, knee, and hip in one or two limbs, paraspastic: both lower limbs), hemispastic (arm and leg on one body side),

Table 1 Some important historical points in spasticity assessment

Is the limb tight all the time or only at certain times?
Does a particular position or movement trigger tightness?
Is the tightness related to spasms?
Does the tightness cause pain?
Have there been episodes of skin compromise due to tightness or spasm?
Does the tightness result in difficulty with cleaning?
Does the tightness result in difficulty donning splints?
Does the tightness limit ability to move limbs, reach for objects, and use the hands?
Does the tightness of the lower limbs result in problems with transferring form one surface to another or with walking?
What treatments for muscle tightness have been tried previously and their outcome?
What are the current medications?
Was there a recent increase in tightness (that may warrant further diagnostic testing to rule out a new neurologic problem)?
Any recent medical problems?

From Francisco GE and Li S. Clinical assessment and management of spasticity and contractures in traumatic brain injury. Chapter 8 *In* Neurological Rehabilitation *Spasticity and Contractures in clinical practice and research.* Pandyan AD, Hermens H, Conway B (2018). https://doi.org/10.1201.9781315374369

Table 2 Practical clinical examination sequence

Examination phase	What to look for	What can be gleaned
Observation	Observe limb posture at rest and how they change with position	Abnormal posture at rest— Sustained muscle contraction (dystonia), contracture Position-dependent postural changes—dynamic tone
Active[a]	How limbs move and how much active range is available Gait characteristics and associated upper limb and trunk postural abnormalities	Functional strength, coordination, spastic co-contraction, contractures, presence of other movement disorders, synkinesis, or associated reactions Pain and discomfort during voluntary movements
Passive	Passive range of motion, strength, muscle tone, velocity-dependent "angle of catch," clonus	Spasticity Rigidity Contracture Clonus Pain and discomfort during passive stretch
Functional activities	Performance of specific tests and tasks (both formal tests, such as Frenchay and improvised tasks such as demonstrating ability to pick up a bottle of water and pour its contents to a cup)	Impact of multiple impairments (e.g., spasticity, weakness) on performance

[a]Active movements, such as sit to stand, transfer, and ambulation, could be part of functional tests

or generalized (more than two limbs involved, e.g., both legs and additional focal or segmental distribution of spasticity in arms, jaw, and trunk (Wissel et al. 2009)).

Spasticity assessment typically consists of a combination of quantitative and qualitative measures. Clinically, the Ashworth scale (AS), the modified Ashworth scale (MAS), and the Tardieu scale (TS) are most commonly used (Tables 3 and 4). Standardization of performance and scoring and summary scores across muscles groups were developed for the AS and resulted in high internal consistency, inter-rater, and test–retest reliability of a summary rating scale (REsistance to PASsive movement scale, REPAS) (Platz et al. 2008). A recent meta-analysis study reports satisfactory scores of inter- and intra-rater reliability in MAS, particularly when used for the upper extremity (Meseguer-Henarejos et al. 2018). The TS has advantages over the MAS because not only it quantifies the muscles' reaction to passive stretch but also it controls for the velocity of the stretch and measures the angle at which the catch, or clonus activity, occurs (Haugh et al. 2006); here, however, issues of reliability still have to be solved for the clinical user (Ansari et al. 2013; Li et al. 2014; Banky et al. 2019). In patients with severe brain injury, the MTS was shown to provide higher test– retest and inter-rater reliability compared to MAS (Mehrholz et al. 2005). This is supported by other investigations (Paulis et al. 2011; Singh et al.

Table 3 Ashworth scale and modified Ashworth scale

Ashworth scale	
0	No increase in tone
1	Slight increase in tone giving a catch when the limb was moved in flexion or extension
2	More marked increase in tone but limb easily moved
3	Considerable increase in tone, passive movement difficult
4	Limb rigid in flexion or extension
Modified Ashworth scale	
0	No increase in muscle tone
1	Slightly increase in tone, manifested by a catch and release at the end of ROM
1+	Slightly increase in tone, manifested by a catch, followed by minimal resistance throughout the remainder (less than half) of the ROM (catch in the first half of ROM)
2	Marked increase in tone through most of the ROM, still easily moved
3	Considerable increase in tone, passive movement difficult
4	Affected part(s) rigid in flexion or extension

Table 4 Tardieu scale

Quality of muscle reaction
0. No resistance
1. Slight resistance
2. Catch followed by a release
3. Fatigable clonus (<10 s)
4. Infatigable clonus (>10 s)
Angle of muscle reaction at different velocities of stretch
V1. As slow as possible
V2. Speed of limb galling under gravity
V3. As fast as possible

Table 5 The Spasticity-Associated Arm Pain Scale (SAAPS) for adults with post-stroke upper limb spasticity: passive range of motion items and ratings

Item	Description
1	Paretic shoulder abduction with elbow flexed to 90°
2	Paretic shoulder external rotation with elbow flexed to 90
3	Elbow stretching/extension
4	Wrist stretching
5	Finger stretching

Score	Observation
0	No pain
1	Pain on repeated movement (maximum of five repetitions)
2	Pain on end-range movement
3	Immediate pain on movement

Verbal and/or physiological responses (pain responses) are rated on a four-point Likert-type scale as 0 ("no pain"), 1 ("pain on repeated movement" (maximum of five repetitions)), 2 ("pain on end-range movement"), or 3 ("immediate pain on movement"). The SAAPS sum score ranges from 0 to 15 points, whereas 0 is the lowest and 15 is the highest pain intensity during passive range of motion in moderate speed of movement

2011). Caution regarding reliability, however, was raised in at least two investigations (Ansari et al. 2008, 2013; Li et al. 2014).

To assess pain associated with arm spasticity following stroke a valid and reliable instrument, the Spasticity-Associated Arm Pain Scale (SAAPS), for adults with post-stroke upper limb spasticity was developed (see Table 5; (Fheodoroff et al. 2017)). Most studies published on spasticity-related pain have used nonspecific pain-assessment scales, e.g., the 11-point box scale (NRS) or visual analog scale (VAS). However, such scales have not been validated in patients with spasticity-related arm pain and may lack the sensitivity to detect change and may also be unsuitable for use in patients in nursing care homes, many of whom have severe cognitive impairment or late-stage dementia (Lichtner et al. 2014; Tyson and Brown 2014). To address these shortcomings when documenting or managing pain in patients with arm spasticity following stroke, the SAAPS was developed and evaluated and showed its sensitivity for detecting and documenting pain and its reduction following BoNT-A treatment in pain associated with arm spasticity following stroke (Fheodoroff et al. 2017).

While it is true that quantitative measures are desirable because of their inherent objectivity and reliability, they may not be practical and may discourage clinicians from assessing and managing spasticity. Quantitative assessment includes biomechanical and electrophysiological assessments. Biomechanical assessment utilizes the concept of velocity-dependent increase in resistance and has advantages of the ability to differentiate neural and nonneural component of spastic hypertonia, thus spasticity vs. contracture (Sinkjaer and Magnussen 1994; Kamper et al. 2003; Li et al. 2006). The measurement of electromyographic activity is able to determine the threshold of stretch reflex, i.e., a physiological evidence of the onset of spasticity (Levin and Feldman 1994; Calota et al. 2008). Advances in quantitative ultrasound imaging have shown some promising pilot data to quantitatively assess spastic muscles (Wu et al. 2017; Gao et al. 2018). Ideal spasticity assessment should include biomechanical and electrophysiological tests, but many of the devices are not available to a typical clinician, and the time needed to perform them properly may impose excessive demands in a busy practice.

Recommendations: It is important to keep in mind that spasticity could be one component of motor impairments and clinical problems following stroke and may contribute to reduction in activities of daily living and quality of life in about 10–12% of chronic stroke survivors. Spasticity should be classified according to the topical distribution as focal, multifocal, segmental, hemispastic, paraspastic, or as generalized spasticity. It should primarily be assessed and documented by standardized validated clinical assessment scales such as the AS or MAS (level of evidence 2a, quality of evidence moderate, B+) or TS (level of evidence 2b, quality of evidence low, 0).

4 Treatment Goal Setting

4.1 Goal Setting

The mere presence of spasticity is not always a reason to initiate treatment. Varying in its severity, spasticity is usually addressed when it presents with marked limitation in range of motion due to abnormally increased muscle tone. Consideration, however, should be given to managing less-than-severe spasticity if it has profound impact on comfort and functioning. An example is a person with pes equinovarus deformity whose ankle plantar flexors and invertors merit only a modified Ashworth Scale score of 1+ at rest, but causes discomfort during walking. Spasticity intervention ought to be considered not only based on severity but also on functional significance and impact on well-being. Thus, the first important step in managing spasticity, and right after problem identification, is laying out the rationale for treatment by identifying goals. Goals, especially patient-centered ones, are a basis for collaboration by patients and clinicians. Together (patient/care giver and clinician), they agree on the desired treatment outcome, which will be based on the extent to which goals were achieved. To assist in developing goals, a useful matrix, SMARTER, can be used (Francisco and Li 2015). This mnemonic stands for goals that are:

- S: Specific (well-defined and targets a specific problem to be addressed).
- M: Measurable (either quantitatively, as for technical goals, or qualitatively as for symptom-directed goals); Meaningful (achievement of goal should be beneficial to the patient or caregiver).
- A: Agreed upon (the patient or caregiver and clinician work toward a common end).
- R: Realistic (will the patient's potential for improvement and available resources support achievement of treatment goal?)
- T: Time-bound (achievement of goal should be within a reasonable amount of time).

- E: Evaluated (at pre-determined points in time, goal achievement and progress in doing so should be performed to determine effectiveness of intervention).
- R: Revised (based on evaluation of goal achievement, new treatment goals may be identified or prior ones revised).

A recent national, multicenter study (Ashford et al. 2016) suggested that goals can be classified into two domains, namely, symptoms and impairment, and activities/function. The former includes pain/discomfort, involuntary movements, and range of movement/contracture prevention. Within the second domain are passive function (e.g., ease of caring for affected limb), active function (using affected limbs to perform tasks), and mobility.

4.2   Goal Attainment Scaling

The most commonly used measure to document treatment goals is goal attainment scaling (GAS), which was originally used in other healthcare settings (Kiresuk and Sherman 1968; Rockwood et al. 1997). GAS tracks the extent to which pre-identified patient-specific treatment goals are achieved using an ordinal scale during the course of treatment. The scoring method is standardized to promote consistent repeatability as the patient and clinician review the progress of goal achievement. In addition, early studies comparing GAS with more traditional outcome measures suggest that GAS is more sensitive. Active patient engagement through GAS may have beneficial impact on achievement of outcomes. Emerging evidence demonstrate that when patients are involved in goal setting, they are more likely to achieve their goals (Turner-Stokes et al. 2015). GAS also shows promise as a means of conveying caregiver burden as it is sensitive in highlighting priority outcomes by patients and caregivers (Turner-Stokes et al. 2010).

Recommendation: An important component of assessment and management decision-making is arriving at treatment goals. Identifying goals that are mutually agreed upon by the patient, caregiver, and clinician a priori should be an important step in spasticity treatment decision-making (level of evidence 2b, quality of evidence moderate, B+). In this context, GAS is a useful tool in negotiating goals, highlighting priority outcomes by patients and caregivers, and tracking their achievement. GAS also encourages patient engagement in goal setting, which has been shown to have a positive relation to achieving the said goals.

5   Pharmacological and Surgical Treatment

5.1   Systemic Medications

Various oral medications with different mechanisms of action have been used to treat spasticity. The most commonly used medications include baclofen, tizanidine, dantrolene and benzodiazepines. Overall, these medications have marginal effect on focal spasticity (Simpson et al. 2009) and marginal to moderate effects on reducing segmental and generalized spasticity (Montane et al. 2004). In a systematic review on contemporary pharmacologic treatments for spasticity of the upper limb after stroke. Olvey et al. (2010) only found one study with a systemic drug (tizanidine) that reported significant reductions in upper limb spasticity after 16 weeks of treatment compared to placebo.

In a Cochrane review on pharmacological interventions other than botulinum toxin for spasticity after stroke, Lindsay et al. (2016) found seven RCTs with a total of 403 participants. Only two of them assessed a systemic drug versus placebo and only one with tizanidine showed significant results. Those two studies included 160 patients and in the meta-analysis of those the antispastic effect of the oral drugs on spasticity showed no significant effects (MAS, Odds Ratio for Response 1.66, 95% KI 0.21–13.07; n.s.). On the other hand, the authors identified a significant risk of adverse events per participant occurring in the treatment group versus placebo group (risk ratio (RR) 1.65, 95% CI 1.12 to 2.42; 160 participants; $I^2 = 0\%$).

The common adverse effects of oral drugs include dose-dependent adverse effects, such as drowsiness and tiredness. Therapeutic efficacy of these medications is only supported by a few placebo-controlled trials with inadequate sample size and lack of functional outcome measurements (Francisco and McGuire 2012; Winstein et al. 2016). Furthermore, likely attributed to these adverse effects or a reflection of limited efficacy, oral medications have poor adherence (Halpern et al. 2013). In general, it is recommended to limit the use of these oral medications for spasticity management (Francisco and McGuire 2012; Winstein et al. 2016). On the other hand, these oral medications as single drug or combination may be a cost-effective treatment option for those who can achieve adequate spasticity management without intolerable adverse effects.

Baclofen, a gamma amino butyric acid (GABA)-B agonist, is a potent inhibitory neurotransmitter. Baclofen has been shown dose-dependent reduction of spasticity and spasms, but has side effects of drowsiness and weakness. Abrupt discontinuation of baclofen may result in a withdrawal syndrome, characterized by rebound spasticity, hallucinations, and seizures (Medaer et al. 1991; Meythaler et al. 2004). Similar to baclofen, benzodiazepines modulate GABAergic transmission by binding GABA-A receptors. Similarly, abrupt discontinuation of benzodiazepines may result in a withdrawal syndrome. Concerns for its side effects, mainly drowsiness, sedation, reduced attention and memory impairment, and the potential for physiological dependence have limited the use of benzodiazepines as first-line treatment for spasticity. The use in post-stroke spasticity management is discouraged and might be reserved to situations when spasticity is accompanied by other conditions that are also amenable to benzodiazepine therapy, such as seizures, anxiety, insomnia, spasms, and other movement disorders (Medaer et al. 1991; Meythaler et al. 2004).

Tizanidine, a central alpha2-adrenergic receptor agonist, reduces spasticity and clonus via inhibiting the facilitatory ceruleospinal tracts and the release of excitatory neurotransmitters from spinal interneurons (Stevenson and Jarrett 2006). In addition to the typical side effects of oral spasmolytics, hepatotoxicity may also occur. Thus, monitoring liver function is important, especially in those patients who concomitantly take hepatically cleared drugs.

Unlike baclofen and tizanidine, dantrolene works directly on skeletal muscle by inhibiting the release of calcium from the sarcoplasmic reticulum during excitation–contraction coupling (Krause et al. 2004). Although it is peripherally acting, dantrolene has also been associated with side effects that appear to be centrally mediated, such as drowsiness, dizziness, fatigue, and weakness, perhaps through alteration of neuronal calcium homeostasis (Flewellen et al. 1983; Katrak et al. 1992). Due to its potential for hepatotoxicity, regular monitoring of liver function is recommended.

Beside baclofen, tizanidine, and dantrolene, other agents have reported to have some effects, including tolperison (Stamenova et al. 2005), gabapentin, clonidine, nabilone (Wissel et al. 2006), and cannabinoids (Whiting et al. 2015).

Summing up the results from studies on oral drugs in PSS, the evidence published from RCTs showed significant risk of side effects and no sufficient data to confirm that systemic antispastic drugs are effective in treating PSS.

Recommendations: Oral systemic medications can be used for segmental and generalized spasticity, but may be associated with dose-dependent adverse effects (level of evidence 2b, quality of evidence low, 0). Selection of type of oral medication depends on individual circumstances and may include combinations. These medications should be titrated slowly, and both clinical benefits and unwanted effects need to be monitored (level of evidence 1a, quality of evidence low, B+ [clinical reasoning]).

5.2   Botulinum Toxin Treatment

Botulinum toxin Type A (BoNT-A) is widely regarded as the treatment of choice for the medical management of focal and multi-focal signs and symptoms of the UMNS including but not limited to hypertonia, spastic dystonia, clonus, and spasms. Systematic studies have also demonstrated improvement in so-called passive function like reducing spasticity-associated pain, hygiene and passive movement of involved limbs, and reduction of mal-positioning of limbs (Brashear et al. 2002a, b) (level of evidence 1b). Demonstration of active functional gains in terms of enhancement of active limb movements in the upper limbs (e.g., reaching or grip and relieve movements with the hand) and increased mobility (e.g., gait speed and gait endurance) has proven to be difficult. But systematic reviews of the outcome of BoNT treatment in spastic upper limbs (Foley et al. 2013; Dong et al. 2017) (level of evidence 1a) and a randomized, controlled, trial in subjects with chronic PSS and traumatic brain injury–related spastic upper limb (Gracies et al. 2015) (level of evidence 1b) reported statistically significant functional improvements in active function of the upper limb.

Controlled studies in the post-acute phase of stroke rehabilitation (less than 3 months following stroke) showed that BoNT-A injected before spasticity became moderate or severe result in improvements in impairment and passive function and reduced occurrence of muscle and/or tendon shortening in long finger flexors (Hesse et al. 2012). The therapeutic outcomes also appeared to be more pronounced and longer lasting (Rosales et al. 2012; Fietzek et al. 2014) (level of evidence 1b). Thus, early BoNT-A intervention seems to have the potential to modify the natural evolution of PSS while a resent systematic review did not indicate higher functional gains or effects on disability (Rosales et al. 2016).

5.2.1   Treatment Outcomes: Upper Limbs

Numerous controlled studies and multiple meta-analyses show a dose-dependent effective reduction of spastic muscle tone, improvement in passive range of motion (PROM) and passive function (measured with the Disability Assessment Scale, DAS) as well as a reduction in carer burden while handling affected limbs, both by single and repeated intramuscular injections of BoNT-A (abobotulinumtoxinA, incobotulinumtoxinA, and onabotulinumtoxinA) in upper limb with increased spastic hypertonia in the chronic stage after stroke and other etiologies ((van Kuijk et al. 2002; Turkel et al. 2006), level of evidence 1a; (Simpson et al. 2008, 2016), level of evidence 1a; (Gracies et al. 2015), level of evidence 1b; (Dong et al. 2017), level of evidence 1a)). In severely affected arms, BoNT-A application supports self-care activities and integration of the spastic arm in everyday life by improving passive function (Baker and Pereira 2015) (level of evidence 1a). Evidence quality for the 11 studies for arm spasticity in a meta-analysis was moderate (GRADE). Significant results of BoNT-A therapy were observed for 4 to 12 weeks post-injection (SMD 0.80, 95% CI 0.55 to 1.06, $P < 0.0001$) and continued for up to 6 months (SMD 0.48, 95% CI 0.34 to 0.62, $P < 0.0001$). Randomized trials included in the systematic review showed a reduced incidence of shortening of finger muscles with improved hand hygiene (Hesse et al. 2012; Rosales et al. 2012) (level of evidence 1b).

In the subacute phase (<3 months) after stroke following BoNT-A use, forearm and leg spasticity significant reductions in velocity-dependent tone increase over more than 3 months could be documented in a systematic review with meta-analysis (3 studies), whereas no greater functional gains and no increase in side effects were shown (Rosales et al. 2016) (level of evidence 1a).

BoNT-A injections may improve active function in some of the patients with arm spasticity (Foley et al. 2013; Gracies et al. 2015; Baker and Pereira 2016, level of evidence 1a). Evidence quality for the six studies for effects on arm activities in a meta-analysis was low to very low (according to GRADE). A small significant result of BoNT-A therapy was documented 4 to 12 weeks post-injection (SMD 0.32, 95% CI 0.01 to 0.62, $P = 0.04$) and only for the Action Research Arm Test (ARAT)— persisted for up to 6 months (MD 1.87, 95% CI 0.53 to 3.21, $P = 0.006$). In a single randomized controlled trial of abobotulinumtoxinA, an increase in active finger and wrist extension with BoNT-A injections into the finger flexors was found and supported the prior statement (Gracies et al. 2015), (level of evidence 1b). For treatment of focal spasticity after stroke, BoNT-A is superior to oral antispastic medication (tizanidine) in terms of both efficacy, measured as reduction in muscle tone with the Modified Ashworth Scale, and adverse events (Simpson et al. 2009) (level of evidence 1b).

Recommendations: BoNT-A therapy should be considered for clinically relevant upper limb PSS that does not sufficiently respond to nonpharmacological treatment. In these cases, it should be entertained when the therapeutic goal is to support passive functions (prevention of contractures; hygiene, washing, dressing) (level of evidence 1a, quality of evidence moderate, B+) and can be used in selected cases to support active function (level of evidence 1a, quality of evidence low, 0).

5.2.2   Treatment Outcomes: Lower Limbs

In chronic ankle flexion spasticity with spastic pes equines and equinovarus gait pattern, significant reduction of muscle tone in the ankle following treatment with abobotulinumtoxinA and onabotulinumtoxinA by intramuscular injections into the calf muscle could be demonstrated after stroke (Pittock et al. 2003; Kaji et al. 2010; Wein et al. 2018) (level of evidence 1b) and after stroke and TBI (Gracies et al. 2017) (level of evidence 1b). Additionally a reduced use of gait tools (orthosis) and an improvement of the Clinical Global Impression Scale in gait were shown ((Pittock et al. 2003; Gracies et al. 2017; Wein et al. 2018), level of evidence 1b). However, no significant improvements in longitudinal gait parameters (e.g., gait speed and gait endurance) of the patients treated with BoNT-A could be achieved in that trials.

One systematic review (mainly by observational studies and case series, 14 studies, 181 patients) also shows a reduction of clonus activity in patients with chronic ankle flexion spasticity as an improvement in a different positive sign of the UMNS that velocity-dependent increase in muscle tone from BoNT treatment (Thanikachalam et al. 2017) (level of evidence 3a).

With respect to the treatment of hip and knee spasticity using BoNT-A injections (abobotulinumtoxinA, onabotulinumtoxinA, and incobotulinumtoxinA), clinical studies were able to show reduction of spastic movement disorders in hip and knee in the chronic stage of spasticity of different etiologies (stroke, traumatic brain injury, multiple sclerosis, and others), and it was also possible to conclude that interventions with BoNT-A showed improving mobility ((Hyman et al. 2000; Rosales and Chua-Yap 2008; Wissel et al. 2017), level of evidence 1b).

In an open dose-escalation study with incobotulinumtoxinA, dose escalation from 400 units to 600 units and 800 units showed increasing numbers of treated upper and lower limb muscles or spastic patterns (combinations of typical spastic muscle activation, e.g., spastic pes equines, pes varus, flexed elbow or wrist, and spastic fist) per escalation level and led to almost double the number of patients, who were able to walk independently without increasing the incidence of side effects at higher dose levels (Wissel et al. 2017) (level of evidence 2b).

Recommendations: BoNT-A therapy can be considered for clinically relevant lower limb PSS (ankle, knee, or hip) that does not sufficiently respond to nonpharmacological treatment (level of evidence 1b, quality of evidence moderate, 0 (functional benefit uncertain)). It is also an option to treat functionally relevant sustained clonus (level of evidence 3a, quality of evidence low, 0).

5.2.3 Treatment Outcomes: Spasticity- or Spasm-Associated Pain

Neuropathic (e.g., spontaneous burning pain in plegic limbs), nociceptive (e.g., knee joint pain when starting walking), spasm-related, and spasticity-associated (stretch- or exercise-induced muscle pain) pain following stroke are all part of the decision-making process with respect to selection of symptomatic treatment and treatments should be tailored accordingly (Finnerup 2017). Reduction of spasm-related and stretch- or exercise-induced spasticity-associated pain in spastic limb segments after injections of upper and lower extremity onabotulinumtoxinA in chronic spasticity was observed in a cohort study with 60 patients with mixed etiologies of spasticity in an open-label observational study and a randomized, placebo-controlled study in 273 patients following stroke and TBI ((Wissel et al. 2000, 2016), level of evidence 2b and 1b). Spasticity-associated stretch- or exercise-induced arm (Fheodoroff et al. 2017) or shoulder pain (Yelnik et al. 2007; Lim et al. 2008) also showed favorable influence by injections of abobotulinumtoxinA, incobotulinumtoxinA, and onabotulinumtoxinA (Fheodoroff et al. 2017, level of evidence 2b; Yelnik et al. 2007; Lim et al. 2008, level of evidence 1b).

Recommendations: BoNT-A therapy can be considered to treat spasm-related and stretch- or exercise-induced spasticity-associated pain in spastic limb segments, both in the upper or lower extremity (level of evidence 1b, quality of evidence low [partially indirect], 0).

5.2.4 Botulinum Toxin A Injection Guidance

It is believed that in order to improve the accuracy of BoNT injection, instrumented guidance using ultrasonography (US), electrical stimulation (ES), and electromyography (EMG) may be superior to a non-guided (e.g., pure anatomic localization) technique. Both ES and US appear to yield superior results over non-guided injection technique when BoNT is injected in wrist and finger flexors (Picelli et al. 2014; Santamato et al. 2014). ES (Chin et al. 2005; Picelli et al. 2012) and US (Picelli et al. 2012) have also been shown to be superior to anatomical guidance and EMG when injecting the triceps surae. A systematic review indicated that instrumented injection guidance is more effective than manual needle placement and showed similar effectiveness of US and ES for upper and lower limb spasticity in stroke (Grigoriu et al. 2015). A more recent investigation did not find a significant difference in clinical results among the various injection techniques when analyzing results of BoNT injections in a setting of an outpatient clinic (Zeuner et al. 2017). Thus, there is still no clear evidence that one injection technique is superior over another, but current literature suggests that for certain muscles instrument-guided injection is superior to pure anatomic localization (deep neck, forearm, and deep calf muscles).

Recommendation: Both US, ES, and EMG guidance can be used and are especially relevant when smaller or deeper muscles are injected (level of evidence 2a, quality of evidence low, 0). For the injection of larger superficial muscles, noninstrumented manual needle placement can be adequate (level of evidence 2a, quality of evidence low, 0).

5.2.5 BoNT-A Products

BoNT-A drugs available are different and not interchangeable. (BoNT-B is also commercially available, but will not be included in this review considering its limited clinical use and scarcity of studies in spasticity. While BoNT-C and BoNT-F have been tried in human studies are up to now exclusive to dystonia.) The currently available BoNT-A drugs in Europe and North America are: abobotulinumtoxinA (Dysport®; Ipsen Ltd., Slough, Berks, UK), incobotulinumtoxinA (Xeomin®; Merz Pharmaceuticals, Frankfurt/M, Germany), and onabotulinumtoxinA (Botox®; Allergan Inc., Irvine, CA, USA). A recent entry in the market, daxibotulinumtoxinA (Revance, USA) is currently being investigated in both dystonia and spasticity. Additional BoNT-A drugs used in other countries (South America, India, and Asia) to manage spastic hypertonia and movement disorders include the Chinese BoNT-A Hengli® (Lanzhou Institute of Biological Products, Lanzhou, Gansu Province, China) and marketed as Prosigne® elsewhere (e.g., Brazil). Neuronox® (Medy-Tox, Ochang, South Korea) is another BoNT-A available in some Asian countries. It is important to note that there has been no published systematic head-to-head comparison of the clinical properties, safety, and efficacy of commercially available formulations of BoNT-A. Hence, clinicians choose a BoNT-A formulation to treat PSS based on availability and experience with particular formulations, and no recommendation can be made regarding choice of a BoNT-A formulation in PSS.

5.2.6 BoNT-A Dosing

Appropriate dosing of BoNT-A is crucial in optimizing treatment outcomes and mitigating dose-related adverse events. Unfortunately, there is scarcity of dose-ranging studies (Simpson et al. 1996; Hyman et al. 2000; Gracies et al. 2015, 2017; Wissel et al. 2017) to allow evidence-based clinical decision-making with regard to dose selection for specific muscles. Hence, clinicians choose doses based on drug-specific summaries of product characteristic in package inserts, clinical experience, availability of toxins, and expert consensus recommendations ((Wissel et al. 2009; Esquenazi et al. 2013; Schramm et al. 2014), level of evidence 3).

Physician surveys suggest that many believe that greater flexibility in dosing might benefit some patients (Bensmail et al. 2014; Wissel 2018). Recently, a prospective, open-label, single-arm, multicenter, dose-titration study using high doses of incobotulinumtoxinA (up to 800 U) did not yield new safety signals (Wissel et al. 2017) (level of evidence 2b). In this particular trial, it was shown that high doses of incobotulinumtoxinA enabled simultaneous treatment of upper and lower limb and was associated with higher treatment goal attainment and no increase in side effect rate.

5.2.7 Adjuvant Therapies to BoNT-A

In a systematic review (without meta-analysis) of nine randomized trials (7 with neuromuscular electrostimulation, 2 with functional electrostimulation, 182 participants), it was shown that adjuvant electrostimulation therapy enhances the effect of BoNT-A injections on spasticity (Intiso et al. 2017) (level of evidence 1a). In two of these studies (both RCTs), spasticity was more responsive to additional electrostimulation after BoNT-A treatment than to additional stretching, but showed comparable effects as taping and lower effects than additional shock wave therapy. Neuromuscular electrostimulation was mostly performed in the studies for 30 min, 1 to 6 times a day for 3 to 5 days after the injection. In another systematic review, 17 studies were included; it was shown that the effect of BoNT-A injections could be improved by various adjuvant therapies (Mills et al. 2016). Thus, an added benefit in the sense of a stronger tonus reduction (MAS ≥ 1) was demonstrated to be proven for concomitant physiotherapy, modified constraint-induced movement therapy (mCIMT), electrostimulation, casting and dynamic splint treatment compared to BoNT-A alone, but not for taping, segmental muscle vibration, cyclic functional electrostimulation, or motorized arm ergometer (Mills et al. 2016) (level of evidence 1a).

Individual examples from selected studies are: After BoNT-A treatment of spastic calf muscles, a 1-week casting and to a lesser extent a 1-week taping showed better results with regard to spasticity reduction, increase of passive range of motion, and increased walking distance per time (6 min walking test) for 3 months after inclusion compared to a 1-week manual stretching by a physiotherapist following injection of BoNT-A (Carda et al. 2011) (level of evidence 1b). In another randomized controlled study for spastic pes equinus, no relevant additional effect of taping could be demonstrated (Karadag-Saygi et al. 2010) (level of evidence 1b).

In a Cochrane review, limited evidence could be provided as to whether and how multi-professional rehabilitation after BoNT-A treatment could improve spasticity in patients following stroke (3 RCS with 91 participants after stroke; (Demetrios et al. 2013), level of evidence 1a). With low-quality studies (GRADE) for mCIMT treatment following BoNT-A treatment, an improvement in active motor function and spasticity reduction could be shown. With very low-quality studies (GRADE) for occupational therapy following BoNT-A treatment improved in elbow mobility using a dynamic elbow extension splint compared to ergotherapy alone could be shown.

Recommendations: Neuromuscular electrostimulation applied for 3 to 5 days after BoNT-A therapy can be considered to enhance treatment effects in treated muscle groups (level of evidence 1a, quality of evidence low (risk of bias), 0). Safety aspects for the medical products used need to be taken into account. Other adjuvant therapies such as casting taping, mCIMT, and dynamic splint treatment can be used as individually indicated (level of evidence 1a, quality of evidence very low (risk of bias, inconsistency), 0). Active motor training and robotic training should be tailored to individual goals (refer to chapters on arm rehabilitation and mobility).

5.3   Neurolysis

Nerve blocks with neurolytic agents (phenol and alcohol) are effective in managing focal spasticity (Petrillo and Knoploch 1988; Chua and Kong 2000; Karri et al. 2017). For neurolysis, concentration of phenol usually ranges for 5% to 7%, while concentration of alcohol varies from 50% to 100%. These agents denature proteins in axons and membranes nonselectively in both afferent and efferent nerve fibers, leading to denervation and degeneration of spindles (Bodine-Fowler et al. 1996). Therefore, it requires precise localization and injection of these agents to the nerve fibers at the trunk, branch, or motor points of the target nerves. Precision localization is usually achieved with guidance of ultrasound imaging and/or electrical stimulation (Karri et al. 2017). Neurolysis usually produce immediate anesthesic effects and a later neurolytic effect on spasticity reduction. The duration depends on the dose, accuracy of injection, and repeated injections, ranging from 3 to 9 months. Unlike BoNT-A injections, nerve blocks can be repeated as early as several days. Common adverse effects include post-injection dysesthesia, localized swelling, and excessive weakness. In a recent retrospective chart review of 293 procedures, phenol neurolysis has a relatively favorable safety profile, including pain (4.0%), swelling and inflammation (2.7%), dysesthesia (0.7%), and hypotension (0.7%) (Karri et al. 2017). Although nerve blocks are widely used to manage spasticity, there is paucity of evidence of efficacy and safety based on randomized controlled studies. In a randomized, double-blind trial which compared phenol neurolysis and BoNT-A injection in the treatment of ankle and foot spasticity after stroke (Kirazli et al. 1998), the authors reported that both interventions were effective in plantar flexor spasticity reduction. The benefits were more significant in the BoNT-A group at weeks 2 and 4 post-injection, while there was no significant difference between two interventions at weeks 8 and 12.

Recommendations: Phenol and alcohol neurolysis can be considered for clinically relevant PSS that does not sufficiently respond to nonpharmacological treatment (and oral medication), especially when BoNT-A treatment is not feasible (level of evidence 2b, quality of evidence low, 0). The possibility of long-term unwanted side effects, especially neuropathic pain following mixed nerve injections, need to be taken into account.

5.4 Intrathecal Baclofen (ITB)

Intrathecal baclofen therapy (ITB) is effective in managing post-stoke spastic hypertonia (Meythaler et al. 2001; Ivanhoe et al. 2006). It is licensed in the European Union to manage severe chronic spasticity in children between ages 4 and 18 years that is recalcitrant to oral spasmolytics and for managing severe spasticity of both cerebral and spinal etiology. In the United States (US), ITB is approved by the US Food and Drug Administration (US FDA) for managing severe spasticity of both cerebral and spinal etiology. Although few randomized, controlled trials of safety and efficacy exist, ITB has high levels of satisfaction among users of 10–24 years' duration (Mathur et al. 2014).

The US FDA recommends initiation of ITB therapy 1-year after disease onset, but a consensus panel of ITB experts suggested that ITB can be considered as early as 3–6 months post-stroke when spasticity is not controlled by other modalities or a patient is unable to tolerate side effects of other treatments (Francisco et al. 2006).

A more recent consensus panel of experts (Saulino et al. 2016) recommended early consideration of ITB to avoid or delay various complications of spasticity and mitigate subsequent functional impairments. The same group commented that ITB should be considered only if other treatments have failed.

Meythaler et al. (2001) demonstrated superiority of ITB over placebo in a small cohort of stroke patients. Twenty-one stroke survivors with severe spasticity received either baclofen or placebo intrathecally. At 6 h post-bolus infusion, the average (mean ± SD) paretic lower limb Ashworth scores of the group that received baclofen decreased significantly from $3.3 ± 1.2$ to $1.4 ± 0.7$ ($P < 0.0001$), spasm score from $1.2 ± 1.2$ to $0.1 ± 0.3$ ($P = 0.0224$), and reflex score from $2.1 ± 1.2$ to $0.1 ± 0.5$ ($P < 0.0001$), compared to the group that received placebo. Seventeen subjects then received an intrathecal pump for continuous baclofen infusion. At 12 months following implantation and with an average daily dose of 268 micrograms per day, the average lower limb Ashworth score of the paretic side decreased from $3.7 ± 1.0$ to $1.8 ± 1.1$ ($P < 0.0001$), the spasm score decreased from $1.2 ± 1.3$ to $0.6 ± 1.0$ ($P = 0.4282$), and the reflex score decreased from $2.4 ± 1.3$ to $1.0 ± 1.3$ ($P < 0.0001$).

The effect of ITB on ambulant stroke survivors is controversial. Small reports (Francisco and Boake 2003; Remy-Neris et al. 2003) showed improvement in gait speed following ITB therapy, but others demonstrated otherwise (Kofler et al. 2009).

A recent randomized, controlled, open-label, multicenter trial also demonstrated superiority of ITB therapy over conventional medical management (cMM) with oral spasmolytics in terms of efficacy (mean Ashworth scale score reduction, -0.99 (ITB) vs. -0.43 (cMM); Hodges-Lehmann estimate -0.667 (95.1% CI -1.0000 to -0.1667); $p = 0.0140$) and pain control (numbers). While more subjects who received ITB reported adverse events (24/25 patients, 96%; 149 events) compared to those who received cMM (22/35, 63%; 77 events), no new safety signals were discovered (Creamer et al. 2018a, b).

Recommendations: ITB can be considered for clinically relevant severe segmental or generalized PSS that does not sufficiently respond to other interventions (level of evidence 1b, quality of evidence moderate, 0 (benefit risk for harm assessment)). ITB treatment ought to be tested, initiated, adjusted, and monitored with long-term support (including emergency work-up when indicated) by physicians experienced with the treatment (level of evidence 1b, quality of evidence moderate, A+ (benefit risk for harm assessment)).

5.5   Surgical Management

Surgical procedures at the spinal cord level, such as interventions in the posterior root entry zone or dorsal rhizotomy, may be introduced in severe cases of spasticity after stroke, which are otherwise untreatable and represent a possibility of avoiding abnormal positions due to a severe spasticity and its complications in care, hygiene, pain, and contractures (review by (Chambers 1997), level of evidence 3a). One positive case report with persistent effects for the partial posterior rhizotomy is available in the literature ((Fukuhara and Kamata 2004), level of evidence 4). Controlled studies on these procedures in children with cerebral palsy are published, and studies in adults following stroke are not available. One major criticism with this surgical procedure is that it may only bring temporal improvements.

Partial neurotomy of the motor branches of the tibial nerve to the triceps surae muscle is an established neurosurgical procedure and leads to reduced spastic muscle tone in pes equinus or equinovarus deformity, and therefore can improve positioning of the foot and can reduce associated pain during walking ((Sindou and Mertens 2000), level of evidence 2b).

Following reports of successful orthopedic surgery with fasciotomy, transfer of muscle attachments, tendon transfer, and even bony surgery to increase upper and lower limb function in persons with low functioning spastic upper and lower limbs following spinal cord injury (Fox et al. 2018) (level of evidence 3) in the last 10 years also in chronic stroke patients with limited upper and lower limb function, those procedures became more available, but no large cohort studies are published. Fascia, tendon and muscle lengthening (e.g., Achilles tendon lengthening, soleus muscle fasciotomy, or lengthening), and tendon transfer surgery (e.g., transfer of the tendon of the flexor carpi ulnaris muscle to the dorsal aspect of the wrist or tibialis posterior split transfer and transpositioning of a part of the tendon to the dorsal aspect of the foot) may help correcting spastic hand or foot posture and help to improve active wrist and foot extension to improve residual function as well as preventing complications due to spastic posturing and development of contracture ((Duquette and Adkinson 2018), level of evidence 4; (Sturbois-Nachef et al. 2019), level of evidence 3). Despite the recognized effectiveness of orthopedic surgery for neuro-orthopedic disorders like chronic stroke patients with spastic contractures, few studies have formally evaluated them. Hence, there is a need for research to provide evidence to support orthopedic surgery for treating such neuro-orthopedic disorders (Genet et al. 2018).

Thumb-in-palm deformity is a well-known cause of disability in the chronic stroke population with upper limb spasticity but no reports on surgical treatments are published. On the other hand, surgical correction of spastic flexion of the thumb due to in juvenile cerebral palsy is established and it was evaluated in a Cochrane review. The authors describe a positive effect noted by patients (patient-related outcome) and the surgeons. The authors of the review critiqued that no standardized surgical procedure is defined, and different assessment methods in evaluation of the results following surgery were used. The authors concluded that based on the data available an evidence-based assessment of this treatment, procedure was not possible (Smeulders et al. 2005) (level of evidence 1a).

Recommendations: In individual cases, after careful examination in the multi-professional team and exhaustion of other reversible treatment options for spastic movement disorder, surgical procedures may be considered as treatment option in chronic spastic movement disorder following stroke (level of evidence 4, quality of evidence very low, 0).

References

Ansari NN, Naghdi S, Hasson S, Azarsa MH, Azarnia S (2008) The modified Tardieu scale for the measurement of elbow flexor spasticity in adult patients with hemiplegia. Brain Inj 22:1007–1012

Ansari NN, Naghdi S, Hasson S, Rastgoo M, Amini M, Forogh B (2013) Clinical assessment of ankle plantarflexor spasticity in adult patients after stroke: inter-and intra-rater reliability of the modified Tardieu scale. Brain Inj 27:605–612

Ashford S, Fheodoroff K, Jacinto J, Turner-Stokes L (2016) Common goal areas in the treatment of upper limb spasticity: a multicentre analysis. Clin Rehabil 30:617–622

Baker JA, Pereira G (2015) The efficacy of Botulinum toxin a on improving ease of care in the upper and lower limbs: a systematic review and meta-analysis using the grades of recommendation, assessment, development and evaluation approach. Clin Rehabil 29:731–740

Baker JA, Pereira G (2016) The efficacy of Botulinum toxin a for limb spasticity on improving activity restriction and quality of life: a systematic review and meta-analysis using the GRADE approach. Clin Rehabil 30:549–558

Banky M, Clark RA, Mentiplay BF, Olver JH, Kahn MB, Williams G (2019) Toward accurate clinical spasticity assessment: validation of movement speed and joint angle assessments using smartphones and camera tracking. Arch Phys Med Rehabil 100(8):1482–1491

Bensmail D, Hanschmann A, Wissel J (2014) Satisfaction with botulinum toxin treatment in post-stroke spasticity: results from two cross-sectional surveys (patients and physicians). J Med Econ 17:618–625

Bodine-Fowler SC, Allsing S, Botte MJ (1996) Time course of muscle atrophy and recovery following a phenol-induced nerve block. Muscle Nerve 19:497–504

Brashear A, Gordon MF, Elovic E et al (2002a) Intramuscular injection of botulinum toxin for the treatment of wrist and finger spasticity after a stroke. N Engl J Med 347:395–400

Brashear A, Zafonte R, Corcoran M et al (2002b) Inter- and intrarater reliability of the Ashworth scale and the disability assessment scale in patients with upper-limb poststroke spasticity. Arch Phys Med Rehabil 83:1349–1354

Calota A, Feldman AG, Levin MF (2008) Spasticity measurement based on tonic stretch reflex threshold in stroke using a portable device. Clin Neurophysiol 119:2329–2337

Carda S, Invernizzi M, Baricich A, Cisari C (2011) Casting, taping or stretching after botulinum toxin type a for spastic equinus foot: a single-blind randomized trial on adult stroke patients. Clin Rehabil 25:1119–1127

CEBM (2009) Oxford center for evidence-based medicine—levels of evidence. In: Last version from March 2009. https://www.cebm.net/2009/06/oxford-centre-evidence-based-medicine-levels-evidence-march-2009/

Chambers HG (1997) The surgical treatment of spasticity. Muscle Nerve Suppl 6:S121–S128

Chin TY, Nattrass GR, Selber P, Graham HK (2005) Accuracy of intramuscular injection of botulinum toxin a in juvenile cerebral palsy: a comparison between manual needle placement and placement guided by electrical stimulation. J Pediatr Orthop 25:286–291

Chua KS, Kong KH (2000) Alcohol neurolysis of the sciatic nerve in the treatment of hemiplegic knee flexor spasticity: clinical outcomes. Arch Phys Med Rehabil 81:1432–1435

Creamer M, Cloud G, Kossmehl P et al (2018a) Intrathecal baclofen therapy versus conventional medical management for severe poststroke spasticity: results from a multicentre, randomised, controlled, open-label trial (SISTERS). J Neurol Neurosurg Psychiatry 89:642–650

Creamer M, Cloud G, Kossmehl P et al (2018b) Effect of Intrathecal baclofen on pain and quality of life in poststroke spasticity. Stroke 49:2129–2137

Demetrios M, Khan F, Turner-Stokes L, Brand C, McSweeney S (2013) Multidisciplinary rehabilitation following botulinum toxin and other focal intramuscular treatment for post-stroke spasticity. Cochrane Database Syst Rev (6):CD009689

Dong Y, Wu T, Hu X, Wang T (2017) Efficacy and safety of botulinum toxin type a for upper limb spasticity after stroke or traumatic brain injury: a systematic review with meta-analysis and trial sequential analysis. Eur J Phys Rehabil Med 53:256–267

Duquette SP, Adkinson JM (2018) Surgical management of spasticity of the forearm and wrist. Hand Clin 34:487–502

Esquenazi A, Albanese A, Chancellor MB et al (2013) Evidence-based review and assessment of botulinum neurotoxin for the treatment of adult spasticity in the upper motor neuron syndrome. Toxicon 67:115–128

Fheodoroff K, Kossmehl P, Wissel J (2017) Validity and reliability of the spasticity-associated arm pain scale. J Pain Manag Med 3:127

Fietzek UM, Kossmehl P, Schelosky L, Ebersbach G, Wissel J (2014) Early botulinum toxin treatment for spastic pes equinovarus—a randomized double-blind placebo-controlled study. Eur J Neurol 21:1089–1095

Finnerup NB (2017) Neuropathic pain and spasticity: intricate consequences of spinal cord injury. Spinal Cord 55:1046–1050

Flewellen EH, Nelson PE, Jones WP, Arens JF, Wagner DL (1983) Dantrolene dose–response in awake man: implications for management of malignant hyperthermia. Anesthesiology 59:275–280

Foley N, Pereira S, Salter K et al (2013) Treatment with botulinum toxin improves upper-extremity function post stroke: a systematic review and meta-analysis. Arch Phys Med Rehabil 94:977–989

Fox IK, Miller AK, Curtin CM (2018) Nerve and tendon transfer surgery in cervical spinal cord injury: individualized choices to optimize function. Top Spinal Cord Inj Rehabil 24: 275–287

Francisco GE, Boake C (2003) Improvement in walking speed in poststroke spastic hemiplegia after intrathecal baclofen therapy: a preliminary study. Arch Phys Med Rehabil 84:1194–1199

Francisco GE, Li S (2015) Spasticity. In: Physical medicine and rehabilitation, 5th edn. Elsevier, Philadelphia

Francisco GE, McGuire JR (2012) Poststroke spasticity management. Stroke 43:3132–3136

Francisco GE, Yablon SA, Schiess MC, Wiggs L, Cavalier S, Grissom S (2006) Consensus panel guidelines for the use of intrathecal baclofen therapy in poststroke spastic hypertonia. Top Stroke Rehabil 13:74–85

Fukuhara T, Kamata I (2004) Selective posterior rhizotomy for painful spasticity in the lower limbs of hemiplegic patients after stroke: report of two cases. Neurosurgery 54:1268–1272. discussion 1272–1263

Gao J, He W, Du LJ et al (2018) Quantitative ultrasound imaging to assess the biceps Brachii muscle in chronic post-stroke spasticity: preliminary observation. Ultrasound Med Biol 44(9):1931–1940

Genet F, Denormandie P, Keenan MA (2018) Orthopaedic surgery for patients with central nervous system lesions: concepts and techniques. Ann Phys Rehabil Med 62(4):225–233

Gracies JM, Brashear A, Jech R et al (2015) Safety and efficacy of abobotulinumtoxinA for hemiparesis in adults with upper limb spasticity after stroke or traumatic brain injury: a double-blind randomised controlled trial. Lancet Neurol 14:992–1001

Gracies JM, Esquenazi A, Brashear A et al (2017) Efficacy and safety of abobotulinumtoxinA in spastic lower limb: randomized trial and extension. Neurology 89:2245–2253

Grigoriu AI, Dinomais M, Rémy-Néris O, Brochard S (2015) Impact of injection-guiding techniques on the effectiveness of Botulinum toxin for the treatment of focal spasticity and dystonia: a systematic review. Arch Phys Med Rehabil 96:2067–2078

Halpern R, Gillard P, Graham GD, Varon SF, Zorowitz RD (2013) Adherence associated with oral medications in the treatment of spasticity. PM R 5:747–756

Haugh A, Pandyan A, Johnson G (2006) A systematic review of the Tardieu scale for the measurement of spasticity. Disabil Rehabil 28:899–907

Hesse S, Mach H, Frohlich S, Behrend S, Werner C, Melzer I (2012) An early botulinum toxin a treatment in subacute stroke patients may prevent a disabling finger flexor stiffness six months later: a randomized controlled trial. Clin Rehabil 26:237–245

Hyman N, Barnes M, Bhakta B et al (2000) Botulinum toxin (Dysport) treatment of hip adductor spasticity in multiple sclerosis: a prospective, randomised, double blind, placebo controlled, dose ranging study. J Neurol Neurosurg Psychiatry 68:707–712

Intiso D, Santamato A, Di Rienzo F (2017) Effect of electrical stimulation as an adjunct to botulinum toxin type a in the treatment of adult spasticity: a systematic review. Disabil Rehabil 39:2123–2133

Ivanhoe CB, Francisco GE, McGuire JR, Subramanian T, Grissom SP (2006) Intrathecal baclofen management of poststroke spastic hypertonia: implications for function and quality of life. Arch Phys Med Rehabil 87:1509–1515

Kaji R, Osako Y, Suyama K, Maeda T, Uechi Y, Iwasaki M (2010) Botulinum toxin type a in post-stroke lower limb spasticity: a multicenter, double-blind, placebo-controlled trial. J Neurol 257:1330–1337

Kamper D, Harvey R, Suresh S, Rymer W (2003) Relative contributions of neural mechanisms versus muscle mechanics in promoting finger extension deficits following stroke. Muscle Nerve 28:309–318

Karadag-Saygi E, Cubukcu-Aydoseli K, Kablan N, Ofluoglu D (2010) The role of kinesiotaping combined with botulinum toxin to reduce plantar flexors spasticity after stroke. Top Stroke Rehabil 17:318–322

Karri J, Mas MF, Francisco GE, Li S (2017) Practice patterns for spasticity management with phenol neurolysis. J Rehabil Med 49:482–488

Katrak PH, Cole AMD, Poulos CJ, McCauley JCK (1992) Objective assessment of spasticity, strength, and function with early exhibition of dantrolene sodium after cerebrovascular accident: a randomised double-blind controlled study. Arch Phys Med Rehabil 73:4–9

Kirazli Y, On AY, Kismali B, Aksit R (1998) Comparison of phenol block and botulinus toxin type a in the treatment of spastic foot after stroke: a randomized, double-blind, trial. Am J Phys Med Rehabil 77:510–515

Kiresuk TJ, Sherman RE (1968) Goal attainment scaling: a general method for evaluating comprehensive community mental health programs. Community Ment Health J 4:443–453

Kofler M, Quirbach E, Schauer R, Singer M, Saltuari L (2009) Limitations of intrathecal baclofen for spastic hemiparesis following stroke. Neurorehabil Neural Repair 23:26–31

Krause T, Gerbershagen MU, Fiege M, Weisshorn R, Wappler F (2004) Dantrolene—a review of its pharmacology, therapeutic use and new developments. Anaesthesia 59:364–373

Lee KB, Hong BY, Kim JS et al (2019) Which brain lesions produce spasticity? An observational study on 45 stroke patients. PLoS One 14:e0210038

Levin MF, Feldman AG (1994) The role of stretch reflex threshold regulation in normal and impaired motor control. Brain Res 657:23–30

Li S, Kamper DG, Rymer WZ (2006) Effects of changing wrist positions on finger flexor hypertonia in stroke survivors. Muscle Nerve 33:183–190

Li F, Wu Y, Li X (2014) Test-retest reliability and inter-rater reliability of the modified Tardieu scale and the modified Ashworth scale in hemiplegic patients with stroke. Eur J Phys Rehabil Med 50:9–15

Lichtner V, Dowding D, Esterhuizen P, Closs SJ, Long AF, Corbett A, Briggs M (2014) Pain assessment for people with dementia: a systematic review of systematic reviews of pain assessment tools. BMC Geriatr 14:138

Lim JY, Koh JH, Paik NJ (2008) Intramuscular botulinum toxin-a reduces hemiplegic shoulder pain: a randomized, double-blind, comparative study versus intraarticular triamcinolone acetonide. Stroke 39:126–131

Lindsay C, Kouzouna A, Simcox C, Pandyan AD (2016) Pharmacological interventions other than botulinum toxin for spasticity after stroke. Cochrane Database Syst Rev 10:CD010362

Malhotra S, Pandyan AD, Rosewilliam S, Roffe C, Hermens H (2011) Spasticity and contractures at the wrist after stroke: time course of development and their association with functional recovery of the upper limb. Clin Rehabil 25:184–191

Mathur SN, Chu SK, McCormick Z, Chang Chien GC, Marciniak CM (2014) Long-term intrathecal baclofen: outcomes after more than 10 years of treatment. PM R 6:506–513.e1

Medaer R, Hellebuyk H, Van Den Brande E, Saxena V, Thijs M, Kovacs L, Dehaen F (1991) Treatment of spasticity due to stroke: a double-blind, cross-over trial comparing baclofen with placebo. Acta Therapeut 17:323–331

Mehrholz J, Major Y, Meissner D, Sandi-Gahun S, Koch R, Pohl M (2005) The influence of contractures and variation in measurement stretching velocity on the reliability of the modified Ashworth scale in patients with severe brain injury. Clin Rehabil 19:63–72

Meseguer-Henarejos AB, SăNchez-Meca J, López-Pina JA, Carles-HernăNdez R (2018) Inter-and intra-rater reliability of the modified Ashworth scale: a systematic review and meta-analysis. Eur J Phys Rehabil Med 54:576–590

Meythaler JM, Guin-Renfroe S, Brunner RC, Hadley MN (2001) Intrathecal baclofen for spastic hypertonia from stroke. Stroke 32:2099–2109

Meythaler JM, Clayton W, Davis LK, Guin-Renfroe S, Brunner RC (2004) Orally delivered baclofen to control spastic hypertonia in acquired brain injury. J Head Trauma Rehabil 19:101–108

Mills PB, Finlayson H, Sudol M, O'Connor R (2016) Systematic review of adjunct therapies to improve outcomes following botulinum toxin injection for treatment of limb spasticity. Clin Rehabil 30:537–548

Montane E, Vallano A, Laporte JR (2004) Oral antispastic drugs in nonprogressive neurologic diseases: a systematic review. Neurology 63:1357–1363

Olvey EL, Armstrong EP, Grizzle AJ (2010) Contemporary pharmacologic treatments for spasticity of the upper limb after stroke: a systematic review. Clin Ther 32:2282–2303

Owens DK, Lohr KN, Atkins D et al (2010) AHRQ series paper 5: grading the strength of a body of evidence when comparing medical interventions—agency for healthcare research and quality and the effective health-care program. J Clin Epidemiol 63:513–523

Paulis WD, Horemans HL, Brouwer BS, Stam HJ (2011) Excellent test-retest and inter-rater reliability for Tardieu scale measurements with inertial sensors in elbow flexors of stroke patients. Gait Posture 33:185–189

Petrillo CR, Knoploch S (1988) Phenol block of the tibial nerve for spasticity: a long-term follow-up study. Int Disabil Stud 10:97–100

Picelli A, Bonetti P, Fontana C et al (2012) Accuracy of botulinum toxin type a injection into the gastrocnemius muscle of adults with spastic equinus: manual needle placement and electrical stimulation guidance compared using ultrasonography. J Rehabil Med 44:450–452

Picelli A, Lobba D, Midiri A, Prandi P, Melotti C, Baldessarelli S, Smania N (2014) Botulinum toxin injection into the forearm muscles for wrist and fingers spastic overactivity in adults with chronic stroke: a randomized controlled trial comparing three injection techniques. Clin Rehabil 28:232–242

Pittock SJ, Moore AP, Hardiman O et al (2003) A double-blind randomised placebo-controlled evaluation of three doses of botulinum toxin type a (Dysport) in the treatment of spastic equinovarus deformity after stroke. Cerebrovasc Dis 15:289–300

Platz T (2017) Practice guidelines in neurorehabilitation. Neurol Int Open 01:E148–E152

Platz T, Vuadens P, Eickhof C, Arnold P, Van Kaick S, Heise K (2008) REPAS, a summary rating scale for resistance to passive movement: item selection, reliability and validity. Disabil Rehabil 30:44–53

Platz T, Wissel J, Donauer E, Vogel M, Tholen R, Lehmler L (2019) S2k-Leitlinie: Therapie des spastischen Syndroms. DGNeurologie (online first/ahead of print). https://doi.org/10.1007/s42451-019-0090-2

Remy-Neris O, Denys P, Daniel O, Barbeau H, Bussel B (2003) Effect of intrathecal clonidine on group I and group II oligosynaptic excitation in paraplegics. Exp Brain Res 148:509–514

Rockwood K, Joyce B, Stolee P (1997) Use of goal attainment scaling in measuring clinically important change in cognitive rehabilitation patients. J Clin Epidemiol 50:581–588

Rosales RL, Chua-Yap AS (2008) Evidence-based systematic review on the efficacy and safety of botulinum toxin-a therapy in post-stroke spasticity. J Neural Transm (Vienna) 115:617–623

Rosales RL, Kong KH, Goh KJ et al (2012) Botulinum toxin injection for hypertonicity of the upper extremity within 12 weeks after stroke: a randomized controlled trial. Neurorehabil Neural Repair 26:812–821

Rosales RL, Efendy F, Teleg ES et al (2016) Botulinum toxin as early intervention for spasticity after stroke or non-progressive brain lesion: a meta-analysis. J Neurol Sci 371:6–14

Santamato A, Micello MF, Panza F et al (2014) Can botulinum toxin type a injection technique influence the clinical outcome of patients with post-stroke upper limb spasticity? A randomized controlled trial comparing manual needle placement and ultrasound-guided injection techniques. J Neurol Sci 347:39–43

Saulino M, Anderson DJ, Doble J, Farid R, Gul F, Konrad P, Boster AL (2016) Best practices for Intrathecal baclofen therapy: troubleshooting. Neuromodulation 19:632–641

Schramm A, Ndayisaba JP, Auf dem Brinke M et al (2014) Spasticity treatment with onabotulinumtoxin a: data from a prospective German real-life patient registry. J Neural Transm (Vienna) 121:521–530

Schünemann H, Brożek J, Guyatt G, Oxman A (2013) GRADE handbook for grading quality of evidence and strength of recommendations. The GRADE Working Group. Updated October 2013. www.guidelinedevelopment.org/handbook

Simpson DM, Alexander DN, O'Brien CF et al (1996) Botulinum toxin type a in the treatment of upper extremity spasticity: a randomized, double-blind, placebo-controlled trial. Neurology 46:1306–1310

Simpson DM, Gracies JM, Graham HK et al (2008) Assessment: Botulinum neurotoxin for the treatment of spasticity (an evidence-based review): report of the therapeutics and technology assessment Subcommittee of the American Academy of neurology. Neurology 70: 1691–1698

Simpson DM, Gracies JM, Yablon SA, Barbano R, Brashear A (2009) Botulinum neurotoxin versus tizanidine in upper limb spasticity: a placebo-controlled study. J Neurol Neurosurg Psychiatry 80:380–385

Simpson DM, Hallett M, Ashman EJ et al (2016) Practice guideline update summary: Botulinum neurotoxin for the treatment of blepharospasm, cervical dystonia, adult spasticity, and headache report of the guideline development Subcommittee of the American Academy of neurology. Neurology 86:1818–1826

Sindou MP, Mertens P (2000) Neurosurgery for spasticity. Stereotact Funct Neurosurg 74:217–221

Singh P, Joshua AM, Ganeshan S, Suresh S (2011) Intra-rater reliability of the modified Tardieu scale to quantify spasticity in elbow flexors and ankle plantar flexors in adult stroke subjects. Ann Indian Acad Neurol 14:23–26

Sinkjaer T, Magnussen I (1994) Passive, intrinsic and reflex-mediated stiffness in the ankle extensors of hemiparetic patients. Brain 117:355–363

Smeulders M, Coester A, Kreulen M (2005) Surgical treatment for the thumb-in-palm deformity in patients with cerebral palsy. Cochrane Database Syst Rev (4):CD004093

Sommerfeld DK, Eek EU, Svensson AK, Holmqvist LW, von Arbin MH (2004) Spasticity after stroke: its occurrence and association with motor impairments and activity limitations. Stroke 35:134–139

Stamenova P, Koytchev R, Kuhn K, Hansen C, Horvath F, Ramm S, Pongratz D (2005) A randomized, double-blind, placebo-controlled study of the efficacy and safety of tolperisone in spasticity following cerebral stroke. Eur J Neurol 12:453–461

Stevenson VL, Jarrett L (2006) Spasticity management: a practical multidisciplinary guide. Informa Healthcare, London

Sturbois-Nachef N, Allart E, Grauwin MY, Rousseaux M, Thevenon A, Fontaine C (2019) Tibialis posterior transfer for foot drop due to central causes: Long-term hindfoot alignment. Orthop Traumatol Surg Res 105:153–158

Thanikachalam V, Phadke CP, Ismail F, Boulias C (2017) Effect of Botulinum toxin on clonus: a systematic review. Arch Phys Med Rehabil 98:381–390

Turkel CC, Bowen B, Liu J, Brin MF (2006) Pooled analysis of the safety of botulinum toxin type a in the treatment of poststroke spasticity. Arch Phys Med Rehabil 87:786–792

Turner-Stokes L, Baguley IJ, De Graaff S, Katrak P, Davies L, McCrory P, Hughes A (2010) Goal attainment scaling in the evaluation of treatment of upper limb spasticity with botulinum toxin: a secondary analysis from a double-blind placebo-controlled randomized clinical trial. J Rehabil Med 42:81–89

Turner-Stokes L, Rose H, Ashford S, Singer B (2015) Patient engagement and satisfaction with goal planning: impact on outcome from rehabilitation. Int J Ther Rehabil 22:210–216

Tyson SF, Brown P (2014) How to measure pain in neurological conditions? A systematic review of psychometric properties and clinical utility of measurement tools. Clin Rehabil 28:669–686

van Kuijk AA, Geurts AC, Bevaart BJ, van Limbeek J (2002) Treatment of upper extremity spasticity in stroke patients by focal neuronal or neuromuscular blockade: a systematic review of the literature. J Rehabil Med 34:51–61

Watkins CL, Leathley MJ, Gregson JM, Moore AP, Smith TL, Sharma AK (2002) Prevalence of spasticity post stroke. Clin Rehabil 16:515–522

Wein T, Esquenazi A, Jost WH, Ward AB, Pan G, Dimitrova R (2018) OnabotulinumtoxinA for the treatment of Poststroke distal lower limb spasticity: a randomized trial. PM R 10:693–703

Whiting PF, Wolff RF, Deshpande S et al (2015) Cannabinoids for medical use: a systematic review and meta-analysis. JAMA 313:2456–2473

Winstein CJ, Stein J, Arena R et al (2016) Guidelines for adult stroke rehabilitation and recovery: a guideline for healthcare professionals from the American Heart Association/American Stroke Association. Stroke 47:e98–e169

Winter T, Wissel J (2013) Behandlung der Spastizität nach Schlaganfall. Konsultationsfassung der DGNR-Leitlinie. Neurol Rehabil 19:285–309

Wissel J (2018) Towards flexible and tailored botulinum neurotoxin dosing regimens for focal dystonia and spasticity—insights from recent studies. Toxicon 147:100–106

Wissel J, Muller J, Dressnandt J, Heinen F, Naumann M, Topka H, Poewe W (2000) Management of spasticity associated pain with botulinum toxin a. J Pain Symptom Manage 20:44–49

Wissel J, Haydn T, Muller J, Brenneis C, Berger T, Poewe W, Schelosky LD (2006) Low dose treatment with the synthetic cannabinoid Nabilone significantly reduces spasticity-related pain: a double-blind placebo-controlled cross-over trial. J Neurol 253:1337–1341

Wissel J, Ward AB, Erztgaard P et al (2009) European consensus table on the use of botulinum toxin type a in adult spasticity. J Rehabil Med 41:13–25

Wissel J, Schelosky LD, Scott J, Christe W, Faiss JH, Mueller J (2010) Early development of spasticity following stroke: a prospective, observational trial. J Neurol 257:1067–1072

Wissel J, Verrier M, Simpson DM, Charles D, Guinto P, Papapetropoulos S, Sunnerhagen KS (2015) Post-stroke spasticity: predictors of early development and considerations for therapeutic intervention. PM R 7:60–67

Wissel J, Ganapathy V, Ward AB et al (2016) OnabotulinumtoxinA improves pain in patients with post-stroke spasticity: findings from a randomized, double-blind, placebo-controlled trial. J Pain Symptom Manage 52:17–26

Wissel J, Bensmail D, Ferreira JJ et al (2017) Safety and efficacy of incobotulinumtoxinA doses up to 800 U in limb spasticity: the TOWER study. Neurology 88:1321–1328

Wu CH, Ho YC, Hsiao MY, Chen WS, Wang TG (2017) Evaluation of post-stroke spastic muscle stiffness using shear wave ultrasound elastography. Ultrasound Med Biol 43:1105–1111

Yelnik AP, Colle FM, Bonan IV, Vicaut E (2007) Treatment of shoulder pain in spastic hemiplegia by reducing spasticity of the subscapular muscle: a randomised, double blind, placebo-controlled study of botulinum toxin A. J Neurol Neurosurg Psychiatry 78:845–848

Zeuner KE, Knutzen A, Kuhl C et al (2017) Functional impact of different muscle localization techniques for Botulinum neurotoxin a injections in clinical routine management of post-stroke spasticity. Brain Inj 31:75–82

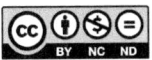

Rehabilitation of Communication Disorders

Rebecca Palmer and Apoorva Pauranik

1 Introduction: The Clinical Problem

Speech, communication and language disorders are many and heterogeneous. The modalities of communication affected include spoken understanding and expression, reading, writing and gesture. The three predominant speech and language disorders that can be acquired post-stroke are as follows:

1.1 Aphasia

Aphasia is a language disorder affecting understanding of spoken language; the ability to express thoughts verbally, including difficulties with word retrieval (anomia), and sentence production; the ability to read and understand written words and sentences and the ability to write including spelling and structuring written sentences. These difficulties result from damage to the left side of the brain in the majority of people. The extent of impairment to each of the four language domains varies from person to person depending on the locations and extent of neurological damage. Flowers et al. (2013) estimated the incidence of aphasia post-stroke to be 30%.

R. Palmer (✉)
School of Health and Related Research (ScHARR), University of Sheffield, Sheffield, UK
e-mail: r.l.palmer@sheffield.ac.uk

A. Pauranik
M.G.M. Medical College, Indore, Madhya Pradesh, India

© The Author(s) 2021
T. Platz (ed.), *Clinical Pathways in Stroke Rehabilitation*,
https://doi.org/10.1007/978-3-030-58505-1_10

1.2   Dysarthria

Dysarthria is a motor speech disorder resulting from impaired movement of the muscles used for the production of speech. The main parameters of speech are respiration, phonation, resonance, articulation and prosody. One or more of these parameters can be affected leading to reduced speech intelligibility and reduced communication effectiveness. These parameters can be impaired in different ways (for example muscles may be more or less paretic, become hypotonic or hypertonic), and they may each be impaired to different extents. This results in different dysarthria profiles (e.g. Darley et al. 1975). Flowers et al. (2013) estimated the incidence of dysarthria post-stroke to be 42%.

1.3   Apraxia

Apraxia of speech (AOS), also known as verbal apraxia or dyspraxia, is also a motor speech disorder. AOS results from a reduction in the ability to co-ordinate the gestures required for speech leading to difficulty producing the right sounds in the right order when speaking. It is characterised by multiple different attempts to articulate words accurately. AOS can occur in isolation, but frequently coincides with expressive aphasia. AOS is acquired with lower frequency following stroke than aphasia or dysarthria.

Aphasia, dysarthria and apraxia are not mutually exclusive, and more than one speech and language disorder may need to be treated.

Communication impairments affect everyday activity, for example the ability to have conversations, make phone calls, listen to the radio, write letters, construct emails and text messages and read for pleasure, for information or for work. They may also affect the use of sign language for people in the deaf community. In turn, they restrict participation: the ability to carry out pre-stroke employment, loss of roles within the family and community and withdrawal from participating in usual activities both outside of and within the family. These changes affect the well-being of both the person with a communication disability and their family/carer with increased frustration, misunderstandings and breakdown/strain on relationships. For the carer, increased responsibilities, mending communication breakdowns and misunderstandings, loss of the person to talk to and dealing with frustration of both the person with the communication difficulty and their own have significant impact on their well-being. It is recognised that the impact of a communication impairment is not always proportional to its severity. For example people with relatively mild dysarthria may be intelligible, but sound different thus challenging their identity and self-confidence. Communication disorders also place a burden on society due to increased dependence, loss of employment of both the individual and the carer who may need to give up work to look after the person and reduced ability to perform previous caring roles, looking after other dependent family members for example.

2   Recommendations for the Assessment and Treatment of Post-Stroke Communication Disorders

Recommendations have been based on evidence from Cochrane reviews in aphasia, dysarthria and AOS and supplemented with evidence from other systematic reviews and recent RCTs. The Cochrane library was searched for reviews of aphasia/dysphasia, dysarthria, apraxia of speech/verbal dyspraxia and motor speech. Twelve reviews were returned and five (those referring to stroke) were used to inform the recommendations. Additional systematic and narrative review evidence is drawn upon in each section where useful in providing additional clinical direction. An information specialist performed searches for reviews in Medline published from 2010 to December 2017 including aphasia OR dysphasia AND speech and language therapy OR therapy OR treatment OR assessment AND stroke AND meta-analysis OR review. A second search was performed replacing aphasia/dysphasia with apraxia of speech OR dysarthria. Thirty-two results were returned for aphasia and 86 for apraxia or dysarthria. A third search was performed for recent RCTs from 2015 to December 2017, replacing the terms meta-analysis OR review with RCT returning 46 results. The first author reviewed the abstracts of all returned papers and excluded non stroke, non-systematic method, known Cochrane reviews, non-treatment or assessment studies, non SLT interventions and non RCT design (for RCT search only). Eleven reviews for aphasia, two reviews for dysarthria and apraxia of speech and eight recent RCTs were identified. Information from selected reviews and RCTs was used if it added information to that already identified in Cochrane reviews. An additional known review of dysarthria treatment was included, published in 2009. Evidence from adequately powered RCTs published between December 2017 and publication of this chapter have also been added.

Levels of evidence for recommendations are indicated using CEMB (levels 1a to 5 according to the 'Oxford Center for Evidence-Based Medicine—Levels of Evidence', last version from March 2009, http://www.cebm.net/Oxford-centre-evidence-based-medicine).

The quality of evidence was rated with four categories according to 'GRADE' ('Grades of Recommendation, Assessment, Development and Evaluation') (Owens et al. 2010):

- High quality: further research is unlikely to affect our confidence in the estimation of the (therapeutic) effect.
- Medium quality: further research is likely to affect our confidence in the estimation of the (therapeutic) effect and may alter the estimate.
- Low quality: further research will most likely influence our confidence in the estimation of the (therapeutic) effect and will probably change the estimate.
- Very low quality: any estimation of the (therapy) effect or prognosis is very uncertain.

The grading of the recommendations according to GRADE (Schünemann et al. 2013) corresponds to the categories 'ought to' (A) (strong recommendation), 'should' (B) (weak recommendation). As a third category had been introduced 'can' (0) (option) (Platz 2017). Recommendation category A is granted for clinically effective interventions with high-quality evidence support; with medium-quality evidence category B and with low- or very low-quality evidence category 0 can be appropriate; deviations might be indicated based on clinical judgement, individually applying reasons are denoted in [brackets]. A+ and B+ denote a strong or weak recommendation in favour on an intervention, A− and B− against its use.

2.1 Clinical Assessment of Communication Disorders

With increasing globalisation, the proportion of people who speak more than one language is rapidly expanding with each language potentially being differently affected (Lekoubou et al. 2015). The clinical profile of aphasia may differ to a variable extent, in the two or more languages used by an individual. Aphasia needs to be assessed in all languages spoken by an individual to assist therapeutic planning.

A systematic review by Hachioui et al. (2017) identified screening tests that have been validated for aphasia, with varying methodological quality and levels of bias. These include the Frenchay Aphasia Screening Test (FAST) (Enderby et al. 1987), Language Screening Test (LAST) (Flamand-Roze et al. 2011), Mississippi Aphasia Screening Test (MAST) (Nakase-Thompson et al. 2005), the Mobile Aphasia Screening Test (also MAST) (Choi et al. 2015), ScreeLing (Doesborgh et al. 2003), Sheffield Screening Test for Acquired Language Disorders (SST) (Al-Khawaja et al. 1996), Semantic Verbal Fluency (SVF) (Kim et al. 2011) and Ullevaal Aphasia Screening Test (UAS) (Thommessen et al. 1999).

Recommendation: Screening tests should be used to identify the presence of aphasia (evidence level 2a, very low quality, B+ (clinical importance)).

No validated screening tools have been published for dysarthria or dyspraxia.

The World Health Organisation endorsed the International Classification of Functioning Disability and Health (ICF) in 2001, recommending assessment of a patient's impairment, activity and participation. For communication, impairment refers to the speech or language disorder itself and the profile of this. Activity refers to having a conversation, reading and writing. Participation refers to carrying out daily activities that are usual for the individual and the degree to which these have been affected by the communication disorder. Additionally, the ICF encourages assessment of the environment (or context) in which the disability is experienced. The quality of life of both patients and their carers/family members is also an important focus of assessment. Detailed assessment should therefore address all areas identified by the ICF.

Commonly used assessments of impairment that have been validated or shown to be reliable include the Western Aphasia Battery (WAB), Boston Diagnostic Aphasia

Examination (BDAE-2) and the Comprehensive Aphasia Test (CAT), Aachen Aphasia Test (AAT), Minnesota Aphasia Test (MAT), Porch Index of Communication Ability (PICA) and the Frenchay Dysarthria Assessment (FDA-2).

Recommendation: Published assessments of speech and language should be used to provide a profile of the speech or language disorder in patients with a positive screening result (evidence level 2b, very low quality, B+ (clinical importance)).

A systematic review by van Dijk et al. (2016) reviewed instruments available for assessing depressive symptoms in people with aphasia. The majority were not sufficiently investigated and those that were generally had low methodological quality. However, the authors recommended the Stroke Aphasia Depression Questionnaire–10, the Stroke Aphasia Depression Questionnaire–H10 and the Signs of Depression Scale as most feasible for use in clinical practice.

Recommendation: Published assessments of depression in aphasia can be considered (level of evidence 2a, very low quality, 0).

Goal setting can help with therapy planning. This is usefully conducted with the person with communication difficulties and their families. Goals can be informed by a screening or detailed assessment in combination with what the patient and family wish to achieve from rehabilitation.

There is a rich literature about imaging in aphasia, including predicting outcome and suggesting individual therapy (Faroqi Shah et al. 2013). For the time being, however, imaging techniques still need to be considered research tools, and while they have the potential to eventually become relevant for clinical management, they are currently investigational.

2.2   Behavioural Therapy Interventions

Behavioural therapy interventions can focus on the ICF levels of impairment, activity and participation. Impairment-based interventions can be carried out in order to underpin improvements in activity and participation level goals.

2.2.1   Aphasia Therapy

Impairment Focus

The Cochrane review of speech and language therapy for aphasia post-stroke (Brady et al. 2016) included impairment-based interventions based on cognitive neuroscience/psycholinguistic models. For example semantic therapies focussing on interpretation of meaning to improve semantic processing; phonological therapies aiming to improve the sound structure of language; sentence mapping matching meaning to sentence structure and narrative therapy to provide a macrostructure for sentences and discourse. Many impairment-based therapies focus on improving specific domains of language such as reading, writing, comprehension and expressive language and more targeted approaches like semantic-based treatment.

Activity/Participation Focus

Constraint-induced aphasia therapy (CIAT) (Pulvermuller et al. 2001), also known as intensive language action therapy (ILAT), is one example of therapy focusing on the activity of using language. The intervention employs constraint, encouraging patients to only use spoken language to communicate during activities such as making requests from other group members.

Functional therapy specifically targets improvement in communication tasks considered to be useful in day-to-day functioning.

Brady et al. (2016) provide evidence from a meta-analysis of RCTs for the effect of speech and language therapy (SLT). Twenty-seven RCTs (1620 participants) assessed SLT versus no SLT. According to these meta-analyses, SLT resulted in clinically statistically significant weak-to-moderate benefit to patients' functional communication (standardised mean difference (SMD) 0.28, 95% confidence interval (CI) 0.06 to 0.49, 10 trials, 376 participants), reading (SMD: 0.29 (0.03 to 0.55); 8 trials, 254 participants), writing (SMD: 0.41 (0.41 to0.67); 8 trials, 253 participants) and expressive language (SMD: 1.28 (0.38 to 2.19); 7 trials, 248 participants). However, there is currently no evidence for one type of therapy being superior to another or of long-term effects of therapy.

Recommendation: Speech and language therapy should be provided to people with aphasia as individually indicated to reduce communication difficulties and enhance functional communication (level of evidence 1a, very low-to-moderate quality, B+).

The activity-based 'constraint-induced therapy' has been the subject of several studies enabling meta-analysis of results for this therapy specifically. In the Cochrane review (Brady et al. 2016), five RCTs (160 participants) compared CIAT to other forms of therapy. The comparisons showed no evidence of greater improvement with CIAT than with other types of therapy in functional outcomes (SMD: 0.15 (−0.21 to 0.50); 3 trials, 126 participants) or aphasia severity (SMD: 0.11 (−0.57 to 0.79); 2 trials, 34 participants), although the quality of evidence for these findings was low and very low, respectively. Zhang et al. performed a more recent systematic review of RCTs of CIAT in 2017. Eight RCTs were found but conclusions were similar to the Cochrane review, in that CIAT may be useful for improving chronic post-stroke aphasia although there is no evidence of superiority to other techniques.

Recommendation: Constraint-induced aphasia therapy can be considered for the treatment of people with aphasia, especially when promotion of verbal communication activity is the aim (level of evidence 1a, very low to low quality, 0).

2.2.2 Dysarthria Therapy

In a Cochrane review of interventions for dysarthria due to stroke including five small RCTs with 234 participants (Mitchell et al. 2017), there was a statistically significant effect of therapy at the level of impairment immediately post-therapy when comparing treatment to another intervention, placebo or control (SMD: 0.47 (0.02 to 0.92, 4 trials, 99 participants)) but no evidence of a persistent effect (SMD 0.07, (−0.91 to 1.06); 2 trials, 56 participants). There was no evidence of effect of therapy at the level of activity or participation immediately post-therapy (activity SMD: 0.29 (−0.07 to 0.66); 3 trials, 117 participants) (participation SMD: −0.24 (−0.94 to 0.45); 1 trial, 32 participants) or of persistent effects (activity SMD: 0.18, (0.18 to 0.55); 3 trials, 116 participants) (participation SMD: −0.11 (−0.56 to 0.33); 2 trials, 79 participants).

Recommendation: People with dysarthria should receive rehabilitation to try to improve their speech impairment. (level of evidence 1a, very low to low quality, B+ (clinical relevance)).

A narrative review of non-randomised studies outlines impairment-based techniques that have demonstrated some qualitative benefit in improving the clarity of speech (Palmer and Enderby 2007). These include articulation exercises practising precision in the production of single sounds, words and sentences; modelling correct pronunciation of words and sentences and providing feedback 'clear' or 'unclear' on repeated attempts; use of visual feedback to increase the use of pitch, loudness and intonation (prosody) and use of the Lee Silverman technique to increase loudness.

At the activity level, compensatory strategies to increase intelligibility through purposeful speech production such as over-articulation or slowing rate of speech can be used. Visual feedback and pacing techniques to slow rate (using a metronome or pointing to the first letter of each word on an alphabet chart) have been described (Palmer and Enderby 2007). Evidence is needed to understand the effectiveness of these therapy options.

Recommendation: Techniques to try and improve clarity of speech described in the literature can be considered (level of evidence 3–4, very low quality, 0).

2.2.3 Apraxia of Speech

The Cochrane review of treatments for apraxia of speech post-stroke found no trials had been conducted (West et al. 2005). In 2015, Ballard et al. conducted a systematic review of studies in AOS and included 26 within-participant experimental designs. The review indicated potential benefit at the level of impairment of articulatory-kinematic and rate-rhythm approaches to treatment, although there is no evidence of effect of AOS interventions on activity and participation.

Kinematic approaches involve motoric practice (repetitive practice of phonemes building in complexity), modelling and repetition (watching listening and speaking with the therapist) and articulatory cuing (involving sound production treatment using minimal pair words and prompt for restructuring oral muscular phonemic targets, e.g. tactile cues for accurate articulation placement (PROMPT). Rate-rhythm approaches use prosodic patterns, e.g. melody, rhythm and stress to improve speech production. In addition, Varley et al. published a small RCT (50 participants) in 2016 and showed single word production benefited from a behavioural speech treatment involving hierarchical exercises from understanding word meanings to imagery of word production to repetition to autonomous word production in words then sentences with the exercises presented on a computer. This was compared to a visuospatial sham treatment.

Recommendation: Behavioural treatment approaches can be used to treat the impairment in AOS (level of evidence 2a, very low quality, 0).

2.3 Biological Therapies

2.3.1 Pharmacological Treatments

A number of drugs have been used to try and improve language recovery after stroke. A Cochrane review of pharmacological treatments (Greener et al. 2001) found 10 RCTs evaluating the effect of six different drugs. There was weak evidence that Piracetam may be effective in the treatment of aphasia (odds ratio: 0.46 (0.3–0.7); 5 trials, 661 participants). Patients who were treated with Piracetam were no more likely (considering statistical significance) than those who took a placebo to experience unwanted effects, including death (odds ratio 1.29, 95% confidence interval for difference 0.9 to 1.7). However, despite not reaching statistical significance, the difference in death rate between groups does give rise to some concerns that there may be an increased risk of death from taking Piracetam. A further review and meta-analysis of Piracetam was conducted by Zhang et al. (2016) showing no overall improvement in aphasia severity but pronounced improvement in written language (SMD: 0.35 (0.04 to 0.66); 7 trials, 261 participants).

Recommendation: On the whole, drugs cannot yet be recommended to augment the effects of behavioural therapy for aphasia. Piracetam can be considered to improve aphasia, notably written language but further investigation of long-term effects and safety are needed (level of evidence 1a, very low quality, 0). Pharmacological licensing issues need to be considered based on regional regulatory affairs.

2.3.2 Non-Invasive Brain Stimulation (NIBS)

Repetitive transcranial magnetic stimulation (rTMS) and transcranial direct current stimulation (tDCS) have been employed in chronic aphasia either to suppress the maladaptive and inhibitory right-hemisphere activity or to stimulate compensatory left-hemispheric peri-lesion areas. Elsner et al. (2015) conducted a Cochrane review and meta-analysis of trials that compared the effect of tDCS to control interventions on correct picture naming and found that tDCS did not enhance picture naming (SMD:0.37 (−0.18 to 0.92); 6 trials, 66 participants). Li et al. (2015) conducted a meta-analysis including four RCTs showing that low-frequency rTMS was beneficial for post-stroke patients in terms of naming (SMD: 0.51 (0.16 to 0.86)) with no adverse effects. In 2016, Shak-Basak et al. conducted a systematic review of between and within-subject studies of rTMS and tDCS and concluded that the magnitude of effect on picture naming was similar: rTMS—SMD: 0.448 (8 trials, 143 participants) and tDCS—SMD: 0.395 (8 studies, 140 participants). However, Al Harbi et al. (2017) identify a range of methodological issues with existing studies and consider evidence to be at the pre-efficacy level with emerging evidence at the efficacy level.

Caution must be exercised as non-invasive brain stimulation (NIBS) may lower the threshold for epileptic seizures, and individual contraindications need to be taken into account (Lefaucheur et al. 2014).

No systematic reviews of non-invasive brain stimulation have been conducted specifically for dysarthria or AOS.

Recommendation: tDCS or rTMS to enhance verbal production in aphasia can be considered (level of evidence 1a, low quality, 0). Licensing of specific medical devices needs to be considered based on regional regulatory affairs and safety standards ought to be followed (level of evidence 1a, level of evidence high, A+).

2.4 Timing, Intensity, Dose and Duration of Therapy

2.4.1 Timing

In a pilot RCT ($N = 59$), people with moderate and severe aphasia were recruited from 3 days post-stroke. Those who received daily impairment-based therapy of 45 min per day scored 15.1 more points ($P = 0.010$) on the aphasia quotient and 11.3 more points ($P = 0.004$) on the functional communication profile than those receiving usual care therapy (which averaged 10.5 min a week) (Godecke et al. 2012).

Recommendation: Early intensive therapy should be considered for people with moderate-to-severe aphasia immediately post-stroke if the individual can tolerate it (level of evidence 2b, low quality, B (clinical relevance)).

Traditionally, it has been thought that recovery from language can reach a 'plateau' which has led to intervention not being offered, if a patient is more than 6 months or a year post-stroke in many places. However, there is evidence to suggest people can improve their communication with therapy in the chronic phase. In a review of 21 RCTs, Allen et al. (2012) found evidence to support the use of computer-based treatments, constraint-induced language therapy, group therapies and training of communication partners more than 6 months post-stroke. Further to this, in a computerised word finding therapy RCT ($n = 278$), Palmer et al. (2019) found that improvement in word finding was not affected by time post-stroke (up to 36 years in this study).

Recommendation: Therapy should be provided to people with aphasia who still wish to have therapy in the chronic phase post-stroke to improve their communication (level of evidence 1a, very low-to-medium quality, B+ (clinical relevance)).

2.4.2 Intensity, Dose and Duration

In the Cochrane review for aphasia (Brady et al. 2016), functional communication was significantly better in people with aphasia that received therapy at a high intensity, i.e. 4 to 15 h a week (MD: 11.75 (4.09 to 19.40); 2 trials, 84 participants), or over a long duration, i.e. 3 to 22 months (SMD: 0.81 (0.23 to 1.40); 2 trials, 50 participants), compared to those who received therapy at a lower intensity, i.e. 1.5 to 5 h a week, or over a shorter period of time, i.e. 2 weeks to 9 months. However, more people stopped attending these highly intensive treatments (of up to 15 h a week) than those who had a less-intensive schedule. People were often more able to tolerate intensive therapy later post-stroke.

An example of intensive speech and language therapy in the chronic stage post-stroke (>6 months) from a high-quality RCT showed significant statistical and clinical benefit of intensive speech and language therapy compared to waiting list controls in 19 rehabilitation centres in Germany (Breitenstein et al. 2017). The intensive therapy was delivered in clinical settings for 10 h or more per week for at least 3 weeks (minimum dose 30 h) and combined one-to-one speech and language therapy, group therapy with an SLT and self-managed computer therapy or pencil and paper linguistic exercises prescribed by an SLT.

Recommendation: People with aphasia who want to improve their language and communication abilities should be offered intensive therapy of a long duration in both the acute and chronic stages post-stroke, if they can tolerate it (level of evidence 1a, medium quality, B+ (clinical relevance)).

There is no Cochrane or systematic review level evidence for timing, intensity, dose or duration of therapy for motor speech disorders acquired after stroke, but neuroplasticity and motor learning principles would suggest that 'more is better' for motor speech as well as aphasia.

2.5   Methods of Therapy Delivery

Speech and language therapy is often delivered by a qualified speech and language therapist in a one-to-one, face-to-face therapy session. However, other methods of delivery exist that may make delivery of therapy more efficient:

2.5.1   Group Therapy

Groups of people with communication disorders can be an advantageous way of providing communication therapy, providing exposure to a range of communication partners. The Cochrane review for aphasia (Brady et al. 2016) concluded that there was no difference in functional outcome (SMD: 0.41 (−0.19 to 1.00); 3 trials, 46 participants) or aphasia severity (SMD: 0.15 (−0.21 to 0.50); 4 trials, 122 participants) between therapy provided in a group or one to one.

2.5.2   Use of Volunteers

The Cochrane review for aphasia (Brady et al. 2016) found little indication of a difference in the effectiveness of therapy facilitated by trained volunteers than therapy delivered by an SLT. The volunteers were trained, had access to therapy materials and were delivering interventions designed and overseen by a qualified speech and language therapist. Volunteers could include family members. In addition, Teasell et al. (2016) found limited evidence that suggests CIAT delivered by trained volunteers may be as effective as delivery by experienced speech and language therapists.

2.5.3 Use of Computers/Telepractice

Computers, tablet computers and smartphones can be used to provide therapy materials for communication practice during a therapy session with either a speech and language therapist or a volunteer or can provide an option for independent or self-managed practice between sessions with a therapist to increase the amount of therapy or to increase the duration of therapy where the amount available from a speech and language therapist is limited. Where internet connections are available, it is often possible for the therapist to monitor the progress of the patient remotely and update therapy exercises. In the Cochrane review of aphasia (Brady et al. 2016), there was no difference shown between therapy delivered on a computer and one-to-one therapy from a speech and language therapist in functional communication (SMD: 0.44 (−0.10 to 0.98); 3 trials, 55 participants). In another systematic review of computerised aphasia therapy, Zheng et al. (2016) conclude that therapy delivered using a computer is more effective than no therapy, and potentially as effective as therapy delivered by a speech and language therapist, although they acknowledge the low quality of the evidence due to including only seven small studies. Marshall et al. (2016) also reported a small quasi-randomised study ($n = 20$) showing potential benefits of using a virtual reality environment for aphasia therapy.

Recommendation: Individual, one-to-one or group therapy from a qualified SLT, computer-mediated therapy and volunteer-supported therapy can all be considered for the provision of speech and language therapy (level of evidence 1a, very low to low quality, 0).

The recommendation for use of computerised aphasia therapy is augmented by an RCT ($n = 278$) of daily self-managed word finding practice on a computer at home, tailored by a speech and language therapist and supported by monthly volunteer/speech therapy assistant visits (Palmer et al. 2019). Word finding improvement was 16.2% (95% CI 12.7 to 19.6; $p < 0.0001$) higher in the computer therapy group than in the usual care group and was 14.4% (10.8 to 18.1) higher than in the attention control group. There were no significant differences between groups in conversational ability however.

Recommendation: Use of self-managed computerised therapy for word finding practice should be considered as a method for delivering repetitive practice to improve word finding ability. However, combination with additional techniques to promote functional use of newly learned vocabulary in conversation need to be considered (level of evidence 1b, medium quality, B+).

2.6   Alternative and Augmentative Communication

Communication aids can be low tech, for example alphabet boards to spell out words, picture charts to point to pictures that indicate wishes or E-tran frames that enable a patient to use eye gaze to communicate. Many high-tech aids and apps are also available using advances in technology. Baxter et al. (2012) reviewed the evidence for high-tech communication aids and concluded that although benefit is reported, existing studies use designs that are at a high risk of bias and that the high level of individual variation in outcome requires a greater understanding of patients who may benefit from high-tech communication aid solutions.

Recommendation: Augmentative and alternative modes of communication can be considered (level of evidence 2a, very low quality, 0).

2.7 Communication Environment

2.7.1 Conversation/Communication Partner Training

Several different approaches to communication partner training exist and training has been provided to usual communication partners, volunteers providing opportunities for conversation and healthcare staff. Systematic reviews (including all study designs) by Simmons-Mackie et al. (2016) conclude there is sufficient evidence that communication partner training can improve partner skill in using strategies to facilitate the communication of people with chronic aphasia, although higher quality randomised trials are needed to strengthen this recommendation.

Recommendation: Communication partner training should be considered to facilitate communication (level of evidence 2a, very low to low quality, B+ (clinical relevance)).

2.8 Psychosocial Interventions to Manage Mood Disorders Secondary to Aphasia

It is recognised that people with aphasia and their carers are at high risk of developing depression (Worrall et al. 2016). A systematic review of rehabilitation interventions to prevent and treat depression in aphasia post-stroke from 45 studies (Baker et al. 2017) suggested that for people without depression, interventions such as goal setting and attainment, psychosocial support and communication partner training may be helpful in preventing depression. People with mild depression may benefit from behavioural therapy, psychosocial support and problem-solving. More research is needed in this area however to make strong recommendations.

Recommendation: A range of techniques to support people with mild symptoms of depression can be considered (level of evidence 2a, very low to low quality, 0). People with moderate-to-severe depression require specialist intervention from mental health services in collaboration with stroke specialists.

3 Top Ten Best Practice Recommendations for Aphasia and Forthcoming Information

In this chapter, the authors discuss the evidence base and recommendations for the assessment and treatment of aphasia, dysarthria and apraxia based on a synthesis of Cochrane reviews, other systematic and narrative reviews of randomised and non-randomised studies, and of definitive RCTs conducted since the Cochrane reviews were published.

The Aphasia United Best Practices Working Group and Advisory Committee developed and published ten best practice recommendations for aphasia that are applicable across multiple countries (Simmons-Mackie et al. 2017). This entailed crafting a set of recommendations drawing from research evidence and stroke guidelines and using a Delphi procedure to obtain consensus on wording from healthcare experts from the United States, Canada, Australia, UK, Ireland, China, Germany, Finland, Sweden, Norway, Denmark, Korea, Greece, Turkey, Japan, Argentina, Israel, South Africa, Russia and India. This chapter would not be complete without making reference to these rigorously developed, internationally applicable recommendations that consider assessment and treatment in the broader context of aphasia management:

1. All patients with brain damage or brain disease should be screened for communication deficits.
2. People with suspected communication deficits should be assessed by a qualified professional (determined by country); Assessment should extend beyond the use of screening measures to determine the nature, severity and personal consequences of the suspected communication deficit.
3. People with aphasia should receive information regarding aphasia, aetiologies of aphasia (e.g. Stroke) and options for treatment. This applies throughout all stages of healthcare from acute to chronic stages.
4. No one with aphasia should be discharged from services without some means of communicating his or her needs and wishes (e.g. using AAC, supports, trained partners) or a documented plan of how and when this will be achieved.
5. People with aphasia should be offered intensive and individualised aphasia therapy designed to have a meaningful impact on communication and life. This intervention should be designed and delivered under the supervision of a qualified professional.
6. Communication partner training should be provided to improve communication of people with aphasia.
7. Families or caregivers of people with aphasia should be included in the rehabilitation process.
8. Services for people with aphasia should be culturally appropriate and personally relevant.
9. All health and social care providers working with people with aphasia across the continuum of care (i.e. acute care to end of life) should be educated about aphasia and trained to support communication in aphasia.
10. Information intended for use by people with aphasia should be available in aphasia-friendly/communicatively accessible formats.

Further insights into factors affecting success of treatments for aphasia are forthcoming from the RELEASE collaboration meta-analysis of individual patient data from aphasia trials internationally (Brady et al. 2020).

References

Al Harbi M, Armijo-Olivo S, Kim E (2017) Transcranial direct current stimulation (Tdcs) to improve naming ability in post stroke aphasia: a critical review. Behav Brain Res 322:7–15

Al-Khawaja I, Wade D, Collin C (1996) Bedside screening for aphasia: a comparison of two methods. J Neurol 243:201–204

Allen L, Mehta S, McClure J et al (2012) Therapeutic interventions for aphasia initiated more than six months post stroke: a review of the evidence. Top Stroke Rehabil 19(6):523–535

Baker C, Worrall L, Rose M, Hudson K, Ryan B, O'Byrne L (2017) A systematic review of rehabilitation interventions to prevent and treat depression in post-stroke aphasia. Disabil Rehabil 19:1–23

Ballard K, Wambaugh J, Duffy J et al (2015) Treatment for acquired apraxia of speech: a systematic review of intervention research between 2004 and 2012. Am J Speech Lang Pathol 24(2):316–337

Baxter S, Enderby P, Evans P, Judge S (2012) Barriers and facilitators to the use of high-technology augmentative and alternative communication devices: a systematic review and qualitative synthesis. Int J Lang Commun Disord 47(2):115–129

Brady M, Kelly H, Godwin J et al (2016) Speech and language therapy for aphasia following stroke. Cochrane Database Syst Rev (5):CD000425

Brady M, Ali M, VandenBerg K, Williams LJ et al (2020) RELEASE: a protocol for a systematic review based, individual participant data, meta- and network meta-analysis, of complex speech-language therapy interventions for stroke-related aphasia. Aphasiology 34(2):137–157

Breitenstein C, Grewe T, Flöel A et al (2017) Intensive speech and language therapy in patients with chronic aphasia after stroke: a randomised, open-label, blinded-endpoint, controlled trial in a health-care setting. Lancet 389:1528–1538

Choi Y, Park H, Ahn K et al (2015) A telescreening tool to detect aphasia in patients with stroke. Telemed E Health 21:729–734

Darley F, Aronson A, Brown J (1975) Motor speech disorders. Saunders, Philadeliphia

Doesborgh S, van de Sandt-Koenderman W, Dippel D et al (2003) Linguistic deficits in the acute phase of stroke. J Neurol 250:977–982

Elsner B, Kugler J, Pohl M, Mehrholz J (2015) Transcranial direct current stimulation (tDCS) for improving aphasia in patients with aphasia after stroke. Cochrane Database Syst Rev (5):CD009760

Enderby P, Wood V, Wade D et al (1987) The Frenchay aphasia screening test: a short, simple test for aphasia appropriate for non-specialists. Int Rehabil Med 8:166–170

Faroqi Shah Y, Kling T, Solomon J, Liu S, Park G, Braun A (2013) Lesion analysis of language production deficits in aphasia. Aphasiology 28:258–277

Flamand-Roze C, Falissard B, Roze E et al (2011) Validation of a new language screening tool for patients with acute stroke: the language screening test (LAST). Stroke 42:1224–1229

Flowers H, Silver F, Fang J et al (2013) The incidence, co-occurrence, and predictors of dysphagia, dysarthria, and aphasia after first-ever acute ischemic stroke. J Commun Disord 46:238–248

Godecke E, Hird K, Lalor E et al (2012) Very early poststroke aphasia therapy: a pilot randomized controlled efficacy trial. Int J Stroke 7(8):635–644

Greener J, Enderby P, Whurr R (2001) Pharmacological treatment for aphasia following stroke. Cochrane Database Syst Rev (4):CD000424

Hachioui H, Visch-Brink E, de Lau L et al (2017) Screening tests for aphasia in patients with stroke: a systematic review. J Neurol 246(2):211–220

Kim H, Kim J, Kim D et al (2011) Differentiating between aphasic and non-aphasic stroke patients using semantic verbal fluency measures with administration time of 30 seconds. Eur Neurol 65:113–117

Lefaucheur JP, Andre-Obadia N, Antal A et al (2014) Evidence-based guidelines on the therapeutic use of repetitive transcranial magnetic stimulation (rTMS). Clin Neurophysiol 125:2150–2206

Lekoubou A, Gleichgerrcht E, McGrattan K et al (2015) Aphasia in multilingual individuals: the importance of bedside premorbid language proficiency assessment. eNeurol Sci 1(1): 1–2

Li Y, Qu Y, Yuan M et al (2015) Low frequency repetitive transcranial magnetic stimulation for patients with aphasia after stroke: a meta-analysis. J Rehabil Med 47(8):678–681

Marshall J, Booth T, Devane N et al (2016) Evaluating the benefits of aphasia of aphasia intervention delivered in virtual reality: results of a quasi-randomised controlled study. PLoS One 11(8):e0160381

Mitchell C, Bowen A, Tyson S et al (2017) Interventions for dysarthria due to stroke and other adult-acquired, non-progressive brain injury. Cochrane Database Syst Rev (1):CD002088

Nakase-Thompson R, Manning E, Sherer M et al (2005) Brief assessment of severe language impairments: initial validation of the Mississippi aphasia screening test. Brain Inj 19:685–691

Owens DK, Lohr KN, Atkins D, Treadwell JR, Reston JT, Bass EB, Chang S, Helfand M (2010) AHRQ series paper 5: grading the strength of a body of evidence when comparing medical interventions--agency for healthcare research and quality and the effective health-care program. J Clin Epidemiol 63:513–523

Palmer R, Enderby P (2007) Methods of speech therapy treatment for stable dysarthria: a review. Adv Speech Lang Pathol 9(2):140–153

Palmer R, Dimairo M, Cooper C, Enderby P, Brady M, Bowen A et al (2019) Self-managed, computerised speech and language therapy for patients with chronic aphasia post-stroke compared with usual care or attention control (big CACTUS): a multicentre, single-blinded, randomised controlled trial. Lancet Neurol 18(9):821–833

Platz T (2017) Practice guidelines in neurorehabilitation. Neurol Int Open 1:E148–E152

Pulvermuller F, Neininger B, Elbert T et al (2001) Constraint induced therapy of chronic aphasia after stroke. Stroke 32:1621

Schünemann H, Brożek J, Guyatt G, Oxman A (2013) GRADE handbook for grading quality of evidence and strength of recommendations. The GRADE Working Group. Updated October 2013. www.guidelinedevelopment.org/handbook

Shak-Basak P, Wurzman R, Purcell J et al (2016) Fields or flows? A comparative meta-analysis of transcranial magnetic and direct current stimulation to treat post stroke aphasia. Restor Neurol Neurosci 34(4):537–558

Simmons-Mackie N, Raymer A, Cherney L (2016) Communication partner training in aphasia: an updated systematic review. Arch Phys Med Rehabil 97(12):2202–2221

Simmons-Mackie N, Worrall L, Murray L et al (2017) The top ten: best practice recommendations for aphasia. Aphasiology 31(2):131–151

Teasell R, Foley N, Salter K et al (2016) The stroke rehabilitation evidence-based review, 17th edn. Canadian Stroke Network, Ottawa

Thommessen B, Thoresen G, Bautz-Holter E et al (1999) Screening by nurses for aphasia in stroke—the Ullevaal aphasia screening (UAS) test. Disabil Rehabil 21:110–115

van Dijk MJ, de Man-van Ginkel JM, Hafsteinsdóttir TB, Schuurmans MJ (2016) Identifying depression post-stroke in patients with aphasia: a systematic review of the reliability, validity and feasibility of available instruments. Clin Rehabil 30(8):795–810. https://doi.org/10.1177/0269215515599665

Varley R, Cowell P, Dyson L et al (2016) Self-administered computer therapy for apraxia of speech: two –period randomized control trial with crossover. Stroke 47(3):822–828

West C, Hesketh A, Vail A et al (2005) Interventions for apraxia of speech following stroke. Cochrane Database Syst Rev (4):CD004298

WHO (2001) International Classification of Functioning, Disability, and Health: ICF. World Health Organization, Geneva

Worrall L, Hoffmann T, Power E, Togher L, Rose M (2016) Reducing the psychosocial impact of aphasia on mood and quality of life in people with aphasia and the impact of caregiving in family members through the aphasia. Trials 17:153

Zhang J, Wei CZ et al (2016) Piracetam for aphasia in post stroke patients: a systematic review and meta-analysis of randomised controlled trials. CNS Drugs 30(70):575–587

Zhang J, Yu J, Bao Y et al (2017) Constraint-induced aphasia therapy in post-stroke aphasia rehabilitation: a systematic review and meta-analysis of randomized controlled trials. PLoS One 12(8):e0183349

Zheng C, Lynch L, Taylor N (2016) Effect of computer therapy in aphasia: a systematic review. Aphasiology 30(2–3):211–244

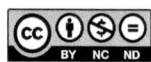

Treating Neurovisual Deficits and Spatial Neglect

Georg Kerkhoff, Gilles Rode, and Stephanie Clarke

1 Neurovisual Disorders After Brain Damage

Neurovisual disorders are frequent function losses after brain damage and occur in about 20–50% of the patients with cerebrovascular disorders (Rowe et al. 2009). In stroke patients >65 years, the incidence rises to 40–60% (Suchoff et al. 2008). Homonymous visual field defects (further abbreviated as VFDs) are present in 20–50% of all neurological patients with stroke (Kerkhoff 1999; Rowe et al. 2009) and also occur frequently in patients with traumatic brain injury, TBI (Kerkhoff 1999). Visual field sparing is <5° on the blind side in 70% of stroke cases with VFDs (Zihl 2011; Kerkhoff 1999). Spontaneous field recovery is present in the first 2–3 months post-lesion in up to 40% of the patients with a stable aetiology such as stroke (Zhang et al. 2006). After 6 months post-lesion, spontaneous recovery is extremely unlikely (Zhang et al. 2006; Zihl 2011).

Patients with VFDs present three types of associated deficits: visual exploration (or scanning) deficits, hemianopic alexia, and visuospatial deficits. With respect to the first point, patients show a time-consuming, inefficient visual search due to loss of overview and unsystematic search strategies. They make many, small amplitude staircase saccades in the blind hemifield and omit targets in the blind field (Kerkhoff

G. Kerkhoff (✉)
Clinical Neuropsychology & Neuropsychological Outpatient Unit, Saarland University, Saarbruecken, Germany
e-mail: kerkhoff@mx.uni-saarland.de

G. Rode
Department of Rehabilitation, Centre Hospitalier Universitaire de Lyon, Lyon, France
e-mail: gilles.rode@chu-lyon.fr

S. Clarke
Service de neuropsychologie et de neuroréhabilitation, Centre Hospitalier Universitaire Vaudois (CHUV), Lausanne, Switzerland
e-mail: Stephanie.Clarke@chuv.ch

© The Author(s) 2021
T. Platz (ed.), *Clinical Pathways in Stroke Rehabilitation*,
https://doi.org/10.1007/978-3-030-58505-1_11

et al. 1992a, 1994; Pambakian et al. 2004; Machner et al. 2009). Second, the central visual field (±5° around the fovea) is crucial for reading because only here visual acuity and form recognition are sufficient for letter recognition ("perceptual reading window"). Hence, slow reading with errors is evident in VFD patients with a field sparing <5° on the blind side of the field, as there is a monotonic relationship between the degrees of visual field sparing on the blind side and reading speed (Kerkhoff 1999). Third, the patient's feeling of the subjective visual straight ahead in space or his/her subjective midline in bisecting horizontal lines and objects is shifted *towards* the blind field. This shift is horizontally in left/right VFDs, vertically in altitudinal upper/lower VFDs, and oblique in quadrantic VFDs and occurs in 90% of the patients (Kerkhoff 1993; Barton and Black 1998; Kuhn; for review see Kerkhoff and Schenk 2011). This spatial shift is also evident in pointing (Hesse et al. 2012) and in daily life (walking through doorways, halving a bread).

Importantly, all three types of visual deficits in VFDs are relevant for daily life: the visual exploration disorder leads to problems in finding objects, persons, or vehicles or colliding with them, especially on the blind side. The reading deficit impairs virtually all activities where reading of letters, numbers, or other symbols is required, and the spatial midline shift affects pointing, walking, halving objects, or drawing. The International Classification of Functioning (ICF) serves as a reference for holistically understanding the different aspects of a pathology (WHO 2001). Figure 1 gives an overview of different neurovisual disorders in the framework of the ICF.

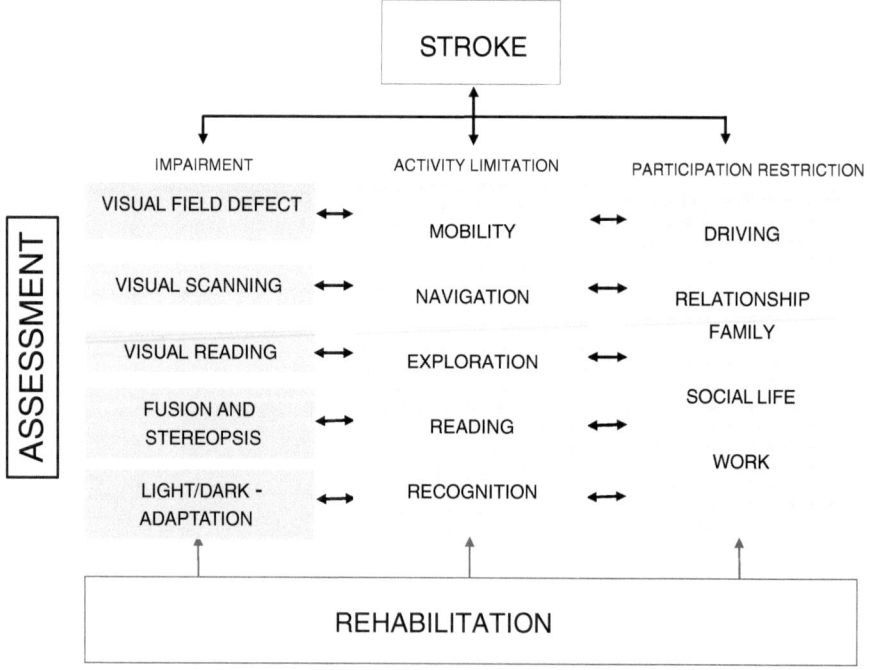

Fig. 1 Neurovisual deficits in the ICF-Framework

Apart from homonymous VFDs and the associated impairments in reading, visual exploration, and spatial midline perception, further low-level (impaired visual acuity and contrast sensitivity, stereopsis and binocular fusion, colour perception, light–dark adaptation, motion perception) as well as high-level (visual object and face agnosia, spatial-perceptual disorders) neurovisual disorders are often found after brain damage (for review see Schaadt and Kerkhoff 2016). Consequently, routine screening of the various types of visual deficits is necessary both for diagnosis and rehabilitation planning.

1.1   Assessment of Neurovisual Disorders

Before starting any assessments, a systematic anamnesis of the most frequently encountered neurovisual deficits should be performed (Table 1) as it reduces the clinician's risk to overlook relevant disorders. Patients with intact awareness can

Table 1 Schema for the anamnesis of neurovisual disorders after acquired brain lesions

Question	Purpose of question, underlying disorder, tests
1. … any changes in vision …?	– Awareness of deficits? Case history?
2. … diplopia …? transiently/permanently?	– Type of gaze palsy? If transient: fusional disorder? Impaired stereopsis?
3. … reading problems …? … syllables/ words missing, change of line, reduced reading span …?	– Hemianopic alexia due to VFD? Differential diagnosis of neglect dyslexia, aphasic alexia, pure alexia, or Balint-Holmes syndrome
4. … problems in estimating depth on a staircase …? … reaching with your unimpaired hand for a cup, hand, door handle …?	– Depth perception? Optic ataxia? Reduced acuity/contrast sensitivity?
5. … bumping into obstacles …? … failure to notice persons …? at which side?	– Visual exploration deficits due to VFD/ Neglect/Balint-Holmes syndrome?
6. … blinding after exposure to bright light …?	– Foveal photopic adaptation?
7. … dark vision …? … that you need more light for reading …?	– Foveal scotopic adaptation?
8. … blurred vision …? transiently/ permanently?	– Contrast sensitivity? Visual Acuity? Fusion?
9. … that colours look darker, paler, less saturated …?	– Colour hue discrimination? Impaired contrast sensitivity?
10. … that faces look darker, paler, unfamiliar …?	– Face discrimination/recognition disorders?
11. … problems in recognizing objects …?	– Object discrimination/recognition disorders?
12. … problems in finding your way in familiar/unfamiliar environments …?	– Topographic orientation deficits? Spatial memory?
13. … visual hallucinations (stars, dots, lines, fog, faces, objects …) or illusions (distorted objects, faces …) …?	– Simple or complex visual hallucinations, illusions? Awareness about illusory character?

Indent the questions in the table into the following phrase: "Did you experience … since your brain lesion?" (Based on Neumann et al. 2016). On the right side, the purpose of each question is illustrated and the putative underlying disorder and tests to be performed. VFD: homonymous visual field defect easily and quickly (<10 min) be questioned with this simple questionnaire, responses to which prove clinically useful and reliable in 95% of cases (Neumann et al. 2016). Moreover, this anamnesis leads the clinician to appropriate diagnostic tests and subsequent treatments.

Subsequently, quantitative tests should be performed. As VFDs are the most frequent neurovisual deficits after brain damage, a quantitative perimetry (using a bowl perimeter) or at least campimetry (on a flat monitor or test plate) should be performed in every case (for details see Biousse and Newman 2009). If time is too short for an apparative perimetry/campimetry, finger perimetry should be performed, by using a coloured pen as a target for identification along the different meridians. This quick (3 min) procedure increases the sensitivity of detecting scotomas by some 20% when compared with using only the examiners fingers (Kerr et al. 2010). After the visual field test, reading should be tested with a standardized reading test (i.e. Radner test), visual scanning, or search with a standardized test, and finally, horizontal and vertical line bisection should be performed to detect a subjective visual midline shift (see Lezak, Howieson, Bigler and Tranel 2004 for appropriate tests). Further, neurovisual tests may be necessary depending on the type of deficit and the patient's subjective complaints. These may include tests of visual object and face recognition, as well as naming tests, in order to disentangle visual object recognition from deficits in object naming (see Schaadt and Kerkhoff 2016, for overview). For these purposes, the VOSP (Visual Object and Space Perception Battery) is suitable to test visual object recognition, the Facial Recognition Test for face perception, and several naming tests including the Boston Naming Test to evaluate naming performance (see Lezak, Howieson, Bigler and Tranel 2004 for further details to these tests and references).

1.2   Therapy of Neurovisual Disorders

The recommendations for treatments given below are based on results from individual trials as stated below, a Cochrane review (Pollock et al. 2012), and two further reviews of that topic (Trauzettel-Klosinski 2011; De Haan et al. 2014).

As spontaneous visual field recovery is very limited during or absent after the first 3–6 months post-stroke (Zhang et al. 2006), the vast majority of VFD patients will suffer from a permanent and stable VFD.

The Cochrane meta-analysis demonstrated that scanning training is more effective than control or placebo at improving reading ability (3 studies, 129 participants; standardized mean difference (SMD) 0.79, 95% confidence interval (CI) 0.29–1.29) and visual scanning (3 studies, 129 participants; SMD 1.14, 95% CI 0.29–2.00) but that scanning may not improve visual field outcomes (2 studies, 110 participants; MD −0.73, 95% CI −3.18 to 1.72). The review reached the following conclusions: "There is limited evidence that supports the use of compensatory scanning training for patients with visual field defects (and possibly coexisting visual neglect) to improve visual field, scanning, and reading outcomes. There is insufficient evidence to reach a conclusion about the impact of compensatory scanning training on functional activities of daily living. There is insufficient evidence to reach general-ized conclusions about the benefits of restitutive or substitutive interventions for patients with visual field defects after stroke". For clarity, we will deal with these treatments in separate sections below in more detail.

1.2.1   Saccadic Compensation (or Scanning) Training

Saccadic compensation training (SCT or scanning) aims at improving the quick and safe visual overview over a visual scene, despite the fact that the field cut will persist in the vast majority of patients with VFDs. This is reached by enlarging saccade amplitude and reducing saccadic reaction time when looking to the blind portion of the visual field (Kerkhoff et al. 1992a, b, 1994). Several observational and smaller randomized controlled trials (RCTs) (Kerkhoff et al. 1992a, b, 1994; Roth et al. 2009; Lane et al. 2010; Mödden et al. 2012; De Haan et al. 2015; Aimola et al. 2014) indicated that these procedures improve visual scanning in VFDs; the effects might, however, at least partially be related to attention training effects (e.g. Lane et al. 2010), which in itself might also be an effective treatment strategy. Moreover, it can be assumed that visual scanning training almost always includes attentive elements, otherwise the training cannot be performed. Moreover, improvements in ADLs were inconsistently shown, e.g. on mobility (De Haan et al. 2015). A cross-modal (visual-auditory) variant of this training is also effec-tive in improving scanning and reading in hemianopia (Keller and Lefin-Rank 2010). Here, visual and auditory targets are presented time-locked in identical locations of the visual field, and the patient has to look to them. This training induces similar improvements as conventional visual scanning training but requires additional technical facilities.

1.2.2   Hemianopic Reading Training

Hemianopic reading training entails the oculomotor compensation of the reading deficit that arises from the loss of parafoveal visual field regions that have a suffi-ciently good visual acuity in order to identify letters and syllables. Most effective strategies of reading training for hemianopic alexia have used an "optokinetic" approach. Here, letters, syllables, words, and numbers are presented in a single text line which float from the right to the left side on a computer screen, while the patient is instructed to read the words in the middle of the screen. The moving character of the words induces pursuit eye movements to the side of motion and an optokinetic nystagmus to the opposite side (Kerkhoff et al. 1992a, b). At least four more or less well-controlled treatment studies have shown that this kind of treatment signifi-cantly improves reading speed, reduces reading errors, and reduces the number of eye fixations during reading (Kerkhoff et al. 1992a, b; Zihl 1995; Spitzyna et al. 2007; Schuett et al. 2008; see review in Schuett 2009). The mean improvement of reading speed when expressed in words per minutes (WPM) read was 38.4 WPM after this type of reading training (see Kerkhoff 2010, page 85). In cultures reading from left to right the motion should be from right to left, in those reading from right to left the motion should be left to right, and in those reading from top to bottom the motion should move upwards.

1.2.3   Compensatory or Restorative Visual Field Training?

In recent years, restorative visual field training has been revived after publication of apparently advantageous results following new training procedures (Kasten et al. 1998). However, numerous subsequent replication studies have failed to find significant visual field enlargements (Nelles et al. 2001; Pambakian et al. 2004; Schreiber et al. 2006; Roth et al. 2009), or found only minimal visual field increases (1°, cf. Mödden et al. 2012). In our view, restorative field training is only promising when lesions are incomplete, and a high degree of residual visual capacities (light, motion, form, or colour perception) is preserved in specific regions of the scotoma (Kerkhoff 2000; Bouwmeester et al. 2007). This residual vision is only present in some 5% of VFD patients and is lacking in the majority of patients. Moreover, restorative visual field training induces only very small or no visual field increases (~1°) and improves visual search or reading only minimally, or not at all (Mödden et al. 2012). Formally assessed, the overall evidence is unclear and thus restorative visual field training cannot generally be recommended for that purpose.

Further, when compared with hemianopic reading training (see above), the effect of restorative visual field training on reading speed is 7 WPM after therapy, compared to 38.4 WPM improvement after reading training (see above, Kerkhoff 2010). Hence, direct reading training is 5 times more effective and less time-consuming than restorative visual field training when we consider reading speed, which is the main handicap of reading in VFDs.

Moreover, compensatory field training (SCT and reading training) leads to a much quicker reduction of visual impairments and needs fewer treatment sessions. Recently, home-based treatments of visual search and reading have been successfully tested in VFDs (Pambakian et al. 2004; Lane et al. 2010; Aimola et al. 2014). These approaches are cost-effective, but require regular advice by the therapist (i.e. by telephone or visit).

In conclusion, SCT and hemianopic reading training improve visual scanning and "visual" activities of daily living in VFD, and they increase functional independence of the patient reliably (Kerkhoff 1999, 2000; Bouwmeester et al. 2007; Spitzyna et al. 2007; Zihl 2011). Therefore, these two types of treatments are based on a consistent body of study evidence of low-to-moderate quality (observational studies and smaller RCTs with one meta-analysis) showing their effectiveness on visual scanning and transfer of treatment gains to some functional domains of ADL such as reading and mobility as reviewed above. Two recent RCTs underlined these findings: Ivanov et al. (2019) treated children with homonymous VFDs and revealed significant improvements after scanning training in visual search behaviour, reported quality of life and ADLs that remained stable for at least 6 weeks after training at follow-up. Rowe et al. (2016) showed that visual search training was more effective than prism glasses and standard care (no training) in improving vision-related quality of life in patients with VFDs. As a consequence, they should be used for treatment of VFD patients (CEBM classification: level 2b to 1a, Grade quality: low to moderate, recommendation: B+) (see Fig. 2).

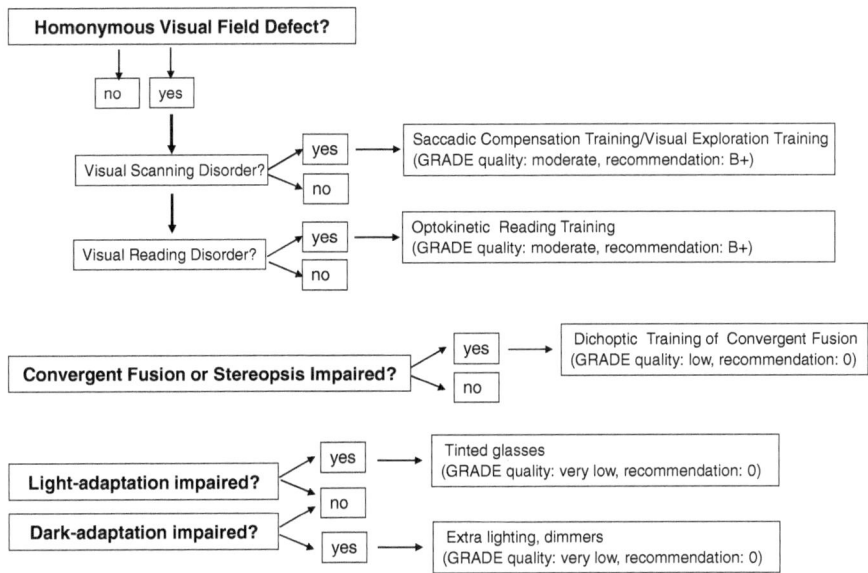

Fig. 2 Clinical pathways for neurovisual rehabilitation

1.2.4 Ineffective or Disadvantageous Therapies in VFDs

Most hemianopic patients get confused when using prisms to substitute the visual field loss. However, small prisms fitted to a spectacle can be useful in some cases. Compensatory head shifts towards the scotoma (either spontaneously adopted by the patient or to instruction) are of no use in the rehabilitation of VFDs because they lead to visual exploration deficits in the ipsilesional visual field, strain of the neck muscles, and delay treatment progress in visual scanning training (Kerkhoff et al. 1992a). Training of "blindsight" (the ability of rare cases of cortical blindness who respond to stimuli in their visual field, e.g. by pointing to them, even if they are not able to consciously perceive them) is probably not useful for the majority of the patients because it does not lead to improved functioning in daily life.

1.2.5 Convergence/Fusion and Stereoscopic Deficits

Apart from VFDs, other neurovisual deficits occur. Impairments in convergent horizontal fusion represent the most frequent oculomotor deficit after brain damage (Kapoor and Ciuffreda 2002). Importantly, they are often associated with visual perceptual deficits such as loss of stereopsis, reduced reading duration, blurred vision, and asthenopic eye symptoms. This is especially relevant for all visual activities in near-space (reading, writing, smartphone and computer use, typing, knitting, and all visuo-motor activities in near-space). Moreover, it has been shown that right-hemispheric vascular lesions cause deficits in stereopsis (Rizzo 1989; Rizzo and Barton 2008). Three recent treatment studies (two controlled group studies, one controlled case series, but none of them randomized controlled) showed that a repetitive binocular fusion treatment using three sorts of dichoptic devices reinstated binocular depth perception, stereopsis, and improved reading duration and reduced asthenopic symptoms in chronic brain damage of cerebrovascular, traumatic, or hypoxic aetiology (Schaadt et al. 2013, 2014). As the available observational studies consistently showed a significant treatment effect in about 90% of treated patients these treatments can be used (CEBM classification: level 2b, Grade quality: low, recommendation: 0) (see Fig. 2).

1.2.6 Visual Light Adaptation Deficits

Some 20–30% of patients with acquired brain damage suffer from feelings of "blinding" and "dark vision" after brain damage (Zihl and Kerkhoff 1990; Jackowski et al. 1996; Kapoor and Ciuffreda 2002; Neumann et al. 2016). The reason for this is an acquired deficit of light and/or dark adaptation of the visual system (not the eye!). Tinted glasses may reduce the feelings of blinding (Jackowski et al. 1996; Kapoor and Ciuffreda 2002), while additional light sources and the use of light dimmers are helpful to cope with dark vision. These treatments do not "heal" the original underlying disorder or light–dark adaptation, but they alleviate the behavioural consequences for the patients and can be used (CEBM classification: level 4, Grade quality: very low, recommendation: 0).

Figure 2 summarizes the clinical procedures described herein as a clinical pathway diagram.

1.2.7 Conclusions

We have reviewed here the available treatments for the most frequent neurovisual disorders after stroke. However, as pointed out in a recent systematic review on 221 publications about homonymous VFDs, most of the available research has so far focused on body functions, less on activities, and almost never on participation (De Haan et al. 2014). One exception to this may be the treatment of reading because it is an integral part of daily life. So, improvement of reading by reading therapy in hemianopic alexia can be viewed as regaining an important daily activity that enables participation in reading books, newspapers, handwritten notices, short notices on a smartphone, or managing internet banking at home, hence participation.

Moreover, very few studies have analyzed how many patients returned to work after neurovisual rehabilitation. This is an important part of participation and this aspect should be included more often in future treatment studies.

2   Spatial Neglect, Extinction, and Anosognosia

Spatial neglect is defined as the inability to respond to sensory stimuli in the contralesional hemispace or body of a neurological patient (Kerkhoff 2001; Husain 2008). In addition to visual, auditory, or tactile neglect, motor neglect often co-occurs as a reduced use of contralesional extremities, i.e. during reaching, standing, or walking. Moreover, neglect patients show a lack of insight into their left-sided sensory and motor deficits termed anosognosia or unawareness. Anosognosia in patients with neglect delays recovery (Gialanella et al. 2005) and both are a major source of long-term disability and associated with an adverse rehabilitation outcome (Jehkonen et al. 2006a, b) and longer hospital stays (Kalra et al. 1997). Return to work seems almost impossible in chronic neglect, even after treatment.

Spontaneous recovery from neglect occurs mostly in the first 3 months after stroke (Nijboer et al. 2013). Some 30–40% of those patients presenting initially with neglect show chronic neglect at 1 year post-lesion (Karnath et al. 2011; Rengachary et al. 2011). The presence of an additional visual field defect reflects larger lesions and predicts chronic neglect as well as severe neglect dyslexia (Ptak et al. 2012). Spatial neglect is most often multimodal (visual, auditory, haptic, olfactory, Kerkhoff 2001). Behavioural recovery is task- and side-specific: while the conspicuous conjugate gaze deviation may be up to 30–40° ipsilesionally in the first weeks, this recovers continuously within 3 months, paralleled by a more symmetrical, wider visual exploration field of the patient (Aimola et al. 2014). Similarly, visual scanning and cancellation tests improve first on the ipsilesional side, later on the contralesional side (Nijboer et al. 2013). Directional hypokinesia (which designates the phenomenon that neglect patients do not reach far enough to their contralesional side with their intact, nonparetic limb/s) shows better spontaneous recovery than visuospatial inattention (Rengachary et al. 2011).

Moreover, left hemineglect is frequently associated with left hemianopia, which is often difficult to disentangle (pseudo-hemianopia). Left hemianopia worsens the severity of visual neglect. Furthermore, hemiparesis/-plegia and hemi-anaesthesia or hypaesthesia are also often present in patients with left neglect. All these associated deficiencies worsen neglect and reduce the functional effects of rehabilitation.

2.1   Assessment of Neglect and Associated Disorders

Assessments should include a visual scanning or exploration task (i.e. crossing out numbers or lines or bells), a standardized text reading task, horizontal and vertical line bisection to detect shifts in the subjective visual midline, and an assessment of anosognosia. The Behavioural Inattention Test (BIT) is a useful test battery to screen for visual neglect in basic and functional tasks (Wilson et al. 1987). Another useful assessment tool for the acute and early post-acute phase is the Catherine Bergego Scale (CBS; Azouvi et al. 2002, 2003, 2006) which assesses visual and body neglect in daily life on a rating scale basis and also anosognosia. Ideally, assessments should *also* include additional tests of visual, tactile, and auditory extinction—especially in the post-acute phase or when only residual neglect is present. This is important as extinction is often chronic and specific extinction tests are most sensitive to detect such residual neglect symptoms and extinction (for assessment see Lezak et al. 2004).

While most neglect tests assess *egocentric* neglect phenomena, *stimulus-centred or word-centred* neglect phenomena may also occur, particularly during reading and visual scanning (Caramazza and Hillis 1990; Hillis et al. 1998) and should be assessed as well. Word-centred neglect phenomena can be detected with a reading test (as in hemianopia, see above) or having the patient read compound words. The apples test is useful to disentangle object-centred and egocentred neglect deficits during a visual search task, where different types of apples have to be cancelled out (Bickerton et al. 2011).

2.2   Rehabilitation of Neglect in the ICF Framework

2.2.1   Effects of Neglect Therapy on Disability to Prove

The latest Cochrane review by Bowen et al. (2013) including 23 randomized clinical trials (628 participants) showed that most studies evaluate the effect of rehabilitation on standardized assessment tests; 15 studies assessed the impact on activities of daily living immediately after rehabilitation and only 6 studies measured these effects at a longer follow-up test after the end of therapy. The currently available results show a significant effect in favour of cognitive rehabilitation, but only on the standardized assessment tests of hemineglect. The effectiveness on the activities of daily life is therefore not rigorously demonstrated.

A limitation in the interpretation of studies is related to the measure of functional impact of cognitive neglect rehabilitation. Indeed, hemineglect is a rarely isolated deficiency, most often associated with multiple sensorimotor and cognitive deficits consecutive to the extent of the brain injury (cf. Kerkhoff 2001). The vast majority of the patients selected in the Cochrane review (last from 2013) had hemineglect due to a stroke of the middle cerebral artery, which was also responsible for left-sided sensory-motor hemiplegia, left-sided hemianopia, and other cognitive deficits such as constructional apraxia, non-lateralized attention deficits, or others. The functional consequences therefore result from all these deficits and not only from hemineglect. Although an improvement of hemineglect is observed after cognitive rehabilitation, it remains in most cases insufficient to decisively reduce the overall measured disability (see Fig. 3).

In addition, the measurement of therapeutic effects on disability is generally carried out by generic assessment scales such as the Barthel Index, the Functional Independence Measure (FIM), or the Activity of Daily Living Scale. A more targeted measurement of the functional consequences of hemineglect can be made by specific scales such as the Catherine Bergego Scale (CBS), provided however that the measured gain is significant in view of the associated deficits and their consequences on the autonomy (Azouvi et al. 2006).

2.2.2   Cognitive Rehabilitation of Hemineglect Based
on the International Classification of Functioning (ICF)

The International Classification of Functioning (ICF) not only is a reference for holistically understanding the different aspects of a pathology (WHO 2001) but also is a model adapted to the development of neurological rehabilitation strategies (Lexell and Brogårdh 2015). Indeed, the four dimensions described by the classification can be considered as targets for neurorehabilitation (Alford et al. 2015) and cognitive rehabilitation of hemineglect. The first dimension, called "body structure/

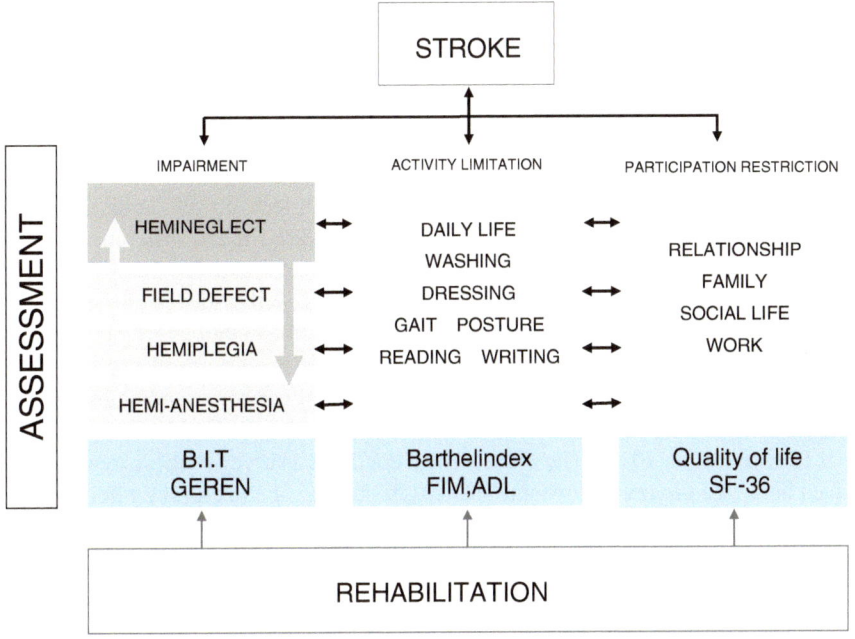

Fig. 3 Spatial neglect and associated deficiencies in the ICF-Framework

lesion", corresponds to brain anatomical structures that are likely to be activated by re-education via brain plasticity mechanisms. The second dimension, "body function/impairment", refers to the recovery of hemineglect (or clinical subtypes) by selective cognitive rehabilitation techniques (bottom-up and top-down strategies, explicit or implicit learning). The third dimension, "activity/limitation", refers to the reduction of disability and the possible functional generalization of therapeutic effects as well as the improvement of activity through compensation methods. Finally, the fourth dimension, "participation/restriction", refers to the reduction of participation restrictions, notably through improved body function, compensation methods, social interventions, and a better recognition of the deficit and its personal and social consequences (see Table 2).

The ICF model can therefore provide a methodological basis for the development of hemineglect cognitive rehabilitation (Rode et al. 2017). For the specialist in neurorehabilitation and the neuropsychologist, an important question will be to determine what is the best judgment criterion for showing the impact of the interventions. This choice should also take into account the recommendations of Evidence-Based Medicine applied to non-drug therapies (Bowen et al. 2013; Yang et al. 2013).

Therapy of Neglect

A Cochrane analysis (Bowen et al. 2013) analyzed randomized controlled treatment studies until mid of 2011 and reached the following conclusions: "Eighteen of the

23 included RCTs compared cognitive rehabilitation with any control intervention (Placebo, attention or no treatment). Meta-analyses demonstrated no statistically significant effect of cognitive rehabilitation, compared with control, for persisting effects on either ADL (5 studies, 143 participants) or standardised neglect f(8 studies, 172 participants), or for immediate effects on ADL (10 studies, 343 participants). In contrast, we found a statistically significant effect in favour of cognitive rehabilitation compared with control, for immediate effects on standardised neglect assessments (16 studies, 437 participants), standardised mean difference (SMD) 0.35, 95 % confidence interval (CI) 0.09–0.62. However sensitivity analyses including only studies with high methodological quality removed evidence of a significant effect of cognitive rehabilitation". As a consequence, the authors gave no clear recommendations for therapy. In the meanwhile, several well-controlled randomized treatment studies have been published that allow some recommendations. Several reviews have described the available treatments in detail (Kerkhoff and Schenk 2012; Bowen et al. 2013). Therefore, only a condensed survey of these treatments is given here (see the text below and Table 3), focussing on the currently documented therapeutic effects on *visual* neglect (which is the most often targeted domain in treatment studies), and also on *nonvisual* (tactile, auditory) neglect, sensory extinction, anosognosia, activities of daily living (ADLs), and motor/postural functions, if such effects have been published (for review see Kerkhoff and Schenk 2012). The references, therapeutic approaches, documented effects, the level of evidence

Table 2 The International Classification of Functioning (ICF), a model adapted to strategies of cognitive rehabilitation of hemineglect

Normal	Pathology	Intervention
Body structure	Lesion	Plasticity (structural, functional)—vicariousness Stimulation of undamaged nervous system structures by neuromodulation (rTMS, tDCS)
Body function	Impairment	Recovery, restoration *Top-down approaches* 　Visual scanning training (VST) 　Attentional Cueing 　Mental practice or imagery *Bottom-up approaches* 　Sensory stimulation (optokinetic, vestibular, proprioceptive, neck vibration) 　Prism adaptation 　Half-field eye patching 　Spatio-motor cueing 　Arm-activation intervention 　Mirror therapy
Activity	Activity limitation	Functional generalization Compensation by equipment (technical help, connects object) Compensation by caregivers or environment
Participation	Participation restriction	Compensation by family, people, society (legal, economic, politic dimensions); Recognition, inclusion

Table 3 Recommendations for different treatments in individual suffering from spatial neglect, extinction, and/or anosognosia

Treatment technique (reference study authors)	Description and putative mechanism	Therapeutic effects in studies						CEBM level of evidence	Quality of evidence (GRADE)	Recommendation
		Visual	Nonvis	Extinct	Anoso	ADL	Motor			
Visual scanning training (VST) (Pizzamiglio et al. 1992; Paolucci et al. 1996; Van Wyk et al. 2014)	Systematization of visual search strategies by cognitive instructions reduces omissions	+	−	−	−	+	−	4 to 2b	Low	0
Optokinetic/smooth pursuit therapy (SPT) (Schröder et al. 2008; Kerkhoff et al. 2013, 2014)	Active, contralesionally smooth pursuit eye movements reduce multimodal neglect by reactivation of ipsi- and contralesional parietal cortices	+	+	?	+	+	?	2b, 1b	Moderate	B
Neck muscle vibration (NMV) (Schindler et al. 2002)	Repetitive NMV realigns subjective straight ahead direction, probably by activation of right perisylvian and insular cortices.	+	+	?	+	+	?	2b	Low	0
Prism adaptation (Rode et al. 2015; Gossmann et al. 2013)	Re-directing gaze towards the neglected hemispace by temporary exposure to prisms inducing a rightward gaze shift. Activates a cerebellar–cortical network.	+	(+)	+	?	(+)	?	2b, 4	Low	0

(continued)

Table 3 (continued)

Treatment technique (reference study authors)	Description and putative mechanism	Therapeutic effects in studies						CEBM level of evidence	Quality of evidence (GRADE)	Recommendation
		Visual	Nonvis	Extinct	Anoso	ADL	Motor			
Visuomotor feedback (Harvey et al. 2003; Rossit et al. 2017)	Patients should lift horizontally extended wooden rods. If lifted too far to the right, the unbalanced rod gives direct feedback to the patient	+	?	?	+	+	+	2b	Low	0
Mirror therapy (Thieme et al. 2013)	Action observation of healthy limb in a mirror promotes recovery of contralesional motor deficits and visuospatial neglect	+	?	?	?	+	+	2b	Low	0
Attention training (Robertson et al. 1995)	Treatment of non-lateralized attention (sustained attention, alertness) reduces neglect and motor deficits	+	?	?	?	+	+	4	Very low, uncertain	
Hemi-field Fresnel prisms (Rossi et al. 1990)	Hemi-field Fresnel press-on prisms shift gaze and attention to the neglected hemispace	+	?	?	?	?	?	2b	Very low (mixed diagnostic group)	
Repetitive transcranial magnetic stimulation (rTMS) (Cazzoli et al. 2012; Koch et al. 2012)	rTMS of left parietal cortex reduces left-sided neglect by reduction of interhemispheric imbalance	+	?	?	+	+	?	2b	Low	0

Treatment	Description						Evidence	Quality	
Transcranial direct current stimulation (tDCS) (Smit et al. 2015; Turgut et al. 2018).	Re-balancing interhemispheric imbalance by tDCS of parietal cortex (right-anodal or left-cathodal)	+	?	?	?	?	4, 1b	Very low, uncertain	
Transcutaneous Electrical Nerve Stimulation (TENS) (Schröder et al. 2008; Pizzamiglio et al. 1996)	Electric stimulation of contralesional neck activates right cerebral hemisphere	+	?	?	(+)	?	1b, 4	Low	0
Arm or hand activation (Kalra et al. 1997), with electric stimulation (Polanowska et al. 2009)	Left-sided motor action shifts attention to the neglected side; concurrent electrical arm stimulation facilitates this	+	?	?	+	+	1b	Low	0
Galvanic vestibular stimulation (GVS) (Wilkinson et al. 2014; Schmidt et al. 2013a, b)	Improves visual neglect, tactile extinction, and arm position sense. Activation of vestibular thalamocortical system and multimodal brain regions	+	+	+	?	?	1b, 2b	Low	0
Drugs (Luvizutto et al. 2015)	Modulation of attention by different drugs	+	?	?	?	?	1a	Very low, uncertain	

Legend: +: yes/effects proven, −: no effects, (+): partial effects, ?: not evaluated/currently not known: Extinct: Extinction, Anoso: Anosogosia, Nonvisual: auditory/haptic or representational neglect; ADL: activities of daily living. Oxford Levels of Evidence: 1a: Systematic review/meta-analysis, 1b: randomized controlled trial (RCT), 2b: cohort study/non-randomized controlled clinical trial or low-quality RCT (e.g. small n, attrition); 3: case-control study; 4: case series

(CEBM), the quality of evidence, and strength of recommendation (GRADE) are presented in Table 3 (see also Platz 2017).

2.3   Description of Treatments for Neglect

While with exception of the Optokinetic/smooth pursuit therapy (SPT), the quality of evidence available is too low to give a weak or strong recommendation, there is nevertheless a variety of therapeutic options that are supported by clinical experience. The résumés presented below are therefore expert opinion.

In *visual scanning training* (VST or exploration training), patients typically look at a visual display (on a table, a computer screen, or a large projection wall) on which different classes of visual stimuli (i.e. stars, circles, numbers, photos from real objects) are shown, and the patient is required to look for a specific class of stimuli ("Search for all stars and point to them", with a stick or laser pointer or on a touch screen). Patients are verbally instructed to look to the neglected side ("cueing of attention"), search systematically row by row as in reading in order to acquire a systematic search strategy. By this, the number of omissions and search time is reduced.

Résumé: VST is the most widely used treatment for neglect and improves selectively *visual* neglect in scanning and related tasks, but has no effect on non-visual neglect. It can easily be realized but requires many sessions to be effective (>40). It is difficult to implement in the early phase (first 2 months after stroke) because it requires some awareness and cooperation on the patient's side.

Optokinetic/smooth pursuit therapy (OKS, SPT): Patients are instructed to make following (pursuit) eye movements to visual stimuli that move slowly towards the neglected field. The stimuli are usually presented on a computer screen or via beamer to a large projection wall via specific software. When the patient has reached with his eyes the neglected side of space, he is instructed to remain there with his eyes for some seconds, before the task is repeated. OKS/SPT can be performed early after stroke at the bedside, or later. Twenty or more sessions (á 30-min) are recommended.

Résumé: OKS/SPT is more effective than scanning therapy and can be implemented earlier. Improvements transfer to a wide variety of visual and non-visual neglect domains and reduce anosognosia.

Neck-muscle vibration (NMV): During NMV therapy, the patient's contralesional neck muscles (hence left neck in left neglect) are vibrated with a conventional vibrator (either battery-driven or not; with a small vibration head, <2 cm diameter, and a vibration frequency >60–80 Hz). This induces activation of muscle spindles and leads to a relocation of gaze (eye and head position) towards a more symmetrical, midline position. The vibrator is usually held by the therapist, which can be demanding for the therapist as he/she will feel the vibration as well and has to do it for at least 20 sessions (á 30 min).

Résumé: NMV is easy to apply but is more demanding for the therapist holding the vibrator. On the other hand, a battery-driven vibrator makes therapy more flexible and mobile, thus therapy can be performed at the bedside, in physio or occupational therapy, or at home.

Prism adaptation (PA): This therapy requires a conventional spectacle on which two prism glasses are mounted inducing a gaze shift to the ipsilesional side (hence to the right in left neglect). This prism goggle is worn by the patient *only* for the period of the prism exposure (not during the day, especially not during walking!). The prism exposure lasts typically for 20–30 min per session, and this should be repeated (several times per week). While the patient wears the prism goggles, he/she carries out visuo-motor tasks. These can be pointing to marked locations on a table, or reaching for objects in daily life (i.e. cups or glasses on a table or in a bookshelf). After this exposure period, the goggles are taken off and the therapeutic after-effect occurs (re-orienting of spatial attention to the neglected side). This can be used for other subsequent therapies (i.e. motor, postural, reading, cognitive …). Twenty or more sessions (á 20–30 min) are recommended.

Résumé: PA is a widely used tool for neglect therapy that works best with a 10° prism (not smaller prism angle!) and is also mobile and relatively easy to apply.

Visuo-motor feedback (VF): The patient has to lift wooden or metal rods with his ipsilesional hand (index finger and thumb), so that their left and right half are balanced and the rod does not fall to one side. As the patient ignores initially the contralesional side of the rod (due to his neglect), he will grasp it more to the right side and consequently the bar will fall to the left side. This "natural" feedback leads to a subsequent adaptation of the patient's lifting behaviour, thus lifting the rods more accurately in the middle part during the course of the therapy. Twenty or more sessions (á 20–30 min) recommended.

Résumé: VF is an easily applicable and low-cost treatment that can be implemented in different settings, including the patient's home. This makes it flexible and mobile.

Mirror therapy (MT): MT is a well-established treatment for therapy of motor impairments (of the hemiparetic arm or leg). It requires a vertically oriented mirror which is placed in front of the patient's breast so that he can view his ipsilesional hand/arm/leg performing different motor tasks. This action observation facilitates motor recovery of the impaired extremity behind the mirror. MT has shown therapeutic effects in patients with left-sided hemiparesis and left-sided visual neglect. Twenty or more sessions (á 20–30 min) recommended.

Résumé: MT is an easily applicable, low-cost therapy which can be used as an add-on treatment (not as a primary neglect therapy) for neglect.

Attention training: Alertness and sustained attention can be trained by various ways: by computer-based training and specific software, by table-top exercises, and also by motor (for instance treadmill) training. Improvements in attention lead to better performance in neglect-specific tasks, especially dual-tasks (i.e. looking and recollecting numbers heard, or looking and walking simultaneously).

Résumé: Attention training can be an element of neglect therapy. However, therapy should not rely solely on computerized training as such improvements are often not stable in the long term.

Hemifield Fresnel Prisms: Press-on (Fresnel) prism foils are attached on the contralesional side of the two glasses of a conventional spectacle sparing the central (macular) visual field region. This induces a gaze shift towards the neglected side (hence opposite to that in prism adaptation, see above).

Résumé: Easy-to-use technique, which should be used only during sitting and when the patient is not involved in transfers or other potentially dangerous activities, as the prism distorts the visual field. The central 10° of each glass should be free from foil to enable unimpaired central vision. Fresnel prisms reduce visual acuity by some 10–20%.

Repetitive transcranial magnetic stimulation (rTMS): During rTMS, a magnetic coil attached to a magnetic stimulator is hold by a medical doctor over the non-lesioned parietal cortex (hence the intact) hemisphere, to re-balance the attentional systems of both hemispheres. Left parietal attentional systems are typically hyperactive in patients with left neglect thus preventing the lesioned right-sided attentional systems from functional recovery. rTMS temporarily dampens the leftward hyperactive systems, thus improving functional recovery. This works without the patient being attentive, but care must be taken not to induce fits. Twenty or more sessions (á 20 min) are recommended.

Résumé: rTMS (or theta burst stimulation) is the most costliest neglect therapy to date and requires medical staff. It can be used earlier than other treatments as the mechanism of action does not require awareness or active cooperation from the patient. An optional add-on treatment when safety criteria are followed.

Transcranial direct current stimulation (tDCS): Similar principle of action as in rTMS, but instead of magnetic pulses, weak electrical currents are delivered via two electrodes over the two parietal lobes. Twenty or more sessions (of 20 min) are recommended.

Résumé: Less costly than rTMS, but often the technique cannot be applied due to exclusion criteria for safety reasons (fits, open scull) or is difficult to apply because of hairy skin thus preventing the flow of electric currents.

Transcutaneous electrical nerve stimulation (TENS): Application of weak electrical currents to the contralesional neck/upper back. Portable, low-cost technique, easily applicable, and no safety problems. Twenty or more sessions (á 20 min) recommended.

Résumé: Suitable as an add-on treatment, probably less suited as a primary and sole neglect therapy. It has good effects also on postural imbalance and non-lateralized attention.

Arm/hand activation with/without peripheral electrical stimulation: The method entails volitional movement of the contralesional limbs (i.e. opening and closing the hand). This can be facilitated by the additional application of electrodes to the neglected limb.

Résumé: Limb activation is often not applicable in the early phase of neglect because of severe hemiparesis or plegia. Later, with concurrent electrical stimulation, it is a useful, low-cost technique that particularly addresses neglect of the neglected extremities which is not targeted by the majority of other neglect treatments (except GVS, see below).

Galvanic vestibular stimulation (GVS): Application of weak electrical current via two electrodes attached behind both ears (over the mastoid bones) activates the vestibular system via the vestibular nerves. This has good therapeutic effects on body-related neglect (tactile extinction, sense of arm position for the neglected limb and visual neglect). Same limitations for safety reasons as in rTMS and tDCS (no fits). Twenty or more sessions (of 20 min) recommended.

Résumé: A suitable add-on treatment, especially for the body-related phenomena of neglect. The same electrical stimulators as used for tDCS can be used.

Drugs: The administration of attention-enhancing drugs is intended to improve non-lateralized attention (alertness), thereby reducing neglect. Moreover, antidepressant drugs can improve attention.

Résumé: Potentially, drugs may be helpful as an add-on treatment (not as a primary neglect therapy). Unfortunately, the therapeutic effects are inconsistent and many potential interactions with other drugs the patient must take have to be considered. Antidepressants given because of post-stroke depression may have an additional positive effect on neglect but should not be the primary reason for their prescription.

2.4   Clinical Decision-Making: Which Therapy, When, Which Dose, and Which Combinations?

While some treatments may be classified as "bottom-up" treatments because they manipulate a specific sensory input channel (i.e. vestibular), others ("top-down") intend to change cognitive strategies (i.e. sustained attention, visual scanning) in order to compensate for neglect. While the knowledge about the exact action profile of these different treatments is still incomplete, some treatment-relevant conclusions can be drawn. First, only a few treatments induce *multimodal* effects in the visual *and* nonvisual modalities, while others improve neglect only in one modality (mostly the visual). Second, not all treatments show transfer effects to ADL and to motor/postural capacities, both of which are very important for gaining functional independence for the patient. Finally, no treatment is currently available that affects all components and modalities of neglect and associated disorders. It is—in our personal opinion—therefore more likely to achieve a better treatment outcome by using several different treatments in combination—either simultaneously or sequentially—than expecting that neglect can be cured by using one specific treatment alone.

According to a recent Cochrane analysis, evaluating the effects of drugs therapy on neglect (Luvizutto et al. 2015), the quality of the evidence from available RCTs was very low. The effectiveness and safety of pharmacological interventions for neglect after stroke are therefore uncertain. Hence, drug therapy cannot be recommended for the treatment of spatial neglect or associated disorders.

For the clinician, the question arises: which of these different treatments should be used, when, how long, and how often? Although many of these questions are currently unanswered by scientific research, some practical recommendations based on the literature and own clinical experience may be given:

- *Early phase after stroke* (first 2 months): Use methods that need less cognitive control, awareness, and cooperation from the patient: rTMS, TENS, OKS/SPT, neck muscle vibration. If feasible, start therapy already at the bedside.
- *Post-acute phase after stroke* (after month 2 post-onset): Add methods that require more active cooperation and participation from the patient during therapy: visual scanning therapy, attention training, mirror therapy, visuo-motor feedback, and arm activation with concurrent electrical stimulation.
- *Late phase after stroke* (>6 months post-onset): Introduce more dual- tasks into therapy because in daily life the patient is often faced with such demands (i.e. looking and talking or walking and looking). This can be done by adding a cognitive task to the primary therapeutic task (i.e. count backwards while scanning for objects on a table-top) or scanning visual scenes on a computer screen. Try therapy with the patient *standing* instead of sitting. Mobility is of utmost importance for most neglect patients (see the chapter by Pèrennou et al., this volume) and the neglect impairs mobility and postural safety. Thus, neglect therapy can be performed during stance looking at stimuli projected (via beamer) on a white wall or while the patient is standing or walking on a treadmill.
- *Seeing straight:* In the first months after stroke, it is important that the patient sees "more straight" instead of ignoring one side and looking always to the ipsilesional side.
- *Systematic scanning strategy:* Later, when the patient can look better to the neglected side, it is important that he can select certain stimuli while ignoring other things. This can be achieved by a systematic scanning strategy taught to the patient (i.e.): "Start looking always on the top left side row by row, scan horizontally row by row. Don't forget the left lower corner, as it is the most often neglected part of the scene (also in daily life)".
- *Multidisciplinary treatments*: Try to implement treatments that span different vocational specialties in your rehab-team: for instance, try to combine physiotherapy with i.e. neck muscle vibration or TENS or attention training in addition with motor therapy for hand function.
- *Motor and Postural Functions*: Left-sided motor functions are often more impaired in patients with neglect than those without neglect (both with hemiparesis or plegia). Specific neglect therapy augments the effects of physiotherapy. Try to combine postural training (i.e. standing during neglect therapy, or with an additional balance pad or on a treadmill with stabilization) with neglect therapy (i.e. visual scanning training, OKS/SPT, attention training).
- *Visuospatial disorders*: Neglect is not a unitary disorder, but rather a multicomponent complex disease with—due to larger lesions—more associated deficits. Often, visuospatial perception (line orientation, subjective visual, or haptic vertical) and visuo-construction are impaired due to parietal lesions. The prior can be

treated for instance with GVS, the latter with specific visuo-constructive therapy. This improves visuo-motor performance in daily life.

- *Exploit after-effects:* Use the known after-effects of several of these treatments (i.e. prism adaptation, OKS/SPT, NMV, rTMS, TENS) for the next therapy afterwards; they facilitate the subsequent therapy.
- *Start early:* Use the morning instead of the afternoon for therapy, patients are more alert. In the early rehab phase, 20–30 min continuous neglect therapy is often the limit and preferable to 1-h sessions.
- *Dose*: More therapy induces more improvements although this remains to be proven scientifically. This can be reached by implementing different neglect therapies into the treatments delivered by different therapists (i.e. nurse, physiotherapist, occupational therapist, neuropsychologist, social worker, recreation therapist, relative at home).
- *Awareness/Anosognosia*: Improved awareness comes gradually (a) by certain treatments (i.e. OKS/SPT or neck muscle vibration, or awareness training) and (b) by improving the patient's and relatives' knowledge about the impairments and treatment progress. This is a joint task of the whole rehab team.
- *As a note of caution, it needs to be added that technical devices may not be licensed for the specific use mentioned; if that was the case, any application would be "off label" and related medico-legal aspects need to be considered.*
- *Late course of the disease:* Moreover, most "therapy knowledge" comes from the first year after stroke. Almost nothing is known about the very late outcome from neglect *several years* after a stroke. There could be later functional recovery, a change of neglect type and/or some adaptation to the deficit. Such aspects should be evaluated in future treatment research.

2.5 Therapy of Sensory Extinction

Sensory extinction may be associated with spatial neglect or dissociate from it (Kerkhoff 2001). In the acute stage, both are often difficult to disentangle. In the chronic stage, extinction is often present although overt neglect signs have vanished. Extinction may persist for years after a stroke and impairs functional independence (i.e. tactile extinction impairs ADLs, visual extinction impairs driving!). Only one treatment has so far shown lasting and significant treatment effects on extinction; Galvanic vestibular stimulation reduced tactile extinction permanently (Schmidt et al. 2013b).

2.6 Therapy of Anosognosia in Neglect

Improving awareness (or reducing anosognosia) is crucial when aiming at a better outcome for patients with neglect and anosognosia. Few studies have shown treatment effects on unawareness after specific therapy. After repetitive neck muscle vibration, ADL functions and unawareness (as assessed from a rating scale) improved significantly (Schindler et al. 2002). Moreover, repetitive optokinetic therapy (SPT) reduced unawareness significantly (again rated from staff), while visual scanning therapy had no effect on unawareness (Kerkhoff et al. 2014). Jenkinson et al. (2011) summarized helpful treatment strategies in anosognosia for hemiplegia, which is often but not always present in the early phase of neglect. These strategies require systematic evaluation in further controlled treatment studies.

2.7 Conclusions

The last two decades have seen a dramatic increase in the number of techniques available for the treatment of unilateral neglect and associated disorders (reviewed in Kerkhoff and Schenk 2012). Many of these techniques were developed from experimental interventions designed to influence the rightward orientation bias of neglect patients. These sensory stimulation techniques have some obvious advantages. They are easy to apply, their effects tend to generalize, and they only require minimal patient compliance—a huge benefit in the case of a disorder that is frequently associated with anosognosia. The induced improvements can last for several weeks when multiple treatment sessions are applied. However, the initial hope for a quick cure for neglect after only one or few treatment sessions has turned out to be unrealistic. Instead, a higher number of treatment sessions are probably necessary to reach functional improvements that last for a sufficiently long time and not only for 1 or 2 weeks. The challenge today is to select the best tool for a given patient and to combine this with other effective treatments to maximize outcome. We have formulated several practical recommendations which can be implemented into neurorehab teams in order to facilitate the transfer of novel knowledge, techniques, and treatments into clinical practice. Finally, we should keep in mind that neglect is not a unitary disorder but rather a complex, multicomponential disease. This requires—like other complex diseases—multiple, coordinated single treatments as we have tried to outline in this chapter.

References

Aimola L, Lane AL, Smith DT, Kerkhoff G, Ford G, Schenk T (2014) Efficacy and feasibility of a home-based computer training for individuals with homonymous visual field defects. Neurorehabil Neural Repair 28:207–218

Alford VM, Ewen S, Webb GR, McGinley J, Brookes A, Remedios LJ (2015) The use of the International Classification of Functioning, Disability and Health to understand the health and functioning experiences of people with chronic conditions from the person perspective: a systematic review. Disabil Rehabil 37:655–666

Azouvi P, Samuel C, Louis-Dreyfus A, Bernati T, Bartolomeo P, Beis J-M, Chokron S, Leclercq M, Marchal F, Martin Y, De Montety G, Olivier S, Perennou D, Pradat-Diehl P, Prairial C, Rode G, Siéroff E, Wiart L, Rousseaux M, French Collaborative Study Group on Assessment of Unilateral Neglect (GEREN/GRECO) (2002) Sensitivity of clinical and behavioural tests of spatial neglect after right hemisphere stroke. J Neurol Neurosurg Psychiatry 73:160–166

Azouvi P, Olivier S, De Montety G, Samuel C, Louis-Dreyfus A, Tesio L (2003) Behavioural assessment of unilateral neglect: study of the psychometric properties of the Catherine Bergego Scale. Arch Phys Med Rehabil 84:51–57

Azouvi P, Bartolomeo P, Beis JM, Perennou D, Pradat-Diehl P, Rousseaux M (2006) A battery of tests for the quantitative assessment of unilateral neglect. Restor Neurol Neurosci 24:273–285

Barton JJS, Black S (1998) Line bisection in hemianopia. J Neurol Neurochir Psychiatr 64(5):660–662

Bickerton W-L, Samson D, Williamson J, Humphreys GW (2011) Separating forms of neglect using the Apples Test: validation and functional prediction in chronic and acute stroke. Neuropsychology 25:567–580

Biousse V, Newman NJ (2009) Neuro-opthalmology illustrated. Thieme, New York

Bouwmeester L, Heutink J, Lucas C (2007) The effect of visual training for patients with visual field defects due to brain damage: a systematic review. J Neurol Neurosurg Psychiatry 78(6):555–564

Bowen A, Hazelton C, Pollock A, Lincoln NB (2013) Cognitive rehabilitation for spatial neglect following stroke. Cochrane Database Syst Rev 2013(7):CD003586

Caramazza A, Hillis AE (1990) Levels of representation, co-ordinate frames, and unilateral neglect. Cogn Neuropsychol 7(5–6):391–445

Cazzoli D, Muri RM, Schumacher R et al (2012) Theta burst stimulation reduces disability during the activities of daily living in spatial neglect. Brain 135:3426–3429

De Haan G, Heutink J, Melis-Dankers BJM, Tucha O, Brouwer W (2014) Spontaneous recovery and treatment effecs in patients with homonymous visual field defects: a meta-analysis of existing literature in terms of the ICF framework. Surv Ophthalmol 59:77–96

De Haan G, Melis-Dankers BJ, Brouwer WH, Bredewoud RA, Tucha O, Heutink J (2015) The effects of compensatory scanning training on mobility in patients with homonymous visual field defects: a randomized controlled trial. PLoS One 10(8):e134459

Gialanella B, Monguzzi V, Santoro R, Rocchi S (2005) Functional recovery after hemiplegia in patients with neglect: the rehabilitative role of anosognosia. Stroke 36:2687–2690

Gossmann A, Kastrup A, Kerkhoff G, Herrero CL, Hildebrandt H (2013) Prism adaptation improves ego-centered but not allocentric neglect in early rehabilitation patients. Neurorehabil Neural Repair 27:534–541

Guyatt GH, Oxman AD, Vist GE, Kunz R, Falck-Ytter Y, Alonso-Coello P, Schünemann JJ (2008) GRADE: an emerging consensus on rating quality of evidence and strength of recommendation. BMJ 336:924–926

Harvey M, Hood B, North A, Robertson IH (2003) The effects of visuomotor feedback training on the recovery of hemispatial neglect symptoms: assessment of a 2-week and follow-up intervention. Neuropsychologia 41:886–893

Hesse C, Lane AR, Aimola L, Schenk T (2012) Pathways involved in human conscious vision contribute to obstacle-avoidance behaviour. Eur J Neurosci 36:2383–2390

Hillis AE, Rapp B, Benzing L, Caramazza A (1998) Dissociable coordinate frames of unilateral spatial neglect: "viewer-centered" neglect. Brain Cogn 37(3):491–526

Husain M (2008) Hemispatial neglect. In: Goldenberg G, Miller BV (eds) Handbook of clinical neurology. Elsevier B.V., Amsterdam, pp 359–372

Ivanov IV, Kuester S, MacKeben M, Krumm A, Haaga M, Staudt M, Cordey A, Gehrlich C, Martus P, Trauzettel-Klosinski S (2019) Effects of visual search training in children with hemianopia. PLoS One 13(7):e0197285

Jackowski MM, Sturr JF, Taub HA, Turk MA (1996) Photophobia in patients with traumatic brain injury—uses of light-filtering lenses to enhance contrast sensitivity and reading rate. NeuroRehabilitation 6:193–201

Jehkonen M, Laihosalo M, Kettunen J (2006a) Anosognosia after stroke: assessment, occurrence, subtypes and impact on functional outcome reviewed. Acta Neurol Scand 114:293–306

Jehkonen M, Laihosalo M, Kettunen JE (2006b) Impact of neglect on functional outcome after stroke: a review of methodological issues and recent research findings. Restor Neurol Neurosci 24:209–215

Jenkinson PM, Preston C, Ellis SJ (2011) Unawareness after stroke: a review and practical guide to understanding, assessing, and managing anosognosia for hemiplegia. J Clin Exp Neuropsychol 33:1079–1093

Kalra L, Perez I, Gupta S, Wittink M (1997) The influence of visual neglect on stroke rehabilitation. Stroke 28:1386–1391

Kapoor N, Ciuffreda KJ (2002) Vision disturbances following traumatic brain injury. Curr Treat Options Neurol 4:271–280

Karnath HO, Rennig J, Johannsen L, Rorden C (2011) The anatomy underlying acute versus chronic spatial neglect: a longitudinal study. Brain 134:903–912

Kasten E, Wüst S, Behrens-Baumann W, Sabel BA (1998) Computer-based training for the treatment of partial blindness. Nat Med 4:1083–1087

Keller I, Lefin-Rank (2010) Improvement of visual search after audiovisual exploration training in hemianopic patients. Neurorehabil and Neural Repair 24:666–673

Kerkhoff G (1993) Displacement of the egocentric visual midline in altitudinal postchiasmatic scotomata. Neuropsychologia 31:261–265

Kerkhoff G, Münßinger U, Meier EK (1994) Neurovisual rehabilitation in cerebral blindness. Arch Neurol 51:474–481

Kerkhoff G (1999) Restorative and compensatory therapy approaches in cerebral blindness—a review. Restor Neurol Neurosci 15(2–3):255–271

Kerkhoff G (2000) Neurovisual rehabilitation: recent developments and future directions. J Neurol Neurosurg Psychiatry 68:691–706

Kerkhoff G (2001) Hemispatial neglect in man. Prog Neurobiol 63:1–27

Kerkhoff G (2010) Evidenczbasierte Verfahren in der neurovisuellen Rehabiliation. Neurol Rehabil 16:82–90

Kerkhoff G, Schenk T (2011) Line bisection in homonymous visual field defects—recent findings and future directions. Cortex 47(1):53–58

Kerkhoff G, Schenk T (2012) Rehabilitation of neglect: an update. Neuropsychologia 6:1072–1079

Kerkhoff G, Munssinger U, Haaf E, Eberle-Strauss G, Stogerer E (1992a) Rehabilitation of homonymous scotomata in patients with postgeniculate damage of the visual system: saccadic compensation training. Restor Neurol Neurosci 4(4):245–254

Kerkhoff G, Münßinger U, Eberle-Strauss G, Stögerer E (1992b) Rehabilitation of hemianopic alexia in patients with postgeniculate visual field disorders. Neuropsychol Rehabil 2(1):21–42

Kerkhoff G, Reinhart S, Ziegler W, Artinger F, Marquardt C, Keller I (2013) Smooth pursuit eye movement training promotes recovery from auditory and visual neglect: a randomized controlled study. Neurorehabil Neural Repair 27:789–798

Kerkhoff G, Bucher L, Brasse M et al (2014) Smooth pursuit "bedside" training reduces disability and unawareness during the activities of daily living in neglect. A randomized controlled trial. Neurorehabil Neural Repair 28:554–563

Kerr NM, Chew SS, Eady EK, Gamble GD, Danesh-Meyer HV (2010) Diagnostic accuracy of confrontation visual field tests. Neurology 74(15):1184–1190

Koch G, Bonnì S, Giacobbe V, Bucchi G, Basile B, Lupo F, Versace V, Bozzali M, Caltagirone C (2012) Theta-burst stimulation of the left hemisphere accelerates recovery of hemispatial neglect. Neurology 78:24–30

Lane A, Smith DT, Elison A, Schenk T (2010) Visual exploration training is no better than attention training for treating hemianopia. Brain 133(6):1717–1728

Lexell J, Brogårdh C (2015) The use of ICF in the neurorehabilitation process. NeuroRehabilitation 36:5–9

Lezak MD, Howieson E, Bigler E, Tranel D (2004) Neuropsychological assessment. Oxford University Press, New York

Luvizutto GJ, Bazan R, Braga GP, Resende LA, Bazan SG, El Dib R (2015) Pharmacological interventions for unilateral spatial neglect after stroke. Cochrane Database Syst Rev 2015(11):CD010882

Machner B, Sprenger A, Sander T, Heide W, Kimmig H, Helmchen C et al (2009) Visual search disorders in acute and chronic homonymous hemianopia: lesion effects and adaptive strategies. Ann N Y Acad Sci 1164:419–426

Mödden C, Behrens M, Damke I, Eilers N, Kastrup A, Hildebrandt H (2012) A randomized controlled trial comparing 2 interventions for visual field loss with standard occupational therapy during inpatient stroke rehabilitation. Neurorehabil Neural Repair 26(5):463–469

Nelles G, Esser J, Eckstein A, Tiede A, Gerhard H, Diener HC (2001) Compensatory visual field training for patients with hemianopia after stroke. Neurosci Lett 306:189–192

Neumann G, Schaadt AK, Reinhart S, Kerkhoff G (2016) Clinical and psychometric evaluations of the cerebral vision screening questionnaire in 461 nonaphasic individuals poststroke. Neurorehabil Neural Repair 30:187–198

Nijboer TC, Kollen BJ, Kwakkel G (2013) Time course of visuospatial neglect early after stroke: a longitudinal cohort study. Cortex 49:2021–2027

Pambakian AL, Mannan SK, Hodgson TL, Kennard C (2004) Saccadic visual search training: a treatment for patients with homonymous hemianopia. J Neurol Neurosurg Psychiatry 75(10):1443–1448

Paolucci S, Antonucci G, Guariglia C, Magnotti L, Pizzamiglio L, Zoccolotti P (1996) Facilitatory effect of neglect rehabilitation on the recovery of left hemiplegic stroke patients—a cross-over study. J Neurol 243:308–314

Pizzamiglio L, Antonucci G, Judica A, Montenero P, Razzano C, Zoccolotti P (1992) Cognitive rehabilitation of the hemineglect disorder in chronic patients with unilateral right brain damage. J Clin Exp Neuropsychol 14:901–923

Pizzamiglio L, Vallar G, Magnotti L (1996) Transcutaeneous electrical stimulation of the neck muscles and hemineglect rehabilitation. Rest Neur Neurosi 10:197–203

Platz T (2017) Practice guidelines in neurorehabilitation. Neurology International Open 1:E148–E152

Polanowska K, Seniow J, Paprot E, Lesniak M, Czlonkowska A (2009) Left-hand somatosensory stimulation combined with visual scanning training in rehabilitation for post-stroke hemineglect: a randomised, double-blind study. Neuropsychol Rehabil 19:364–382

Pollock A, Zazelton C, Henderson CA, Angilley J, Dhillon B, Lanthorne P, Livingstone K, Munro FA, Heather O, Row F, Shahani U (2012) Interventions for visual field defects in patients with stroke. Stroke 43:e37–e38

Ptak R, Di PM, Schnider A (2012) The neural correlates of object-centered processing in reading: a lesion study of neglect dyslexia. Neuropsychologia 50:1142–1150

Rengachary J, He BJ, Shulman GL, Corbetta M (2011) A behavioral analysis of spatial neglect and its recovery after stroke. Front Hum Neurosci 5:29

Rizzo M (1989) Astereopsis. In: Boller F, Grafman J (eds) Handbook of neuropsychology. Elsevier, Amsterdam, pp 415–427

Rizzo M, Barton JJS (2008) Central disorders of visual function. In: Miller NR, Newman NJ, Biousse V, Kerrison JB (eds) Walsh and Hoyt'a clinical neuro-opthalmology: the essentials. Lippincott Williams & Wilkins, Philadelphia, pp 263–284

Robertson IH, Tegnér R, Tham K, Lo A, Nimmo-Smith I (1995) Sustained attention training for unilateral neglect: theoretical and rehabilitation implications. J Clin Exp Neuropsychol 17:416–430

Rode G, Lacour S, Jacquin-Courtois S, Pisella L, Michel C, Revol P, Alahyane N, Luauté J, Gallagher S, Halligan P, Pélisson D, Rossetti Y (2015) Long-term sensorimotor and therapeutical effects of a mild regime of prism adaptation in spatial neglect. A double-blind RCT essay. Ann Phys Rehabil Med 58:40–53

Rode G, Pisella L, Petitet P, O'Shea J, Huchon L, Jacquin-Courtois S, Rossetti Y (2017) Quelles stratégies de rééducation dans la négligence spatiale unilatérale ? In: Roussel M, Godefroy O, de Boissezon X (eds) Troubles neurocognitifs vasculaires et post-AVC. De l'évaluation à la prise en charge. De Boeck Supérieur, Paris, pp 97–110

Rossi PW, Kheyfets S, Reding MJ (1990) Fresnel prisms improve visual perception in stroke patients with homonymous hemianopia or unilateral visual neglect. Neurology 40:1597–1599

Rossit S, Benwell CSY, Szymanek L, Learmonth G, McKernan-Ward L, Corrigan E, Muir K, Reeves I, Duncan G, Birschel P, Roberts M, Livingstone K, Jackson H, Castle P, Harvey M

(2017) Efficacy of home-based visuomotor feedback training in stroke patients with chronic hemispatial neglect. Neuropsychol Rehabil 23:1–20

Roth T, Sokolov AN, Mesias A, Roth P, Weller M, Trauettel-Klosinski S (2009) Comparing explorative saccade and flicker training in hemianopia: a randomized controlled study. Neurology 72:324–331

Rowe F, Brand D, Jackson CA, Price A, Walker L, Harrison S et al (2009) Visual impairment following stroke: do stroke patients require vision assessment? Age Ageing 38(2):188–193

Rowe FJ, Conroy EJ, Bedson E, Cwiklinski E, Drummond A, Garcia-Finana M, Howard C, Pollock A, Shipman T, Dodridge C, MacIntosh C, Johnson S, Noonan C, Barton G, Sackley C (2016) A pilot randomized controlled trial comparing effectiveness of prism glasses, visual search training and standard care in hemianopia. Acta Neurol Scand 2017(136):310–321

Schaadt AK, Kerkhoff G (2016) Vision and visual processing deficits. In: Husain M, Schott J (eds) Oxford textbook of cognitive neurology & dementia. Oxford University Press, Oxford, pp 147–160

Schaadt AK, Schmidt L, Reinhart S, Adams M, Garbacenkaite R, Leonhardt E, Kuhn C, Kerkhoff G (2013) Perceptual relearning of binocular fusion and stereoacuity after brain injury. Neurorehabil Neural Repair 28(5):462–471

Schaadt AK, Schmidt L, Kuhn C, Summ M, Adams M, Garbacenkaite R, Leonhardt E, Reinhart S, Kerkhoff G (2014) Perceptual relearning of binocular fusion after hypoxic brain damage: four controlled single-case treatment studies. Neuropsychology 28(3):382–387

Schindler I, Kerkhoff G, Karnath H-O, Keller I, Goldenberg G (2002) Neck muscle vibration induces lasting recovery in spatial neglect. J Neurol Neurosurg Psychiatry 73:412–419

Schmidt L, Keller I, Artinger F, Stumpf O, Kerkhoff G (2013a) Galvanic vestibular stimulation improves arm position sense in spatial neglect: a sham-stimulation-controlled study. Neurorehabil Neural Repair 27:497–506

Schmidt L, Utz KS, Depper L et al (2013b) Now you feel both: galvanic vestibular stimulation induces lasting improvements in the rehabilitation of chronic tactile extinction. Front Hum Neurosci 7:90

Schreiber A, Vonthein R, Reinhard J, Trauzettel-Klosinski S, Connert C, Schiefer U (2006) Effect of visual restitution training on absolute homonymous scotomas. Neurology 67:143–145

Schröder A, Wist ER, Hömberg V (2008) TENS and optokinetic stimulation in neglect therapy after cerebrovascular accident: a randomized controlled study. Eur J Neurol 15:922–927

Schuett S (2009) The rehabilitation of hemianopic dyslexia. Nat Rev Neurol 5:427–437

Schuett S, Heywood C, Kentridge W, Zihl J (2008) Rehabilitation of hemianopic alexia: are words necessary for relearning oculomotor control? Brain 131:3156–3168

Smit M, Schutter DJLG, Nijboer TCW, Visser-Meily JMA, Kappelle LJ, Kant N, Penninx J, Dijkerman HC (2015) Transcranial direct current stimulation to the parietal cortex in hemispatial neglect: a feasibility study. Neuropsychologia 74:152–161

Spitzyna GA, Wise RJ, McDonald SA, Plant GT, Kidd D, Crewes H et al (2007) Optokinetic therapy improves text reading in patients with hemianopic alexia: a controlled trial. Neurology 68(22):1922–1930

Suchoff IB, Kapoor N, Ciuffreda KJ, Rutner D, Han E, Craig S (2008) The frequency of occurrence, types, and characteristics of visual field defects in acquired brain injury: a retrospective analysis. Optometry 79(5):259–265

Thieme H, Mehrholz J, Pohl M, Behrens J, Dohle C (2013) Mirror therapy for improving motor function after stroke. Stroke 44:e1–e2

Trauzettel-Klosinski S (2011) Current methods of visual rehabilitation. Deutsches Ärzteblatt International (English) 108:871–878

Turgut N, Miranda M, Kastrup A, Eling P, Hildebrandt H (2018) tDCS combined with optokinetic drift reduces egocentric neglect in severely impaired post-acute patients. Neuropsychol Rehabil 28(4):515–526

Van Wyk A, Eksteen CA, Rheeder P (2014) The effect of visual scanning exercises integrated into physiotherapy in patients with unilateral spatial neglect poststroke: a matched-pair randomized control trial. Neurorehabil Neural Repair 28:856–873

WHO (2001) International classification of functioning, disability and health. World Health Organization, Geneva.

Wilkinson D, Zubko O, Sakel M, Coulton S, Higgins T, Pullicino P (2014) Galvanic vestibular stimulation in hemi-spatial neglect. Front Integr Neurosci 8:4

Wilson B, Cockburn J, Halligan P (1987) Development of a behavioral test of visuospatial neglect. Arch Phys Med Rehabil 68:98–102

Yang NYH, Zhou D, Chnung RCK, Li-Tsang CWP, Fong KNK (2013) Rehabilitation interventions for unilateral neglect after stroke: a systematic review from 1997 through 2012. Front Hum Neurosci 7:1–11

Zhang X, Kedar S, Lynn JJ, Newman NJ, Viousse V (2006) Natural history of homonymous hemianopia. Neurology 66:901–905

Zihl J (1995) Eye movement patterns in hemianopic dyslexia. Brain 118:891–912

Zihl J (2011) Rehabilitation of visual disorders after brain injury, 2nd edn. Psychology Press, New York

Zihl J, Kerkhoff G (1990) Foveal photopic and scotopic adaptation in patients with brain damage. Clin Vis Sci 2:185–195

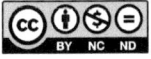

Cognition, Emotion and Fatigue Post-stroke

Caroline M. van Heugten and Barbara A. Wilson

1   Introduction

Stroke can have physical as well as cognitive, emotional and social consequences. Depending on the time of measurement, cognitive impairments are present in 50–70% of stroke survivors (e.g. Rasquin et al. 2002, 2004; Nys et al. 2005; Barker-Collo and Feigin 2006). In the first 2 weeks almost every stroke patient (92%) is impaired in at least one cognitive domain (Linden et al. 2005). Memory, executive functions, speed of information processing, language and visuo-spatial abilities are the most affected domains. The latter two have been discussed in chapters "Rehabilitation of Communication Disorders" and "Treating Neurovisual Deficits and Spatial Neglect", respectively.

Cognitive deficits have a negative impact on long-term outcomes such as independent functioning, community integration and quality of life (Nys et al. 2005; Duits et al. 2008; Van der Zwaluw et al. 2011; Barker-Collo et al. 2010; Wagle et al. 2011). Early identification of cognitive deficits is therefore necessary (van Dijk and de Leeuw 2012) and treatment should be offered accordingly (Langhorne et al. 2011; Albert and Kesselring 2012).

The same is true for emotional consequences after stroke. Depressive symptoms also have a profound influence on outcome and occur frequently. These symptoms range from 5 to 54% in the acute phase and remain present in 23–25% after 6

C. M. van Heugten (✉)
Brain Injury Center Limburg, Maastricht, The Netherlands

Department of Neuropsychology & Psychopharmacology, Faculty of Psychology & Neuroscience, Maastricht University, Maastricht, The Netherlands

School for Mental Health and Neuroscience, Faculty of Health, Medicine and Life Sciences, Maastricht University Medical Center, Maastricht, The Netherlands
e-mail: caroline.vanheugten@maastrichtuniversity.nl

B. A. Wilson
The Oliver Zangwill Centre, Ely, UK

© The Author(s) 2021
T. Platz (ed.), *Clinical Pathways in Stroke Rehabilitation*,
https://doi.org/10.1007/978-3-030-58505-1_12

months, when anxiety is present in 19–23% (Whyte and Mulsant 2002; Aben et al. 2002; De Wit et al. 2008; Kouwenhoven et al. 2011). Prevalence rates decrease over time but after 2 years major depression is seen in 20% of the stroke patients (Van Mierlo et al. 2015). In research and clinical practice, more attention is paid to depression but anxiety is almost as common and the two symptoms often occur together. Irritability, agitation, eating disturbances and apathy are also commonly found post-stroke (Angelelli et al. 2004).

Another common and debilitating but also less visible problem after stroke is fatigue. A recent meta-analysis showed that prevalence estimates vary from 25 to 85% on the basis of the Fatigue Severity Scale with a pooled prevalence estimate of 50% (Cumming et al. 2016). Post-stroke fatigue is an independent predictor of disability and burden of care and should therefore be taken into account when formulating post-stroke rehabilitation treatment goals (Mandliya et al. 2016).

Patients usually receive further rehabilitation treatment after suffering a major stroke (Winstein et al. 2016), while full recovery is assumed in a transient ischemic attack (TIA), and minor stroke patients are discharged home without further rehabilitation or follow-up treatment (Edwards et al. 2006). However, previous studies in TIA and minor stroke patients found high prevalence of dysfunction across all domains of health, of which cognitive and emotional problems and fatigue were most notable (Arts et al. 2008; Muus et al. 2010; Radman et al. 2012; Moran et al. 2014)—and mostly specific to stroke (van der Kemp et al. 2017; De Graaf et al. 2018; Fens et al. 2013). These symptoms may be overlooked with conventional clinical measures such as the neurological examination or the Barthel Index, despite the fact that they can be a major contributor to an impaired performance in activities of daily living including decreased participation and a diminished quality of life (QOL) (Edwards et al. 2006; Duncan et al. 1997; Suenkeler et al. 2002; Verbraak et al. 2012).

2   Best Evidence Synthesis

Best evidence synthesis relevant to clinical decision-making (with reference to Cochrane reviews, meta-analyses and RCTs as well as selected guidelines) including (when applicable).

The evidence on therapy presented in this chapter is gathered by a systematic search in December 2017 using the following steps. First, the Cochrane database of systematic reviews was consulted to select the most recent reviews on cognition, emotion and fatigue post-stroke. In addition, the search terms from these reviews were used to find additional, more recent studies. In case no recent Cochrane review was available, PubMed was searched using the filter 'review' and a combination of the search terms 'stroke' and the topic of interest. Furthermore, studies were added on the basis of the authors' own knowledge of relevant studies in this field. The evidence on assessment is mostly based on the authors' own knowledge because Cochrane reviews are not available in this field.

2.1   Assessment: Brief Overview, Key Instruments

2.1.1   Screening for Cognitive Problems

Given the high prevalence of cognitive and emotional consequences including fatigue after stroke and the negative impact on daily life functioning and social participation, it is important to screen every stroke patient for problems in these areas. Early screening can support the discharge destination and can help to plan the most adequate rehabilitation treatment and inform the patient and his or her caregivers about the possible consequences of these impairments in daily life and future functioning.

Cognitive screening early after stroke is recommended in many stroke guidelines and has even been determined as a key quality indicator of stroke services (Hachinski et al. 2006). Extensive neuropsychological assessment is recommended at later stages, but in the first days after stroke this is not feasible because patients may not be medically stable, can be fatigued easily and arousal levels may fluctuate. Screening for cognitive consequences should be conducted using a sensitive instrument specifically for stroke. From three systematic reviews in recent years (Stolwyk et al. 2014; Van Heugten et al. 2015; Burton and Tyson 2015), the Montreal Cognitive Assessment (MoCA) was identified as the most reliable, sensitive and feasible instrument for cognitive screening after stroke. A cutoff score of 26 is commonly used in stroke patients. In a recent study, it was shown that even in a mild stroke population ($n = 324$) 66.4% of the patients was cognitively impaired on the basis of the MoCA at 2 months post-stroke, with a significant improvement leaving 51.9% impaired at 6 months (Nijsse et al. 2017b). All reviews on cognitive screening instruments state that the widely used Mini Mental State Examination (MMSE) should no longer be used for this purpose because it was originally designed for screening of dementia and is therefore not sufficiently sensitive for consequences of stroke. Also for TIA and mild stroke patient, the MoCA can be used (Sivakumar et al. 2014).

Cognitive impairment may arise due to damage to strategic areas of the brain, even in patients who do not have motor or communication deficits. Especially in the group of so-called 'walking and talking' patients (i.e. good outcome in terms of motor and communication functioning), cognitive problems may be missed (van Dijk and de Leeuw 2012; Mark 2012). A routine follow-up visit, which is often dedicated to secondary prevention, should therefore also include cognitive screening.

Additionally, people may experience subjective cognitive complaints which are not necessarily related to objective cognitive functioning. Subjective cognitive complaints are very common after stroke, may increase over time and have a negative impact on outcome (van Rijsbergen et al. 2014). The use of stroke-specific instruments that measure subjective cognitive complaints, such as the Checklist for Cognition and Emotion (CLCE-24; van Heugten et al. 2007), are preferred (van Rijsbergen et al. 2015). Patients and their informal caregivers may disagree about the presence, nature and severity of these problems (van Rijsbergen et al. 2014), which is why it is advisable to also ask the primary caregiver about potential problems in these areas. The CLCE-24 can also be used to assess the experience of cognitive changes by the patient's caregiver.

A 5-min cognitive screening such as the MoCA should be the absolute minimum, and cognitive assessment should only be restricted to this global form of initial assessment in the acute phase post-stroke and in later phases when no other means or capacity of neuropsychologists is available. The National Institute of Neurological Disorders and Stroke—Canadian Stroke Network Vascular Cognitive Impairment already proposed a 30-min and 60-min protocol for neuropsychological assessment as part of their harmonization standards (Hachinski et al. 2006). There may be cultural differences and therapist preferences for the use of specific instruments, but more extensive neuropsychological assessment in addition to a 5-min cognitive screening should be common practice after stroke. The choice for suitable neuropsychological instruments can be made by trained neuropsychologists; instruments specifically validated for stroke patients are preferred.

2.1.2   Screening for Emotional Problems and Fatigue

Screening for mood disorders should involve both depression and anxiety screening, and the Hospital Anxiety and Depression Scale (HADS) has been found to be the only available tool to accurately screen for both (Burton and Tyson 2015). A cutoff value of 7 for both subscales on depression (HADS-D) and anxiety (HADS-A) is commonly used. The Stroke Aphasic Depression Questionnaire—Hospital version (SADQ-H) has good psychometric properties and can also be used for stroke patients with aphasia (Burton and Tyson 2015; van Dijk et al. 2016).

The most widely used measure to screen for post-stroke fatigue is the Fatigue Severity Scale (FSS; Cumming et al. 2016). A cutoff value of 3 or 4 is commonly used. The FAS is also used after stroke. A cutoff of 24 provides the best sensitivity/specificity values for the FAS (Cumming and Mead 2017).

2.1.3   Further Neuropsychological Assessment

Further neuropsychological assessment on cognitive, emotional, behavioural and social consequences should follow, especially when the screening has identified impaired functioning and also when there is a discrepancy between objective cognitive test results and subjective cognitive experiences by patients and caregivers. Neuropsychological rehabilitation or vocational rehabilitation should start with a thorough analysis of mental functions to assess both impaired and intact cognitive functions to identify strengths and weaknesses. Additionally, the impact of cognitive impairments on daily life functioning should be determined. Ideally, all levels of the framework of the International Classification of Functioning (ICF, WHO) are considered in a full neuropsychological assessment. In addition to assessment on the level of functions, activities and participation, the personal and external factors should be taken into account as well. In several studies, in the past few years, it has been shown that personal factors, especially psychological factors such as coping styles and personality traits influence the outcome after stroke (van Mierlo et al. 2014). In a large longitudinal cohort study on stroke patients we showed that more neuroticism, pessimism, passive coping and helplessness, and less extraversion, optimism, self-efficacy, acceptance, perceived benefits and proactive coping were associated with the presence of depressive symptoms at 2 months post-stroke (Van Mierlo et al. 2015). In the subsequent multivariate analyses, we showed that more helplessness and passive coping, and less acceptance and perceived benefits were independently significantly associated with the presence of depressive symptoms. Neuroticism at 2 months post-stroke appeared to be an independent predictor for both depression and anxiety at 1-year post-stroke in the same cohort (Kootker et al. 2016). Similarly, more proactive coping was related to less cognitive complaints at 2 months post-stroke (Nijsse et al. 2017a).

A treatment plan should be formulated at the start of rehabilitation allowing not only the planning of treatment but also the execution and evaluation. A stepwise approach is suggested by Wilson et al. (2003), which can be recommended to guide the treatment planning process. For an overview of all elements of a comprehensive neuropsychological assessment, we would like to refer to the chapter by Malec (2017) in the international handbook on neuropsychological rehabilitation (Wilson et al. 2017).

2.2 Therapy (Training, Technology, Medication): This Is the Major Focus

2.2.1 Cognitive Rehabilitation

After a stroke, spontaneous recovery can result in changes in structure and function of the brain, which is one form of neuroplasticity, but changes can also occur as a result of development, learning and environmental stimulation. Restoration of impaired cognitive functions will occur automatically to a certain extent but treatment is needed to further stimulate behavioural and brain changes. Restorative treatments are directed at the level of functions and have mostly short-term and only limited effects while long-lasting improvements in daily life functioning and societal participation should be the main goals of (neuro) rehabilitation.

Restorative approaches to cognitive rehabilitation are being investigated both in pre-clinical and clinical studies. In pre-clinical studies, cognitive enhancement approaches are tested in animal models such as enriched environment, early-onset multimodal stimulation, neuro-stimulating, pharmacotherapy or neuro-modulation (i.e. nervus vagus stimulation) but effects are small, mechanisms are not fully understood and generalization to humans is very difficult (e.g. Wogensen et al. 2015; Neren et al. 2016; Kochanek et al. 2015; Mala and Rasmussen 2017). One approach that raised renewed attention is the stimulation of cognitive functioning through physical exercise (i.e. multimodal stimulation). A recent meta-analysis showed that physical activity has small but significant positive effects on post-stroke cognition, even in the chronic phase (Oberlin et al. 2017). A total of 14 studies representing 736 participants showed an overall positive effect of physical activity on cognitive performance (Hedges' g (95% confidence interval) = 0.30 (0.14–0.47)). Combined aerobic and strength training programs generated the largest effects.

Improving the functionality of the whole brain in order to enhance the experience-dependent brain changes is the most probable explanation for these findings.

Clinical studies aimed at cognitive recovery focus on pharmacotherapy, computer-based cognitive retraining (CBCR) and non-invasive brain stimulation (NIBS). Pharmacotherapy studies aimed at cognition functions in stroke patients are scarce, and a recent meta-analysis showed that there is insufficient evidence to evoke effects of central nervous system drugs on enhancing global cognition (Yeo et al. 2017). CBCR has become very popular in the last 10–15 years, both in clinical practice and among the public. The idea that cognitive functioning can be improved or decline can be prevented or even reversed by regularly playing computer games is attractive, but effects are limited to the trained tasks while near- and far-transfer effects to untrained tasks and daily life functioning are small or lacking (van Heugten et al. 2016; van Heugten 2017). The number of studies on NIBS is growing rapidly, and new techniques are being developed. A recent Cochrane review on transcranial direct current stimulation (tDCS) for improving activities of daily living (ADL), and physical and cognitive functioning, in people after stroke showed that there are many ongoing studies (Elsner et al. 2016). A moderate effect of tDCS for improving ADL was found at the end of the intervention period (9 studies, 396 participants; standardized mean difference (SMD) 0.24, 95% confidence interval (CI) 0.03–0.44) and at follow up (6 studies, 269 participants; SMD 0.31, 95% CI 0.01–0.62), but not on cognitive functioning. In stroke patients, NIBS studies focus mainly on neglect, aphasia and (working) memory deficits. However, most studies are conducted within experimental settings to show the proof of principle without evaluating long-term effects or improvements in daily life functioning (van Heugten 2017). Recently, it has been suggested that NIBS can be applied as an adjuvant approach to rehabilitation (Wessel et al. 2015). The idea is that it augments the effects of behavioural training by increasing cortical excitability, neuronal plasticity and that it interacts with learning and memory.

Compensatory approaches to cognitive rehabilitation are shown to be the most effective to improve cognitive functioning after stroke and are most often applied in clinical practice (Wilson et al. 2017). In these circumstances, recovery is not achieved by restoring or substituting impaired cognitive functions but by offering patients' strategies to compensate for their impairments at task level. However, most evidence comes from studies on patients with acquired brain injury in which stroke patients are included as one of the major patient groups besides traumatic brain injury (Cicerone et al. 2000, 2005, 2011; Van Heugten et al. 2012). A meta-analysis in which only randomized controlled trials with stroke patients were included concluded that there was insufficient evidence or only evidence of insufficient quality to support recommendations for clinical practice (Gillespie et al. 2015). The Cochrane reviews on cognitive rehabilitation for post-stroke apraxia (West et al. 2008), executive dysfunctioning following stroke (Chung et al. 2013), prevention and treatment of post-stroke fatigue (Wu et al. 2015) and occupational therapy for cognitive impairments post-stroke (Hoffmann et al. 2010) came to the same conclusion about the lack of high-quality RCTs or positive outcomes. Recent Cochrane reviews have added to this evidence.

In the Cochrane review on cognitive rehabilitation for memory deficits following stroke, 13 RCTs including 514 participants were selected (das Nair et al. 2016). The authors conclude that memory rehabilitation has beneficial effects on subjective measures of memory in the short term (7 RCTs, n = 215; SMD 0.36, 95% CI 0.08–0.64, P = 0.01, moderate quality of evidence), but long-term effects could not be substantiated statistically beyond trend level (3 RCTs, n = 149; SMD 0.31, 95% CI −0.02 to 0.64, P = 0.06, low quality of evidence). The results do not show any significant effect of memory rehabilitation on objective memory tests, mood, functional abilities or quality of life. The authors conclude that more robust, well-designed high-quality trials are necessary.

A similar conclusion was drawn by Loetscher and Lincoln (2013) in their Cochrane review on attention deficits following stroke including 6 RCTs with 223 patients in total. A statistically significant effect was found in favour of cognitive rehabilitation when compared with control for immediate effects on measures of divided attention (SMD 0.67, 95% CI 0.35–0.98; P value <0.0001; 4 trials, 165 participants) but no significant effects on global attention (2 studies, 53 participants; P value = 0.06), or other attentional domains (6 studies, 223 participants; P value ≥0.16) or functional outcomes (3 studies, 109 participants; P value ≥0.21). Meta-analyses demonstrated no statistically significant effect of cognitive rehabilitation for persisting effects on global measures of attention (2 studies, 99 participants; standardized mean difference (SMD) 0.16, 95% confidence interval (CI) −0.23 to 0.56; P value = 0.41), standardized attention assessments (2 studies, 99 participants; P value ≥0.08) or functional outcomes (2 studies, 99 participants; P value ≥0.15).

Taking only Cochrane reviews on stroke patients into account, however, has the danger of throwing away the baby with the bathwater. Many evidence-based cognitive rehabilitation programs are available and used in clinical practice all over the world (Wilson et al. 2017). Evidence is often based on samples of mixed aetiologies including stroke patients among other patient groups (mostly traumatic brain injury). In a series of systematic reviews on evidence-based cognitive rehabilitation by Cicerone et al. (2000, 2005, 2011), practice standards, guidelines and options are formulated on the basis of studies in patients with acquired brain injury. Compensatory strategy training and the use of external aids have been shown to be effective for memory deficits, reduced speed of information processing (Time Pressure Management), executive dysfunctioning (Goal Management Training in combination with problem solving therapy) and apraxia.

Moreover, cognitive impairments hardly ever occur in isolation, which is why in clinical practice many multidomain cognitive rehabilitation programs are offered. Limited evidence shows that these programs are effective in attaining individual goals related to daily life functioning which remained in the long term (Brands et al. 2013; Rasquin et al. 2010). Typically, these programs are low-intensive and consist of a combination of psycho-education and compensatory strategy training. Often, these programs are offered in groups to strengthen the effects of peer support.

2.2.2 Pharmacological and Psychological Interventions for Depression and Anxiety After Stroke

Both pharmacological and psychological treatments to prevent depression after stroke (Hackett et al. 2008a, b) have been investigated. Fourteen trials involving 1515 participants were included in a Cochrane review of which 10 trials involved pharmacological agents and did not show significant effects on preventing depression. The psychological interventions showed small but significant positive effects on mood including problem-solving therapy and motivational interviewing.

The Cochrane review on treatment of depression after stroke (Hackett et al. 2008a, b) included 16 trials in which 13 pharmacological agents were investigated and four trials in which the effect of psychological treatment was examined. In most trials, selective serotonin reuptake inhibitors (SSRIs) were applied and also tricyclic antidepressants (TCAs) were investigated. Moderate significant effects were found on remission of depression (pooled OR 0.47; 95% CI 0.22–0.98) and also small improvements of scores on depression questionnaires (pooled OR 0.22; 95% CI 0.09–0.52). There was, however, also a significant increase of neurological and gastro-intestinal side effects. There was no significant improvement in cognitive and ADL functioning nor a reduction of disabilities. Mead et al. (2012) investigated the effect of SSRIs on stroke recovery. In the meta-analysis, 52 trials randomizing 4059 patients to SSRI or control were included, and a positive effect was found on neurological deficits (SMD −1.00, 95% CI −1.26 to −0.75; 29 trials, 2011 participants), ADL dependence, level of disabilities (SMD 0.91, 95% CI 0.60–1.22; 22 trials, 1343 participants), anxiety (SMD −0.77, 95% CI, −1.52 to −0.02; 8 trials, $n = 413$) and depression (SMD was −1.91 (95% CI, −2.34 to −1.48; 39 trials, 2728 participants)), however, with considerable variability across trials and substantial risks for bias. For disability, neurological deficits and depression, the effects had been larger when depression was present among participants. The results of this review tentatively support the use of SSRIs in stroke survivors with depression and provide evidence for clinically relevant positive treatment effects not only in the emotional domain.

The psychological interventions in the review of Hackett et al. (2008a, b) involved problem-solving therapy in combination with counselling, cognitive behavioural therapy, motivational interviewing and a combination of support and education, but no significant effects were found. Later studies on behavioural interventions for post-stroke depression show more positive results. The CALM (Communication and Low Mood) intervention for stroke patients with aphasia was effective in improving mood (Thomas et al. 2013) and was cost-effective over a period of 6 months in comparison to care as usual (Humphreys et al. 2015). In a study by Mitchell et al. (2009) patients ($n = 101$) received a short psychosocial intervention in addition to antidepressants which led to lower depression scores and better remission both in the short and the long term. Home-based supportive care also has a positive effect on mood in home-dwelling stroke patients (Huang et al. 2017). Recently, a scientific statement on post-stroke depression was published (Towfighi et al. 2017), summarizing seven studies on brief psychosocial interventions for reducing depression showing a positive effect. Neuro-modulation, stroke liaison workers and self-management programs did not have a positive effect. A meta-analysis on the effect of physical exercise on depression in neurological disorders showed a positive effect of physical exercise, preferably those meeting physical activity guidelines, on the reduction of depressive symptoms (26 trials, 1324 participants; effect size 0.28 95% confidence interval 0.15–0.41) (Adamson et al. 2015). A higher effect size (0.38) was found for studies that met physical activity guidelines versus those that did not (0.19). It has to be noted though that only 2 of the 26 trials included stroke patients.

Only three trials have been conducted in which treatment of anxiety post-stroke was investigated according to the most recent Cochrane review (Knapp et al. 2017). Due to small sample sizes, methodological concerns and adverse effects, recommendations for clinical practice cannot be given. In case of emotionalism after stroke (i.e. unwanted laughing or crying), a Cochrane review including seven trails showed that antidepressants can reduce the frequency and severity of crying or laughing episodes (7 studies, 239 participants). On the basis of five trials (213 participants), a large effect was found in a 50% reduction of emotionalism but with a wide confidence interval showing a small positive effect and in one study even a negative effect (Hackett et al. 2010). There is not one specific pharmacological agent.

2.2.3 Managing Post-stroke Fatigue

The effects of treatment of post-stroke fatigue are still limited. In the most recent Cochrane review, 12 trials with 703 participants were selected, but only 6 trails could be used for the meta-analysis (Wu et al. 2015). Five pharmacological interventions and two non-pharmacological interventions (fatigue education and mindfulness-based stress reduction) were investigated, but effects were small and the studies were not without risk of bias. Since post-stroke fatigue is multifactorial in nature with physical, cognitive, mental components and individual differences in the way people cope with fatigue, there is not one treatment that will fit all patients' needs (Visser-Keizer et al. 2015; Malley 2017). Psychosocial treatment and physical activity seem promising for the management of post-stroke fatigue but high-quality effect studies are necessary (Kutlubaev et al. 2015).

2.2.4 Comprehensive Neuropsychological Rehabilitation

The direct consequences of a stroke may also lead to secondary psychosocial problems, which hinder independent functioning and participation in society. The complexity of these problems requires comprehensive rehabilitation programs. Comprehensive neuropsychological (holistic) rehabilitation is aimed at cognitive, emotional, behavioural and social consequences after stroke, taking into account the personal and environmental factors as well. The evidence is still limited but findings suggest that such programs can improve community integration, functional independency and productivity, even many years after the injury (Cicerone et al. 2011). These programs can be divided into neurobehavioural interventions, residential community reintegration and day treatment programs (Geurtsen et al. 2010). Day treatment programs have the highest level of evidence leading to a reduction in psychosocial problems, a higher level of community integration and an increase in employment. These programs are typically group-based and offer a combination of individual and group therapy. One of the essential components of such programs is psycho-education about the brain injury and its consequences both for patients and caregivers. Every stroke patient and their primary caregivers should receive information about the potential consequences of stroke.

A Cochrane review on information provision after stroke included 21 trials involving 2289 patients and 1290 carers (Forster et al. 2012). This review shows that information improves patients' (SMD 0.29, 95% CI 0.12–0.46) and more so caregivers' knowledge (SMD 0.74, 95% CI 0.06–1.43) and aspects of satisfaction (odds ratio (OR) 2.07, 95% CI 1.33–3.23, $P = 0.001$) and reduces patient depression (mean difference (MD) −0.52, 95% CI −0.93 to −0.10). The best way to provide information is not clear yet, but active involvement of patients and carers has a higher effect on patient mood.

The Holistic Approach to Rehabilitation

Kurt Goldstein can probably be regarded as the grandparent of holistic rehabilitation arguing that we should look at the whole aspects of a situation and not one isolated part such as word finding difficulties (Goldstein 1919, 1942; Boake 1996). Both Goldstein and later Ben-Yishay (1996) recognized that it is futile to separate the cognitive, social, emotional and functional aspects of brain injury given that how we feel affects how we think, remember, communicate, solve problems and behave. This is the core of the holistic approach. As Ben-Yishay and Prigatano said in 1990, holistic rehabilitation "…consists of well integrated interventions that exceed in scope, as well as in kind, those highly specific and circumscribed interventions which are usually subsumed under the term 'cognitive remediation'" (Ben-Yishay and Prigatano 1990, p. 40).

Diller (1976), Ben-Yishay (1978) and Prigatano (1986) pioneered the holistic approach which is now seen as one of the most effective ways of providing cognitive rehabilitation to survivors of brain injury. This approach is now much in evidence (Wilson et al. 2009). Holistic programs are concerned with increasing a client's awareness, alleviating cognitive deficits, developing compensatory skills and providing vocational counselling. All such programs provide a mixture of individual and group therapy. They differ from the combined approach primarily in their recognition of the importance of treating emotional problems at the same time as treating the cognitive and social difficulties. Thus, inherent in the holistic approach are theories and models of emotion, which are becoming increasingly important in cognitive rehabilitation, as evidenced, for example by a special issue of the journal Neuropsychological rehabilitation focussing entirely on biopsychosocial approaches in neuropsychological rehabilitation (Williams and Evans 2003).

Ben-Yishay and Prigatano (1990) provide a model of hierarchical stages in the holistic approach through which the patient must work in rehabilitation. These are, in order, engagement, awareness, mastery, control, acceptance and identity. Holistic programs, explicitly or implicitly, tend to work through Ben-Yishay's hierarchical stages and are concerned with (1) increasing the individual's awareness of what has happened to him or to her, (2) increasing acceptance and understanding of what has happened, (3) providing strategies or exercises to reduce cognitive problems, (4) developing compensatory skills and (5) providing vocational counselling. All holistic programs include both group and individual therapy.

For a further overview of all aspects of neuropsychological rehabilitation after stroke and other forms of brain injuries, we would like to refer to the International Handbook of Neuropsychological Rehabilitation (Wilson et al. 2017).

2.2.5 Technical Aids

The use of assistive technology (AT) to compensate for cognitive impairments has become a common element of neuropsychological rehabilitation (Gillespie et al. 2012). In the area of attention, AT can be used to direct attention and support to sustain attention, for instance by tonal cues or automated text messages. Such mobile phone reminders and alarms/timers can also be used as reminders to support episodic memory (Jamieson et al. 2017). Additionally, time and planning management functions are common forms of AT which are nowadays available on any smartphone. In a meta-analysis including seven group studies, the authors concluded that there is strong evidence for the efficacy of prospective prompting memory devices ($d = 1.27$, $p < 0.01$; 147 participants) (Jamieson et al. 2015). AT can also be used to assist organization and provide step-by-step support during task performance.

3   Clinical Pathway/Evidence-Based Recommendations (What, When, Why?)

Since our recommendations for screening and neuropsychological assessment of post-stroke cognitive impairment and emotional disorders are not systematically based on evidence, they are not presented with ratings of quality of evidence and strength of recommendations, but rather reflect expert opinion.

The evidence, quality ratings and conclusions are summarized in Table 1.

The therapeutic recommendations given below are based on the evidence that had systematically been searched and presented above. The quality of this evidence has been grouped into four categories according to "GRADE" ("Grades of Recommendation, Assessment, Development and Evaluation") (Owens et al. 2010):

- High quality: further research is unlikely to affect our confidence in the estimation of the (therapeutic) effect.
- Medium quality: further research is likely to affect our confidence in the estimation of the (therapeutic) effect and may alter the estimate.
- Low quality: further research will most likely influence our confidence in the estimation of the (therapeutic) effect and will probably change the estimate.
- Very low quality: any estimation of the (therapy) effect or prognosis is very uncertain.

Table 1 Evidence from Cochrane reviews and other systematic reviews and meta-analyses

Treatment	Outcome	Review/ meta-analysis	N studies/n participants	Quality	Effects	Conclusion
Cognition: restorative approaches						
Pharmacotherapy: SSRIs	Global cognition	Yeo et al. (2017)	5/295	Low	SMD 0.23, 95% CI −0.01 to 0.46	Insufficient evidence for use of SSRIs to enhance global cognition
tDCS to improve cognitive and ADL functioning	ADL post-treatment	Elsner et al. (2016)	9/396	Moderate	SMD 0.24 (CI: 0.03–0.44)	tDCS can be considered to enhance ADL post-treatment. It is uncertain whether cognitive functioning can be improved
	ADL at follow up	Elsner et al. (2016)	6/269	Moderate	SMD 0.31 (CI: 0.01–0.62)	tDCS can be considered to enhance ADL in the long term
Physical activity (PA)	Cognitive performance	Obernin (2017)	14/736	Low to moderate	Hedges g 0.30 (CI: 0.14–0.47)	PA can be considered to enhance cognitive functioning
Cognition: compensatory approaches						
Apraxia training	Disability due to motor apraxia	West et al. (2008)	3/132	Low	No pooled data available	Insufficient evidence for therapeutic interventions for motor apraxia
Executive dysfunctioning training	Global executive functioning	Chung et al. (2013)	13/770 (340 stroke)	Low	No data on the primary outcome available	Insufficient evidence for cognitive rehabilitation for executive dysfunctioning
Memory training	Subjective memory functioning short term	das Nair et al. (2016)	7/215	Moderate	SMD 0.36, 95% CI 0.08–0.64	Memory rehabilitation can be considered to enhance subjective memory functioning in the short term
	Subjective memory functioning long term	das Nair et al. (2016)	3/149	Low	SMD 0.31, 95% CI −0.02–0.64	Memory rehabilitation might enhance subjective memory functioning in the long term

Attention training	Divided attention post-treatment	Loetscher and Lincoln (2013)	4/165	Low	SMD 0.67, 95% CI 0.35–0.98	Attention rehabilitation can be considered to enhance divided attention in the short term
Occupational therapy (OT)	Specific cognitive abilities	Hoffmann et al. (2010)	1/33	Low	No data	Insufficient evidence for OT on cognitive abilities
Fatigue						
Treatment of fatigue	Post-stroke fatigue	Wu et al. (2015)	7/244	Low	SMD −1.07, 95% CI −1.93 to −0.21	Insufficient evidence to prevent or treat fatigue
Depression and anxiety						
Pharmacotherapy for depression	Remission of depression	Hackett et al. (2008a, b)	12/1121	Moderate	pooled OR 0.47; 95% CI 0.22–0.98	There was evidence of a moderate benefit of pharmacotherapy in terms of a complete remission of depression, but also for an increase of adverse events
	Proportion of patients with a 50% reduction on mood scores (response)	Hackett et al. (2008a, b)	12/1121	Low to moderate	Pooled OR 0.22, 95% CI 0.09–0.52	There was some evidence of benefit of pharmacotherapy in terms of a reduction (improvement) in scores on depression rating scales, but also an increase of adverse events
SSRIs for stroke recovery	Depression	Mead et al. (2012)	39/2728	Moderate	SMD −1.91 (95% CI −2.34 to −1.48)	SSRIs can be considered to improve depression
SSRIs for anxiety	Anxiety	Mead et al. (2012)	8/413	Moderate	−0.77 (95% CI −1.52 to −0.02)	SSRIs may improve anxiety
Pharmacotherapy, relaxation, psychotherapy	Anxiety	Knapp et al. (2017)	3/196	Low	No pooled data	Insufficient evidence for treatment of anxiety

(continued)

Table 1 (continued)

Treatment	Outcome	Review/ meta-analysis	N studies/n participants	Quality	Effects	Conclusion
Physical exercises	Depression	Adamson et al. (2015)	26/1324	Low	ES 0.28 (95% CI 0.15–0.41)	Physical exercises may reduce depression but this is not specific to stroke
Information provision						
Information provision	Patient knowledge	Forster et al. (2012)	21/2289	Moderate	SMD 0.29, 95% CI 0.12–0.46	Information provision improves patient knowledge to some extent
	Caregiver knowledge	Forster et al. (2012)	21/2289	Moderate	SMD 0.74, 95% CI 0.06–1.43	Information provision improves carer knowledge
	Patient depression	Forster et al. (2012)	21/2289	Moderate	MD −0.52, 95% CI −0.93 to −0.10	Information provision improves patient depression, but this is not clinically significant
	Patient satisfaction	Forster et al. (2012)	21/2289	Moderate	Odds ratio (OR) 2.07, 95% CI 1.33–3.23, $P = 0.001$	Information provision improves patient satisfaction
Assistive Technology						
Cognitive prosthetic technology	Everyday memory	Jamieson et al. (2014)	7/147	Low to moderate	$d = 1.27$, $p < 0.01$	Prosthetic technology can improve performance on everyday tasks requiring memory

The grading of the recommendations according to GRADE (Schünemann et al. 2013) corresponds to the categories "ought to" (A) (strong recommendation), "should" (B) (weak recommendation). As a third category had been introduced "can" (0) (option) (Platz 2017). Recommendation category A is granted for clinically effective interventions with high-quality evidence support; with medium-quality evidence category B and with low- or very low-quality evidence category 0 can be appropriate. A+ and B+ denote a strong or weak recommendation in favour on an intervention, A− and B− against its use.

The recommendations following from the evidence are summarized in Table 2.

3.1 Cognitive Screening in Hospital

Every stroke patient should be screened for cognitive and emotional consequences following stroke. Objective cognitive screening should be conducted before the patient is discharged from the hospital to support the decision on the discharge destination and further rehabilitation treatment. Cognitive screening can best be

Table 2 Recommendations for the management of cognition, emotion and fatigue post-stroke

Management	Phase	Recommendation
Screening and Assessment		
Cognitive screening	Acute	Every stroke patient should be screened for cognitive and emotional consequences following stroke before hospital discharge to support the decision on the discharge destination and further rehabilitation treatment
Cognitive assessment	Post-acute	If cognitive deficits are not present upon early global cognitive screening or not checked at all, cognitive functioning should be assessed again at a later stage. If communication disorders exist, the method of information extraction must be modified accordingly for valid conclusions to be made
Cognitive assessment	First year	Both objective and subjective cognitive and emotional screening should always be performed during follow-up visits
Neuropsychological assessment	Rehabilitation and community reintegration	At the start of rehabilitation, and also when support is needed for community reintegration, an extensive neuropsychological assessment should be conducted
Treatment and Management		
Information provision	All phases	All patients and caregivers should receive information about the (potential) cognitive and emotional consequences, including fatigue, following stroke (level of evidence 1a, low quality, recommendation B+)

(continued)

Table 2 (continued)

Management	Phase	Recommendation
Referral to specialist services for cognitive, emotional and behavioral consequences	From post-acute onwards	Patients and caregivers should be referred to relevant follow-up care and neuropsychological rehabilitation within their stroke service (level of evidence 5, very low quality, recommendation B+) There is no time limit to these programs which means that patients may also be supported many years after the injury (level of evidence 5, very low quality, recommendation B+) General practitioners should be informed about the regional healthcare options for these problems
Cognitive rehabilitation	From post-acute onwards	Compensatory strategy training and the use of external and technical aids should be offered to help stroke patients to deal with cognitive impairments (level of evidence 1b, low quality, recommendation B+).
Neuropsychological rehabilitation aimed at cognitive, emotional, behavioral and social consequences	From post-acute onwards	Neuropsychological rehabilitation can be offered by experienced clinical or neuropsychologists working within a multidisciplinary team (level of evidence 5, very low quality, recommendation 0). Both low-intensity and high-intensity (holistic) group programs can be considered
Antidepressants	Chronic phase	SSRIs should be considered when depressive complaints or emotionalism are long lasting and become chronic while adverse effects should be monitored continuously (level of evidence 1a, moderate quality, recommendation B+)
Psychotherapy	All phases	Problem-solving therapy and motivational interviewing can be considered to prevent depressive symptoms post-stroke (level of evidence 2b, low quality, recommendation 0)

Classification of evidence level (1a to 5 according to the "Oxford Center for Evidence-Based Medicine – Levels of Evidence", last version from March 2009, http://www.cebm.net/Oxford-centre-evidence-based-medicine). Rating of quality of evidence (very low to high) and categories of recommendations (0, B+, A+) according to GRADE ("Grades of Recommendation, Assessment, Development and Evaluation"); for explanation see text
These ratings are only given for evidence-based recommendation for interventions (not for screening and assessment: expert opinion)

performed using the Montreal Cognitive Assessment (MoCA) because this is the most sensitive instrument for this purpose. A cutoff value of 24 is recommended. The Mini Mental State Examination (MMSE) should not be used because it was not designed for this purpose and is therefore not sufficiently sensitive. If cognitive deficits are found, referral for neuropsychological rehabilitation should follow. If cognitive deficits are not present upon early global cognitive screening or not checked at all, cognitive functioning should be assessed again at a later stage because cognitive deficits are easily missed during hospital admission when the patient has good functional outcome in terms of motor and language functioning (i.e. the walking and talking patient).

3.2 Cognitive and Emotional Screening at Routine Follow-Up

Most stroke patients are invited to visit a neurological outpatient clinic for a neurological follow-up and secondary prevention purposes. We recommend that both objective and subjective cognitive and emotional screening are always performed during these visits, which can be completed by a specialized stroke nurse. Cognitive deficits are easily missed during hospital admission. Cognitive functioning may not have been assessed before. Additionally, global cognitive screening may not be enough to pick up cognitive problems which arise from the more complex daily life challenges and return to prior activities such as work. For this reason, subjective cognitive complaints should be surveyed as well. Patients and their informal caregivers may differ in their experiences of cognitive consequences, which is why problems in cognitive functioning experienced by the primary caregiver should also be taken into account in the assessment. The stroke-specific Checklist for Cognition and Emotion (CLCE-24) can be used for this purpose.

Screening for emotional problems can be done with the Hospital Anxiety and Depression Scale (HADS), which is the only sensitive tool that also incorporates anxiety. The recommended cutoff value for each subscale (i.e. depression and anxiety) is seven. Post-stroke fatigue can best be screened with the Fatigue Severity Scale (FSS) using four as the cutoff point.

Most of these screening instruments can be used by specialized stroke nurses who have been trained in using and interpreting these instruments. Screening for the less-visible neuropsychological consequences of stroke should be done on a regular basis. If patients and caregivers do not report problems spontaneously, this does not necessarily mean that they are not present. If cognitive and emotional problems are experienced which interfere with daily life functioning, referral for neuropsychological rehabilitation should follow. At the start of rehabilitation, and also when support is needed for community reintegration, an extensive neuropsychological assessment should be conducted.

3.3 Neuropsychological Rehabilitation

All patients and caregivers should receive information about the potential cognitive and emotional consequences, including fatigue, following stroke because it improves patients' and caregivers' knowledge and reduces the level of depression in patients (level of evidence 1a, low quality, recommendation B+). Active and personalized information provision is preferred. Information can be given by any experienced member of the treatment team and should be repeated as often as necessary and possible.

Cognitive problems may arise at a later stage when the patient is discharged home and environmental demands are increasing. Resuming to prior activities, especially returning to work, may lead to problems which were not detected earlier. Patients and caregivers should be referred to relevant follow-up care and neuropsychological rehabilitation within their stroke service (level of evidence 5, very low quality, recommendation B+). General practitioners should be informed about the regional healthcare options for these problems.

Compensatory strategy training and the use of external and technical aids should be offered to help stroke patients with cognitive impairments to improve their daily life functioning (level of evidence 1b, low quality, recommendation B+). Psycho-education and strategy training can easily be combined in low-intensity group-based programs aimed at individualized patient-centred goals. Regional low-frequency or national high-intensity (holistic) outpatient neuropsychological rehabilitation programs may be indicated because of the complex interplay between cognitive, emotional and social consequences. There is no time limit to these programs which means that patients may also be supported many years after the injury (level of evidence 5, very low quality, recommendation B+). New problems may occur in the chronic phase after stroke when environmental demands are changing or increasing. Chronicity does not necessarily imply stability. Neuropsychological rehabilitation can be offered by experienced clinical or neuropsychologists working within a multidisciplinary team in which occupational therapists will address the link to the patient's daily life functioning and societal participation (level of evidence 5, very low quality, recommendation 0).

Clinicians should be aware of the influence of post-stroke fatigue on daily life functioning and societal participation. Although evidence is limited, psychosocial treatment and physical activity seem promising for the management of post-stroke fatigue (level of evidence 5, very low quality, recommendation 0).

In the first months, post-stroke antidepressant pharmacotherapy is only recommended if the process of rehabilitation is hindered by emotional problems. Increasing motivation for and participation in rehabilitation is the target for treatment. SSRIs should be considered when depressive complaints or emotionalism are long lasting and become chronic while adverse effects should be monitored continuously (level of evidence 1a, moderate quality, recommendation B+). Problem-solving therapy and motivational interviewing can be considered to prevent depressive symptoms post-stroke (level of evidence 2b, low quality, recommendation 0). Psycho-education should always be offered to both prevent and reduce anxiety, stress and depressive complaints in both patients and caregivers (level of evidence 1a, moderate quality, recommendation B+).

3.4   New Developments

There is no effective treatment for deficits in social cognition or emotion regulation yet, but professionals should be aware of problems in these areas, especially in relation to caregiver burden.

Restorative approaches such as pharmacotherapy, CBCR and NIBS can be offered to improve cognitive functioning but effects are limited to cognitive functions in testing situations (level of evidence 2b to 1a, low quality, recommendation 0). These forms of rehabilitation are primarily focused on alleviating cognitive impairment while neuropsychological rehabilitation is aimed at a broader spectrum of human functioning, also taking into account emotional, behavioural and social functioning, with the ultimate goal to optimize the participation and quality of life of both patients and caregivers. Although promising, restorative approaches in rehabilitation should always be offered only in combination with comprehensive neuropsychological rehabilitation programs aimed at improving daily life functioning and societal participation.

References

Aben I, Denollet J, Lousberg R, Verhey F, Wojciechowski F, Honig A (2002) Personality and vulnerability to depression in stroke patients: a 1-year prospective follow-up study. Stroke 33:2391–2395

Adamson BC, Ensari I, Motl RW (2015) Effect of exercise on depressive symptoms in adults with neurologic disorders: a systematic review and meta-analysis. Arch Phys Med Rehabil 96(7):1329–1338

Albert SJ, Kesselring J (2012) Neurorehabilitation of stroke. J Neurol 259(5):817–892

Angelelli P, Paolucci S, Bivona U, Piccardi L, Ciurli P, Cantagallo A, Antonucci G, Fasotti L, Di Santantonio A, Grasso MG, Pizzamiglio L (2004) Development of neuropsychiatric symptoms in poststroke patients: a cross-sectional study. Acta Psychiatr Scand 110(1):55–63

Arts MLJ, Kwa VIH, Dahmen R (2008) High satisfaction with an individualised stroke care programme after hospitalisation of patients with a TIA or minor stroke: a pilot study. Cerebrovasc Dis 25:566–571

Barker-Collo S, Feigin V (2006) The impact of neuropsychological deficits on functional stroke outcomes. Neuropsychol Rev 16:35–64

Barker-Collo S, Feigin V, Parag V, Lawes C, Senior H (2010) Auckland stroke outcomes study. Part 2: cognition and functional outcomes 5 years post stroke. Neurology 75:1608–1615

Ben-Yishay Y (ed) (1978) Working approaches to remediation of cognitive deficits in brain damaged persons (Rehabilitation Monograph). New York University Medical Center, New York

Ben-Yishay Y (1996) Reflections on the evolution of the therapeutic milieu concept. Neuropsychol Rehabil 6(4):327–343

Ben-Yishay Y, Prigatano GP (1990) Cognitive remediation. In: Rosenthal M, Griffith ER, Bond MR, Miller JD (eds) Rehabilitation of the adult and child with traumatic brain injury, 2nd edn. F. A. Davis, Philadelphia, pp 393–409

Boake C (1996) Editorial: historical aspects of neuropsychological rehabilitation. Neuropsychol Rehabil 6:241–243

Brands IM, Bouwens SF, Wolters Gregório G, Stapert SZ, van Heugten CM (2013) Effectiveness of a process-oriented patient-tailored outpatient neuropsychological rehabilitation programme for patients in the chronic phase after ABI. Neuropsychol Rehabil 23(2):202–215

Burton L, Tyson SF (2015) Screening for cognitive impairment after stroke: a systematic review of psychometric properties and clinical utility. J Rehabil Med 47(3):193–203

Chung CS, Pollock A, Campbell T, Durward BR, Hagen S (2013) Cognitive rehabilitation for executive dysfunction in adults with stroke or other adult non-progressive acquired brain damage. Cochrane Database Syst Rev (4):CD008391

Cicerone KD, Dahlberg C, Kalmar K, Langenbahn DM, Malec JF, Bergquist TF, Felicetti T, Giacino JT, Harley JP, Harrington DE, Herzog J, Kneipp S, Laatsch L, Morse PA (2000) Evidence-based cognitive rehabilitation: recommendations for clinical practice. Arch Phys Med Rehabil 81(12):1596–1615

Cicerone KD, Dahlberg C, Malec JF, Langenbahn DM, Felicetti T, Kneipp S, Ellmo W, Kalmar K, Giacino JT, Harley JP, Laatsch L, Morse PA, Catanese J (2005) Evidence-based cognitive rehabilitation: updated review of the literature from 1998 through 2002. Arch Phys Med Rehabil 86(8):1681–1692

Cicerone KD, Langenbahn DM, Braden C, Malec JF, Kalmar K, Fraas M, Felicetti T, Laatsch L, Harley JP, Bergquist T, Azulay J, Cantor J, Ashman T (2011) Evidence-based cognitive rehabilitation: updated review of the literature from 2003 through 2008. Arch Phys Med Rehabil 92(4):519–530

Cumming TB, Mead G (2017) Classifying post-stroke fatigue: Optimal cut-off on the fatigue assessment scale. J Psychosom Res 103:147–149

Cumming TB, Packer M, Kramer SF, English C (2016) The prevalence of fatigue after stroke: a systematic review and meta-analysis. Int J Stroke 11(9):968–977

das Nair R, Cogger H, Worthington E, Lincoln NB (2016) Cognitive rehabilitation for memory deficits after stroke. Cochrane Database Syst Rev 9(9):CD002293

de Graaf JA, van Mierlo M, Post M, Achterberg W, Kapelle J, Visser-Meily J (2018) Long-term restrictions in participation in stroke survivors under and over 70 years of age. Disabil Rehabil 40(6):637–645

De Wit L, Putman K, Baert I, Lincoln LB, Angst F, Beyens H et al (2008) Anxiety and depression in the first six months after stroke. A longitudinal multicentre study. Disabil Rehabil 30:1858–1866

Diller L (1976) A model for cognitive retraining in rehabilitation. Clin Psychol 29:13–15

Duits AA, Munnecom T, van Heugten CM, Van Oostebrugge RJ (2008) Cognitive and emotional consequences in the early phase after stroke: complaints versus performance. JNNP 79(2):143–146

Duncan PW, Samsa GP, Weinberger M, Goldstein LB, Bonito A, Witter DM, Enarson C, Matchar D (1997) Health status of individuals with mild stroke. Stroke 28(4):740–745

Edwards DF, Hahn M, Baum C, Dromerick AW (2006) The impact of mild stroke on meaningful activity and life satisfaction. J Stroke Cerebrovasc Dis 15:151–157

Elsner B, Kugler J, Pohl M, Mehrholz J (2016) Transcranial direct current stimulation (tDCS) for improving activities of daily living, and physical and cognitive functioning, in people after stroke. Cochrane Database Syst Rev 3(3):CD009645

Fens M, van Heugten C, Beusmans G, Limburg M, Haeren R, Kaemingk A, Metsemakers J (2013) Not as transient: patients with transient ischaemic attack or minor stroke experience cognitive and communication problems; an exploratory study. Eur J Gen Pract 19:11–16

Forster A, Brown L, Smith J, House A, Knapp P, Wright J, Young J (2012) Information provision for stroke patients and their caregivers. Cochrane Database Syst Rev 11(11):CD001919

Geurtsen GJ, van Heugten CM, Martina JD, Geurts AC (2010) Comprehensive rehabilitation programmes in the chronic phase after severe brain injury: a systematic review. J Rehabil Med 42(2):97–110

Gillespie A, Best C, O'Neill B (2012) Cognitive function and assistive technology for cognition: a systematic review. J Int Neuropsychol Soc 18:1–19

Gillespie DC, Bowen A, Chung CS, Cockburn J, Knapp P, Pollock A (2015) Rehabilitation for post-stroke cognitive impairment: an overview of recommendations arising from systematic reviews of current evidence. Clin Rehabil 29(2):120–128

Goldstein K (1919) Die Behandlung, Fürsorge und Begutachtung der Hirnverletzten. Zugleich ein Beitrag zur Verwendung psychologischer Methoden in der Klinik. F.C.W. Vogel, Leipzig

Goldstein K (1942) After-effects of brain injuries in war: their evaluation and treatment. Grune & Stratton, New York

Hachinski V, Iadecola C, Petersen RC, Breteler MM, Nyenhuis DL, Black SE, Powers WJ, DeCarli C, Merino JG, Kalaria RN, Vinters HV, Holtzman DM, Rosenberg GA, Wallin A, Dichgans M, Marler JR, Leblanc GG (2006) National Institute of Neurological Disorders and Stroke-Canadian Stroke Network vascular cognitive impairment harmonization standards. Stroke 37(9):2220–2241

Hackett ML, Anderson C, House A, Halteh A (2008a) Interventions for preventing depression after stroke. Cochrane Database Syst Rev (3):CD003689

Hackett ML, Anderson CS, House A, Xia J (2008b) Interventions for treating depression after stroke. Cochrane Database Syst Rev (4):CD003437

Hackett ML, Yang M, Craig S, Anderson C, Horrocks J, House A (2010) Pharmaceutical interventions for emotionalism after stroke. Cochrane Database Syst Rev (2):CD003690

Hoffmann T, Bennett S, Koh CL, McKenna K (2010) Occupational therapy for cognitive impairment in stroke patients. Cochrane Database Syst Rev 2010(9):CD006430

Huang HC, Huang YC, Lin MF, Hou WH, Shyu ML, Chiu HY, Chang HJ (2017) Effects of home-based supportive care on improvements in physical function and depressive symptoms in patients with stroke: a meta-analysis. Arch Phys Med Rehabil 98(8):1666–1677

Humphreys I, Thomas S, Phillips C, Lincoln N (2015) Cost analysis of the communication and low mood (CALM) randomised trial of behavioural therapy for stroke patients with aphasia. Clin Rehabil 29(1):30–41

Jamieson M, Cullen B, McGee-Lennon M, Brewster B, Evans J (2015) The efficacy of cognitive prosthetic technology for people with memory impairments: a systematic review and meta-analysis. Neuropsychol Rehabi 24(3–4):419–444

Jamieson M, Cullen B, McGee-Lennon M, Brewster B, Evans J (2017) Technological memory aid use by people with acquired brain injury. Neuropsychol Rehabil 27(6):919–936

Knapp P, Campbell Burton C, Holmes J, Murray J, Gillespie D, Lightbody E, Watkins C, Chun H-Y, Lewis S (2017) Interventions for treating anxiety after stroke. Cochrane Database Syst Rev 2017(5):CD008860

Kochanek P, Jackson T, Ferguson N, Carlson S, Simon D et al (2015) Emerging therapies in traumatic brain injury. Semin Neurol 35(1):83–100

Kootker JA, van Mierlo ML, Hendriks JC, Sparidans J, Rasquin SM, de Kort PL, Visser-Meily JM, Geurts AC (2016) Risk factors for symptoms of depression and anxiety one year poststroke: a longitudinal study. Arch Phys Med Rehabil 97(6):919–928

Kouwenhoven SE, Kirkevold M, Engedal K, Kim HS (2011) Depression in acute stroke: prevalence, dominant symptoms, and associated factors. A systematic literature review. Disabil Rehabil 33:539–556

Kutlubaev MA, Mead GE, Lerdal A (2015) Fatigue after stroke--perspectives and future directions. Int J Stroke 10(3):280–281

Langhorne P, Bernhardt J, Kwakkel G (2011) Stroke rehabilitation. Lancet 377(9778): 1693–1702

Linden T, Samuelson H, Skog I, Blomstrand C (2005) Visual neglect and cognitive impairment in elderly patients late after stroke. Acta Neurol Scand 111:163–168

Loetscher T, Lincoln NB (2013) Cognitive rehabilitation for attention deficits following stroke. Cochrane Database Syst Rev 2013(5):CD002842

Mala H, Rasmussen C (2017) The effect of combined therapies on recovery after acquired brain injury: systematic review of preclinical studies combining enriched environment, exercise, or task-specific training with other therapies. Restor Neurol Neurosci 35:25–64

Malec J (2017) Assessment for neuropsychological rehabilitation planning. In: Wilson BA, Winegardner J, van Heugten C, Ownsworth T (eds) Neuropsychological rehabilitation: the international handbook. Routledge Taylor & Francis Group, Cambridge, pp 36–48

Malley D (2017) Managing fatigue in adults after acquired brain injury. In: Wilson BA, Winegardner J, van Heugten C, Ownsworth T (eds) Neuropsychological rehabilitation: the international handbook. Routledge Taylor & Francis Group, Cambridge, pp 391–402

Mandliya A, Das A, Unnikrishnan JP, Amal MG, Sarma PS, Sylaja PN (2016) Post-stroke fatigue is an independent predictor of post-stroke disability and burden of care: a path analysis study. Top Stroke Rehabil 23(1):1–7

Mark RE (2012) Good recovery after stroke may hide widespread cognitive deficits. Eur J Neurol 19(7):e61

Mead GE, Hsieh C, Lee R, Kutlubaev MA, Claxton A, Hankey GJ, Hackett ML (2012) Selective serotonin reuptake inhibitors for stroke recovery. Cochrane Database Syst Rev 11(11):CD009286

Mitchell PH, Veith RC, Becker KJ, Buzaitis A, Cain KC, Fruin M et al (2009) Brief psychosocial-behavioral intervention with antidepressant reduces poststroke depression significantly more than usual care with antidepressant: living well with stroke: randomized, controlled trial. Stroke 40(9):3073–3078

Moran GM, Fletcher B, Feltham MG, Calvert M, Sackley C, Marshall T (2014) Fatigue, psychological and cognitive impairment following transient ischaemic attack and minor stroke: a systematic review. Eur J Neurol 21:1258–1267

Muus I, Petzold M, Ringsberg KC (2010) Health-related quality of life among Danish patients 3 and 12 months after TIA or mild stroke. Scand J Caring Sci 24:211–218

Neren D, Johnson M, Legon W, Bachour S, Lang G, Divani A (2016) Vagus nerve stimulation and other neuromodulation methods for treatment of traumatic brain injury. Neurocrit Care 24:308–319

Nijsse B, van Heugten CM, van Mierlo ML, Post MW, de Kort PL, Visser-Meily JM (2017a) Psychological factors are associated with subjective cognitive complaints 2 months post-stroke. Neuropsychol Rehabil 27(1):99–115

Nijsse B, Visser-Meily JM, van Mierlo ML, Post MW, de Kort PL, van Heugten CM (2017b) Temporal evolution of poststroke cognitive impairment using the montreal cognitive assessment. Stroke 48(1):98–104

Nys G, Van Zandvoort MJ, De Kort PL, Jansen BP, Van der Worp HB, Kapelle LJ, De Haan EH (2005) Domain-specific cognitive recovery after first-ever stroke: a follow-up study of 111 cases. J Int Neuropsychol Soc 11(7):795–806

Oberlin LE, Waiwood AM, Cumming TB, Marsland AL, Bernhardt J, Erickson KI (2017) Effects of physical activity on poststroke cognitive function: a meta-analysis of randomized controlled trials. Stroke 48(11):3093–3100

Owens DK, Lohr KN, Atkins D, Treadwell JR, Reston JT, Bass EB, Chang S, Helfand M (2010) AHRQ series paper 5: grading the strength of a body of evidence when comparing medical interventions--agency for healthcare research and quality and the effective health-care program. J Clin Epidemiol 63:513–523

Platz T (2017) Practice guidelines in neurorehabilitation. Neurol Int Open 1:E148–E152

Prigatano GP (1986) Personality and psychosocial consequences of brain injury. In: Prigatano GP, Fordyce DJ, Zeiner HK, Roueche JR, Pepping M, Wood BC (eds) Neuropsychological rehabilitation after brain injury. The Johns Hopkins University Press, Baltimore, pp 29–50

Radman N, Staub F, Aboulafia-Brakha T, Berney A, Bogousslavsky J, Annoni JM (2012) Poststroke fatigue following minor infarcts. A prospective study. Neurology 79:1422–1427

Rasquin S, Verhey F, Lousberg R, Winkens I, Lodder J (2002) Vascular cognitive disorders: memory, mental speed and cognitive flexibility after stroke. J Neurol Sci 203–204:115–119

Rasquin S, Lodder J, Ponds R, Einkens I, Jolles J, Verhey FR (2004) Cognitive functioning after stroke: a one-year follow up study. Dement Geriatr Cogn Disord 18(2):138–144

Rasquin SM, Bouwens SF, Dijcks B, Winkens I, Bakx WG, van Heugten CM (2010) Effectiveness of a low intensity outpatient cognitive rehabilitation programme for patients in the chronic phase after acquired brain injury. Neuropsychol Rehabil 20(5):760–777

Schünemann H, Brożek J, Guyatt G, Oxman A (2013) GRADE handbook for grading quality of evidence and strength of recommendations. The GRADE Working Group. Updated October 2013. www.guidelinedevelopment.org/handbook

Sivakumar L, Kate M, Jeerakathil T, Camicioli R, Buck B, Butcher K (2014) Serial Montreal cognitive assessments demonstrate reversible cognitive impairment in patients with acute transient ischemic attack and minor stroke. Stroke 45(6):1709–1715

Stolwyk RJ, O'Neill MH, McKay AJ, Wong DK (2014) Are cognitive screening tools sensitive and specific enough for use after stroke?: a systematic literature review. Stroke 45(10): 3129–3134

Suenkeler IH, Nowak M, Misselwitz B, Kugler C, Schreiber W, Oertel WH, Back T (2002) Timecourse of health-related quality of life as determined 3, 6 and 12 months after stroke: relationship to neurological deficit, disability and depression. J Neurol 249:1160–1167

Thomas SA, Walker MF, Macniven JA, Haworth H, Lincoln NB (2013) Communication and low mood (CALM): a randomized controlled trial of behavioural therapy for stroke patients with aphasia. Clin Rehabil 27(5):398–408

Towfighi A, Ovbiagele B, El Husseini N, Hackett ML, Jorge RE, Kissela BM, Mitchell PH, Skolarus LE (2017) Posstroke depression: A scientific statement for healthcare professionals from the american heart assocaition/american stroke association. 48(2):e30–e43

van der Kemp J, Kruithof WJ, Nijboer TCW, van Bennekom CAM, van Heugten C, Visser-Meily JMA (2017) Return to work after mild-to-moderate stroke: work satisfaction and predictive factors. Neuropsychol Rehabil 29(4):638–653

Van der Zwaluw C, Valentijn S, Mark-Nieuwenhuis R, Rasquin S, van Heugten C (2011) Cognitive functioning in the acute phase post stroke: a predictor for discharge destination? J Stroke Cerebrovasc Dis 20(6):549–555

van Dijk EJ, de Leeuw FE (2012) Recovery after stroke: more than just walking and talking again If you don't look for it, you won't find it. Eur J Neurol 19(2):189–190

van Dijk MJ, de Man-van Ginkel JM, Hafsteinsdóttir TB, Schuurmans MJ (2016) Identifying depression post-stroke in patients with aphasia: a systematic review of the reliability, validity and feasibility of available instruments. Clin Rehabil 30(8):795–810

Van Heugten C (2017) Novel forms of cognitive rehabilitation. In: Wilson BA, Winegardner J, van Heugten C, Ownsworth T (eds) Neuropsychological rehabilitation: the international handbook. Routledge Taylor & Francis Group, Cambridge, pp 425–433

van Heugten C, Rasquin S, Winkens I, Beusmans G, Verhey F (2007) Checklist for cognitive and emotional consequences following stroke (CLCE-24): development, usability and quality of the self-report version. Clin Neurol Neurosurg 109(3):257–262

Van Heugten C, Gregório GW, Wade D (2012) Evidence-based cognitive rehabilitation after acquired brain injury: a systematic review of content of treatment. Neuropsychol Rehabil 22(5):653–673

Van Heugten CM, Walton L, Hentschel U (2015) Can we forget the Mini-Mental State Examination? A systematic review of the validity of cognitive screening instruments within one month after stroke. Clin Rehabil 29(7):694–704

van Heugten CM, Ponds RW, Kessels RP (2016) Brain training: hype or hope? Neuropsychol Rehabil 26(5–6):639–644

van Mierlo ML, Schröder C, van Heugten CM, Post MW, de Kort PL, Visser-Meily JM (2014) The influence of psychological factors on health-related quality of life after stroke: a systematic review. Int J Stroke 9(3):341–348

Van Mierlo M, van Heugten C, Post M, de Kort P, Visser-Meily J (2015) Psychological factors determine depressive symptomatology after stroke. Arch Phys Med Rehabil 96(6):1064–1070

van Rijsbergen MW, Mark RE, de Kort PL, Sitskoorn MM (2014) Subjective cognitive complaints after stroke: a systematic review. J Stroke Cerebrovasc Dis 23(3):408–420 van Rijsbergen MW, Mark RE, de Kort PL, Sitskoorn MM (2015) Prevalence and profile of post-stroke subjective cognitive complaints. J Stroke Cerebrovasc Dis 24(8):1823–1831

Verbraak ME, Hoeksma AF, Lindeboom R, Kwa VIH (2012) Subtle problems in activities of daily living after a transient ischemic attack or an apparently fully recovered non-disabling stroke. J Stroke Cerebrovasc Dis 21:124–130

Visser-Keizer AC, Hogenkamp A, Westerhof-Evers HJ, Egberink IJ, Spikman JM (2015) Dutch multifactor fatigue scale: a new scale to measure the different aspects of fatigue after acquired brain injury. Arch Phys Med Rehabil 96(6):1056–1063

Wagle J, Fanrer L, Flekoy K, Bruun Willer T, Sandvik L, Fure B, Stensrod B, Engedal K (2011) Early post-stroke cognition in stroke rehabilitation patients predicts functional outcome at 13 months. Dement Geriatr Cogn Disord 31:379–387

Wessel MJ, Zimmerman M, Hummel FC (2015) Non-invasive brain stimulation: an intervenjtional tool for enhancing behavioral training after stroke. Front Hum Neurosci 9:265

West C, Bowen A, Hesketh A, Vail A (2008) Interventions for motor apraxia following stroke. Cochrane Database Syst Rev 2008(1):CD004132

Whyte EM, Mulsant BH (2002) Post stroke depression: epidemiology, pathophysiology, and biological treatment. Biol Psychiatry 52:253–264

Williams WH, Evans JJ (2003) Biopsychosocial approaches in neurorehabilitation. Special issue. Neuropsychol Rehabil 13(1–2):1–325

Wilson BA, Herbert CM, Shiel A (2003) Behavioral approaches in neuropsychological rehabilitation: Optimising rehabilitation procedures. Psychology Press, Hove

Wilson BA, Evans JJ, Gracey F, Bateman A (2009) Neuropsychological rehabilitation: theory, models, therapy and outcomes. Cambridge University Press, Cambridge

Wilson BA, Winegardner J, van Heugten CM, Ownsworth T (2017) Neuropsychological rehabilitation: the international handbook. Routledge Taylor & Francis Group, Cambridge

Winstein CJ, Stein J, Arena R, Bates B et al (2016) Guidelines for adult stroke rehabilitation and recovery: a guideline for healthcare professionals from the American Heart Association/American Stroke Association. Stroke 47(6):e98–e169

Wogensen E, Mala H, Mogensen J (2015) The effects of exercise on cognitive recovery after acquired brain injury in animal models: a systematic review. Neural Plast 2015:830871

Wu S, Kutlubaev Mansur A, Chun H-Y, Cowey E et al (2015) Interventions for post-stroke fatigue. Cochrane Database Syst Rev 2015(3):CD007030

Yeo S, Lian Z, Mao J, Yau W (2017) Effects of central nervous system drugs on recovery after stroke: a systematic review and meta-analysis of randomized controlled trials. Clin Drug Investig 37:901–928

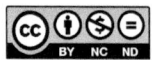

Driving After Stroke

Hannes Devos, Carol A. Hawley, Amber M. Conn,
Shawn C. Marshall, and Abiodun E. Akinwuntan

1   Introduction

From childhood to older ages, there remains a constant, societal fascination with driving. At each stage of life, the autonomy of a motor vehicle provides for independence, freedom and is even in many ways a symbol of success and vitality. Throughout the world, motor vehicles have been entrenched in our lifestyle, our communities, and even our entertainment. In 2013, across 180 countries, there were 947 million registered passenger cars and numbers continue to grow (World Health Organisation 2016). It is from this perspective that persons who have sustained a stroke often find that their inability to return to driving is a major barrier or disappointment along the road to recovery.

From the patient and family perspective, driving allows for independence in the community and the ability to leave the home. Driving is essentially a daily skill taken for granted where 87% of Americans over the age of 16 have a driver's license (Federal Highway Administration 2011). In the United Kingdom, there are 45.5 million licensed drivers representing 74% of the adult population (Driver and Vehicle Licensing Agency 2015). Contrarily, only 25% of the adult Chinese

H. Devos · A. M. Conn · A. E. Akinwuntan
School of Health Professions, University of Kansas Medical Center, Kansas City, KS, USA
e-mail: hdevos@kumc.edu; aakinwuntan@kumc.edu

C. A. Hawley (⊠)
Mental Health and Wellbeing, Division of Health Sciences, Warwick Medical School,
University of Warwick, Coventry, UK
e-mail: C.A.Hawley@warwick.ac.uk

S. C. Marshall
University of Ottawa, Ottawa, ON, Canada

Ottawa Hospital Research Institute, Ottawa, ON, Canada

Bruyere Research Institute, Ottawa, ON, Canada
e-mail: smarshall@toh.ca

© The Author(s) 2021   243
T. Platz (ed.), *Clinical Pathways in Stroke Rehabilitation*,
https://doi.org/10.1007/978-3-030-58505-1_13

population have driver's licenses; however, this represents over 303 million drivers (National Bureau of Statistics 2016). From a clinical perspective, patients who have recovered from the effects of stroke will often ask about driving, or not recognize that driving ability could be affected. Inability to return to driving can have a negative impact on overall health in relation to isolation from community and resources (Waller 1991).

The role of jurisdictions is to keep roadways safe for all drivers. From an administrative perspective, there is an emphasis on public safety versus a focus on having individuals return to driving post-stroke. The evidence for increased crash risk post-stroke is inconclusive (Charlton et al. 2010; Devos et al. 2011). However, there is little doubt that ability to drive for many persons following stroke is clearly affected due to severe impairments that affect patients at an even more basic level of ability to provide self-care. Many countries have policies in relation to need for physician reporting and subsequent assessment prior to return to driving (Charlton et al. 2010). Administrative and financial barriers of paying for assessments are factors that may make it challenging for a patient post-stroke to return to driving.

From the perspective of the healthcare providers, there is often a balance between patient safety and autonomy that must be considered. While patients may want to return to driving post-stroke, there are clear impairments that can affect driving ability. Stroke impairments can be myriad, affecting everything from vision such as diplopia or visual field defects to motor impairments such as hemiparesis or ataxia as common examples. The less well-recognized impairments of visual neglect, cognition impairments, and even behavioral changes post-stroke can also have significant impact on driving ability. In this context, depending on the healthcare provider's jurisdiction, some states, provinces, and countries have reporting laws requiring physicians and other healthcare providers to identify persons who may be at risk to drive due to health reasons. This need to report can often have negative effects on the physician–patient relationship (Jang et al. 2007; Marshall and Gilbert 1999).

The impact of impairments from stroke on an individual can have significant implications for return to driving. This scenario is often counter to the more common scenario for physicians who may need to determine when health impacts for older drivers are at a point where driving cessation needs to be considered. Following stroke in most instances, patients are immediately unable to drive. Through recovery, they may reach a point where their abilities, while not fully recovered, may be at a stage where they are able to resume driving safely. Visual, physical, cognitive, and behavioral impairments post-stroke may all impact the ability to return to driving. It is often the healthcare provider who must make decisions if the patient has recovered enough to resume driving or be further assessed for their potential to return to driving.

While these health factors can affect the ability to drive, it is not only health that plays a role in the ability to return to driving. Using Michon's hierarchical model of driving (Fig. 1), driving can be broken down into stages each with inherent risks (Michon 1985). At the strategic level, drivers make general plans about their driving about destination, routes, identifying driving conditions such as weather and then

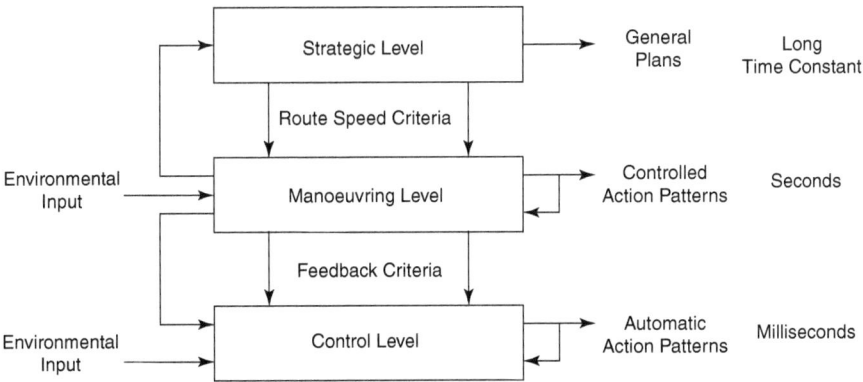

Fig. 1 Michon's hierarchical model of driving (Michon 1985). (Reproduced with permission)

formulating a plan. At this stage, the driver is accepting the risks associated with the driving task. The next level is the tactical level where the driver maneuvers in relation to the driving task and is essentially taking risk. For example, a driver exceeds the speed limit in inclement weather or performs maneuvers such as tailgating or aggressive passing. These actions may put the driver or others at increased risk of collision. In the final operational level of Michon's model, the driver is dealing with acute danger or risk and must take action to avoid a collision. The ability to avoid collision in this instance relies on factors such as reaction time, agility, and past experience of how to successfully control the vehicle in relation to actions such as steering and braking.

Often patients who have had a stroke have significant past driving experience; however, driving experience and ability are highly variable, and confidence may be high since driving is almost an overlearned and automatic task with most elements considered routine. For example, professional drivers or persons who have specialized driving training such as police or ambulance drivers would most likely have a higher skill set for driving compared to individuals who primarily use driving on a leisure or commuting basis. Many people are confident in their driving ability; however, as collision rates for young drivers demonstrate, experience and risk taking do play a role in driving risk (National Research Council US 2007).

Ultimately, return to driving post-stroke is seen by patient and family as both an indicator of recovery and an even more needed ability to compensate for newly reduced mobility. Clinicians typically are expected to advocate for return to driving but must do so responsibly for both the safety of the patient and the society. Many patients will be able to return to driving post-stroke, and the decisions faced by clinicians will be to determine when the patient has reached the ability to be considered for return to driving and what evaluations or rehabilitation interventions can be reliably used. The aim for both patient and healthcare provider is to have a safe return to driving, if possible, in the most expedient manner. The determination of this is critical for patient safety, autonomy, and health.

2 Evidence-Based Practice in Driving Screening, Assessment, and Interventions

A PubMed database search conducted on November 27, 2018 using the medical subject headings (MeSH) key terms "automobile driving" and "stroke" revealed 105 studies on driving after stroke. Research on this topic has seen an exponential increase in the last decade, with more than half (58) of the research articles being published since 2010. This growing body of evidence may assist healthcare professionals in the evidence-based practice (EBP) of assessing fitness-to-drive after stroke. EBP is a clinical decision-making process within a specific healthcare setting that integrates the best available scientific evidence with the best available clinical expertise from a multidisciplinary team of healthcare providers (Sackett et al. 1996). EBP considers internal and external influences on practice and encourages critical thinking in the judicious application of such evidence to the care of individual patients, a patient population, or a system (Newhouse et al. 2005).

In this section, we will provide an evidence-based overview of three critical issues related to driving after stroke: (1) screening; (2) assessment; and (3) interventions. Later, we will show how the evidence drives clinical decision-making for fitness-to-drive after stroke using an actual case scenario.

2.1 Screening for Fitness-to-Drive

The goal of a clinical screening tool is to identify individuals who meet the legal criteria for driving, but exhibit functional deficits that may adversely affect their fitness-to-drive. A fail performance on the screening battery warrants a more detailed assessment at a specialized driving clinic. The clinical utility of these screening tools depends on their efficacy in predicting on-road driving outcomes, the administration time, the ease of use, and the costs to purchase the tools. Although most screening tools lack face validity, some batteries have been developed particularly for fitness-to-drive screening after stroke. The Stroke Drivers Screening Assessment (SDSA) is one of such screening tools that was originally developed in the United Kingdom (Nouri and Lincoln 1993), but has successfully been adopted for use in other European countries (Selander et al. 2010; Lundberg et al. 2003), Australia (George and Crotty 2010), Israel (Lincoln et al. 2016), Korea (Park et al. 2013), and the United States (Akinwuntan et al. 2013). The SDSA consists of four subtests: (1) Dot Cancellation, (2) Directions, (3) Compass, and (4) Road Sign Recognition. A prediction equation algorithm that includes the results of each of the subtests shows the likelihood of passing or failing an on-road driving assessment (Selander et al. 2010; Lundberg et al. 2003; Nouri and Lincoln 1993; Akinwuntan et al. 2013; Park et al. 2013). However, these prediction equations suffer from methodological limitations such as subject and cultural bias and have rarely been validated in independent cohorts. No information is available on the prediction rates of the SDSA and other screening tools in developing countries.

One way to bypass these limitations is to pool all evidence on screening tools for fitness-to-drive after stroke. In our PubMed search, we identified four systematic reviews listing the most accurate screening tools for fitness-to-drive after stroke (Hird et al. 2014; Murie-fernandez et al. 2014; Devos et al. 2011; Marshall et al. 2007). None of the proposed screening tools are perfect in predicting on-road driving performance. Yet, four tests emerged from the systematic reviews to best predict the likelihood of failing an on-road driving assessment: (1) the Compass and (2) Road Sign Recognition tests of the SDSA; (3) the Trail Making Test (TMT) B; and (4) the Rey-Osterrieth Complex Figure (ROCF). Table 1 shows the psychometric properties, cutoff values, approximate administration time, training required, and approximate cost of these four tests. We also assigned the Oxford Centre for Evidence-Based Medicine–Levels of Evidence (OCEBM Levels of Evidence Working Group 2011) and Grades of Recommendation (Schünemann et al. 2013; Platz 2017) for each of the four tests. The description of the levels and quality of evidence and grades of recommendations is detailed in chapter "Clinical Pathways in Stroke Rehabilitation: Background, Scope, and Methods" (Chap. 2). The Compass, Road Sign Recognition, and Trail Making Test B showed acceptable sensitivity at the expense of specificity.

2.2 Assessment of Fitness-to-Drive

Compared to the screening process, an assessment of fitness-to-drive is a more formal, elaborate procedure that typically involves clinical (off-road) assessments of motor, cognitive, and visual abilities prior to a practical on-road driving test. The procedure for assessment of fitness-to-drive varies across countries depending on the legal framework, the licensing systems, and the resources available. Fitness-to-drive assessments take many shapes depending on location and include: medical tests, purpose-built driving assessment centers, clinical off-road and practical on-road comprehensive tests performed by driving assessors, healthcare workers, and/or driving licensing agencies. The driving-related functions commonly tested after stroke include: memory, attention, visuospatial perception, spatial neglect, sensory and motor functions, and vision (e.g., hemianopia). These assessments are usually conducted by physicians, psychologists, occupational therapists, or physical therapists with specialized training in fitness-to-drive assessments. Both the clinical off-road and on-road assessment protocols reported in the literature differ between studies, usually due to the country in which the study was conducted (Devos et al. 2011). Although there is still no commonly accepted standardized and validated battery to determine the fitness-to-drive of stroke survivors, many studies have identified some common cognitive, visual, and motor skills that predict performance on an on-road driving test (Ranchet et al. 2016; Devos et al. 2014; Aslaksen et al. 2013; Ponsford et al. 2008).

Apart from being the assessment used officially in countries around the world for licensing novice drivers, the on-road test is the only assessment that bears similarity and face validity to real-world driving. As such, the on-road assessment was used as

Table 1 Clinical utility of the screening tools[a]

Tool	Reliability[b]	Validity[c]	OCEBM LOE	GOR	Cutoff score[d]	Sensitivity (95% CI)	Specificity (95% CI)	PPV (95% CI)	NPV (95% CI)	Admin time	Training required	Equipment	Cost
Compass	r_s = 0.73 (Lincoln and Fanthome 1994)	ES = 1.06 (0.74–1.39) (Devos et al. 2011)	1a	B+	25	85% (74–93%)	54% (43–65%)	56% (50–62%)	84% (74–91%)	5 min	Minimal	Board and cards	$200[e]
Road Sign Recognition	r_s = 0.67 (Lincoln and Fanthome 1994)	ES = 1.22 (1.01–1.44) (Devos et al. 2011)	1a	B+	8.5	84% (72–92%)	54% (44–65%)	56% (50–62%)	83% (73–90%)	3 min	Minimal	Board and cards	$200[e]
Trail Making Test B	r = 0.67 (Tucker et al. 1981)	ES = 0.81 (0.48–1.15) (Devos et al. 2011)	1a	B+	90s	80% (66–90%)	62% (42–79%)	78% (69–85%)	64% (49–77%)	5 min	Minimal	Paper and pencil	$50 for 100 copies
Rey-Osterrieth Complex Figure	ICC = 0.94 (Tupler et al. 1995)	ES = 0.80 (Akinwuntan et al. 2007)	1a	0	N/R	N/R	N/R	N/R	N/R	No time limit	Minimal	Paper and pencil	Free

CI confidence interval; *ES* effect size, calculated as the absolute difference in mean values on the test of interest between the pass and fail groups, divided by the pooled variance; *GOR* grades of recommendation; *ICC* intra-class coefficient; *LOE* levels of evidence; *OCEBM* Oxford Centre for Evidence Based Medical scale; *r* Pearson correlation coefficient; *PPV* positive predictive value; *NPV* negative predictive value; r_s Spearman rho correlation

[a]Information was partly extracted from references Devos et al. (2011) and Burns et al. (2018)

[b]Test–retest reliability

[c]Criterion validity against on-road driving outcome

[d]From Devos et al. (2011)

[e]Cost of the SDSA battery provided by publisher on 12/2017

the criterion for assessing driving performance in most studies reported on driving after stroke (Nouri and Lincoln 1993; Lundqvist et al. 2000; Akinwuntan et al. 2006). Yet, the use of the on-road assessment as the best indicator of fitness-to-drive of stroke survivors remains controversial. Some of the concerns include lack of repeatability of traffic events, reduced access to dual operated vehicle, the inability to assess driving ability during hazardous traffic situations or inclement weather conditions, the large variation in traffic demands and routes, different scoring systems, and low inter-rater reliability due to inconsistencies in judging the on-road driving performance by experts. These concerns prompted researchers to investigate the usefulness of novel assessment methods, including driving simulation technology, as indicators of the true driving capabilities of stroke survivors (Blane et al. 2017; Hird et al. 2015; Kobayashi et al. 2016; Park 2015). Many recent studies have reported on the use of driving simulators in the assessment of fitness-to-drive of stroke survivors (Akinwuntan and Devos 2017).

2.3 Interventions for Fitness-to-Drive

The body of literature on interventions to improve driving after stroke is sparse (George et al. 2014). The authors of this Cochrane review concluded that based on four randomized controlled trials and 245 participants, there was insufficient evidence that a driving rehabilitation program was effective in improving driving skills after stroke.

It is nevertheless reasonable to assume that any training is better than no training at all. Different methods of training can be categorized as (1) non-contextual training using paper and pencil, computerized-video or specialized equipment or (2) contextual training in a simulator or on the road. Hence, the related evidence will be summarized next.

2.3.1 Non-contextual Training

Non-contextual training is a remedial form of training that targets the visual, motor, and cognitive deficits underlying impaired on-road driving performance in stroke survivors. Although the benefits from the training program are purported to generalize to improvements in on-road driving performance, there is little evidence to support the claim.

Cognitive training using specialized equipment such as the Useful Field of View® (UFOV) or Dynavision® generally show benefits of training on on-road driving skills after stroke in non-randomized or pilot randomized controlled trials (RCTs) (Klavora and Warren 1998; Mazer et al. 2001). However, in the only RCT comparing the effect of 18 sessions of Dynavision® training ($n = 13$) with a non-active control group ($n = 13$), no differences in pass rates on the on-road test (77% vs. 46%; $p = 0.23$) were found after training (Crotty and George 2009). Although the study was likely underpowered due to the small sample size, a difference in pass percentages of 31% in favor of the Dynavision® training group appears clinically relevant. Likewise, Mazer et al. (2003)

compared 20 sessions of visual attention training using the UFOV training (n = 47) with traditional computerized visuoperceptual training (n = 50). Although no differences on on-road driving were found between the UFOV (39%) and control intervention (33%; p = 0.53), stroke survivors with right-sided lesions (52%) were almost twice more likely to pass the road test after UFOV training compared to those with left-sided lesions (29%) (Mazer et al. 2003).

In addition, cognitive skills that were specifically targeted in the intervention program show greater improvement compared to a control intervention. Crotty and George (2009) demonstrated a significant improvement in the Dynavision® group compared to the control group on visual neglect task (p = 0.007) and a response time task (p = 0.03; no measures of central tendency reported). Mazer et al. (2003) could not corroborate a differential effect of UFOV® training with other visuoperceptual training on any of the cognitive outcomes.

2.3.2   Contextual Training

With the advent of more realistic graphic images, higher fidelity of the driving simulator steering wheel and pedals, and the improving flexibility of interactive programming language, the use of driving simulators has sparked great interest in the scientific and clinical community to retrain driving-related skills after stroke. One RCT found that 15 h of training in a driving simulator was superior to a non-contextual training program that included paper-and-pencil route finding activities and board games in 73 stroke survivors. Participants who received simulator training were more likely to succeed on a formal on-road driving test at 3 months after training compared to those who received non-contextual training (73% versus 42%; p = 0.03) (Akinwuntan et al. 2005). The encouraging benefits of simulator training were confirmed in a more recent trial that compared 16 h of training in the driving simulator (n = 23) with no training (n = 22) (Mazer et al. 2015). Following completion of training, 6 out of 7 (86%) participants with moderate stroke-related deficits who were trained in the driving simulator passed an on-road test whereas only 1 out of 6 (17%) in the control group passed the same on-road test (p = 0.03, effect size = 0.63). However, there were no differences for those with severe impairments (Mazer et al. 2015).

It is logical to assume that training of driving skills on a real road, in a real car, in real traffic, will result in most generalization of benefits from training to driving performance in real traffic. In a small study that included 15 participants with stroke who initially failed an on-road test, 13 eventually passed the test after 6–12 h of on-road driving training. However, authors doubt if the on-road training program led to improvement in driving skills since there were no associated improvements in any visuo-cognitive functions. The authors surmised that the natural recovery of stroke, awareness of driving difficulties, or familiarization with the test process led to passing the driving test after the intervention program (Soderstrom et al. 2006).

3   Adaptive Driver Assistance Systems and Car Modifications

There is emerging research on the impact of Advanced Driver Assistive Systems (ADAS) for older adults with and without medical conditions (Shaheen and Niemeier 2001; Davidse 2006; Davidse et al. 2009). These studies show that some ADAS systems, including but not limited to—*lane departure warnings, lane keeping support, automated cruise control, collision avoidance systems, pedestrian crash avoidance mitigation, night vision systems, driver fatigue warning systems, turning assist, surround view, and traffic sign recognition*—could extend the older drivers' mobility and have the capacity to improve road safety. In a driving simulator study, Dotzauer et al. (2013) studied the effects of an intersection ADAS on driving in healthy older adults. Equipped with ADAS, drivers allocated more attention to the center of the road and crossed intersections in shorter time, but also engaged in higher speeds and accepted more risk in taking left turns against oncoming vehicles. To our knowledge, no studies have evaluated the use of ADAS to improve driving safety in drivers with stroke.

The other areas of technological aids for driving are disability vehicle adaptations that are used to maintain or improve the functional capabilities of an individual with disabilities. Common examples of this are a spinner steering driving knob which enables one-handed steering and a left-side accelerator that can assist someone with hemiparesis to resume driving of an automatic transmission vehicle.

4   Clinical Pathway

Rules for fitness-to-drive vary between countries, states, and provinces. It is important for healthcare providers to familiarize themselves with the specific licensing requirements and clinical guidelines for driving after stroke in their own locality. Figure 2 below offers a framework for driving assessment and intervention after mild stroke which is based on best evidence and practice.

Our review of evidence examined screening, assessment, and interventions. Based on this evidence, Fig. 3, along with the following broad-based recommendations, presents a clinical algorithm for fitness-to-drive to aid decision-making. The description of the levels and quality of evidence and grades of recommendations is detailed in chapter "Clinical Pathways in Stroke Rehabilitation: Background, Scope, and Methods" (Chap. 2).

1. Determine that the patient meets the jurisdiction's minimum requirement for driving (if any) (level of evidence/quality of evidence: not applicable (regulatory), A+).
2. If there are specific requirements for driving after stroke in the jurisdiction, refer to it and ensure the patient meets the requirements (level of evidence/

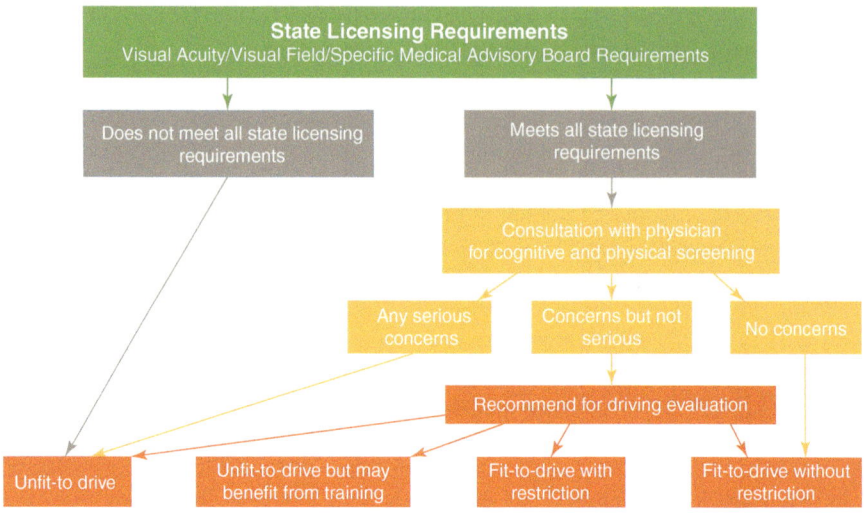

Fig. 2 Framework for driving assessment and intervention after stroke based on best evidence and practice. (Permission to use from Burns et al. 2018)

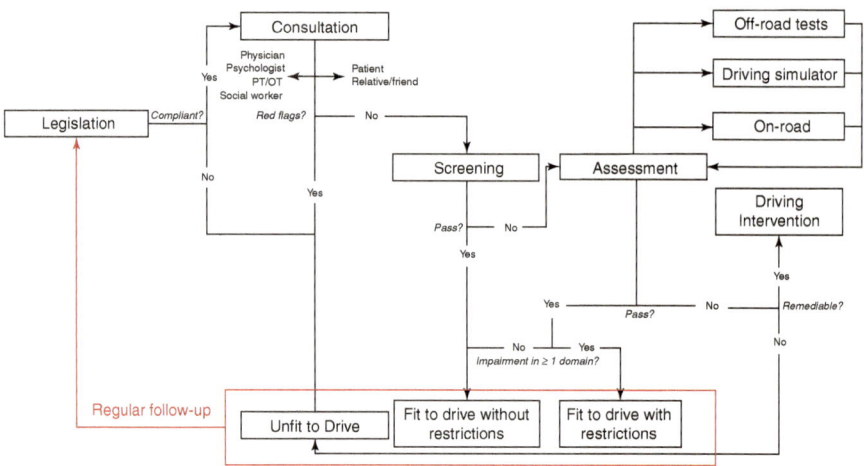

Fig. 3 Clinical decision rule for fitness-to-drive after stroke. (Permission to use from De Baets et al. (2018). Complex Case Management. Physical Management for Neurological Conditions)

quality of evidence: not applicable (regulatory), A+). Clinical guidelines for stroke and driving in several countries stipulate a preclusion period of 4 weeks post event (Austroads 2016; Canadian Medical Association 2017; Driver and Vehicle Licensing Agency 2018), although some countries mandate a driving ban up to 6 months after stroke (Devos et al. 2012).

3. If the patient does not meet one or more of the jurisdiction's prescribed requirements, the patient ought to be advised to allow more time for better recovery and/or discuss alternative transportation methods (level of evidence 5, quality of evidence very low, A+).

4. Red flags ought first to be assessed, i.e. risk of recurring stroke, risk of epileptic seizures or severe neglect, and others listed below (level of evidence 5, quality of evidence very low, A+). Red flags are usually exclusion criteria that preclude patients from driving legally. These vary between countries and jurisdictions. It should be noted that this is a non-exhaustive list and healthcare providers should consult medical guidelines for fitness-to-drive which apply locally.

   (a) Uncontrolled medical status.
   (b) Uncontrolled epilepsy.
   (c) Severe neglect.
   (d) Hemianopia that patients cannot compensate for.
   (e) Marked cognitive or behavior impairment such as impulsivity, aggression, anosognosia and severe dementia.

5. Then, screening tools such as the ones presented in Table 1 should be used to determine patients whose functional deficit(s) is(are) reason(s) for concerns (level of evidence 1a, quality of evidence moderate, B+).

6. If the outcome of the screening shows concerns, the patient should be referred for a comprehensive fitness-to-drive assessment with a driving rehabilitation specialist, if available (level of evidence 1a, quality of evidence moderate, B+).

7. The off-road part of the fitness-to-drive assessment (e.g., Table 2) ought to include tests of monocular and binocular visual acuities and visual field; cognitive testing to ascertain general cognitive status also needs to be done; finally, basic motor testing of strength, coordination, and range of motion should be assessed. However, there is no consensus on the selection of tests to include in the assessment (level of evidence 5, quality of evidence very low, A+).

8. If the outcome of the off-road assessment shows some, but no serious concern, the patient should be referred for a practical on-road test (if available) to confirm the suitability to resume driving with or without restrictions (level of evidence 5, quality of evidence very low, B+). The driving assessment expert will determine if the patient has enough compensatory skill to be declared fit-to-drive with or without restrictions or fit-to-drive with vehicle aids or will benefit from driving-specific rehabilitation or unfit-to-drive. Not all countries use conditional licensing, and in these cases, driving may only resume if the patient is fit to drive.

9. If driving-specific rehabilitation is warranted, contextual training in a driving simulator is preferred for maximum generalization of benefit, although non-contextual training has also shown moderate benefit (level of evidence 1a, quality of evidence low (imprecision, inconsistency), B+). Retraining can also be offered in the form of lessons with a driving instructor in a dual controlled vehicle (level of evidence 4, quality of evidence very low, 0).

10. If the patient is found unfit to drive, alternative transportation methods should be discussed with the patient (level of evidence 5, quality of evidence very low, A+).

Table 2 Results of Mr. Smith's Driving Assessment (areas of concern are italicized in table)

Physical/sensory	
Range of motion of the neck/ torso	*Reduced bilaterally, neck and torso*
Range of motion of the major joints of upper and lower limbs	110-degree shoulder level (left torn rotator cuff), 100-degree/ slightly reduced hip flexion bilaterally, reduced left ankle flexion. Within functional range for driving
Strength in limbs	4/5 left, 5/5 right
Cylindrical and pincer grip	Within functional range for driving
Balance with static sitting/ dynamic sitting, and static standing/dynamic standing	Romberg negative: balance within functional range for driving
Barthel Index Score	95/100
Rapid Pace Walk test	7.1 s (>7.5 s = $2.5 \times$ risk, >9 s = $3 \times$ risk) (Mielenz et al. 2017)
Brake reaction test (using driving simulator)	3.57 s, inside of the corresponding age-based average normal value on the same task (Akinwuntan et al. 2009)
Other; coordination, vehicle transfers, proprioception, sensation, tremor, response speed, tone, pain	All normal
Visual assessment using a visual screening apparatus, no visual aids used with test.	
[a]Far acuity, contrast sensitivity, glare recovery, [a]peripheral horizontal visual field	Satisfactory
Stereopsis (depth)	60%, Level 3, unsatisfactory
Cognitive/Perceptual	
SDSA Dot cancellation Directions [b]Compass [b]Road Sign Recognition Prediction of pass or fail	− Time 721 s, 12 errors, 1 false positive 28/32 22/32 (cut off score is 25, Devos et al. 2011) 9/12 (cut of score is 8.5, Devos et al. 2011) Difference Value: + 0.951 pass (Akinwuntan et al. 2013)
Trail Making Test A	51 s (age-based norm value = 42 ± 15 s) (Tombaugh 2004)
[b]Trail Making Test B	*150 s (age-based norm value = 101 ± 44 s)* (Tombaugh 2004)
[b]Rey-Osterrieth Complex Figure (copy)	30/36 (age-based norm value = 31 ± 4) (Fastenau et al. 2010)
MoCA	*25/30, lost 1 point for recall, 2 for attention, and 2 for visuospatial/executive (≤ 26 = possible impairment)* (Nasreddine et al. 2005)
Maze test	Time seconds 38, risk category: safe risk (<60 s) (Barco et al. 2014)

Table 2 (continued)

Physical/sensory	
Useful Field of View (UFOV)	–
Processing speed	*14.8 ms suggestive of normal processing speed*
Divided attention	*258 ms suggesting some difficulty with divided attention*
Selective attention	*500 ms suggesting severe difficulty with selective attention*
Category risk report	*Risk category: moderate risk, 3* (Visual Awareness Research Group 2009)
Other; Insight, communication, endurance, praxis	*Reduced insight into driving limitations*
On-road Practical Test	
Competencies	Demonstrated following competencies: pedal/steering control, follow distance, gap selection, lane position, mirror/indicator use, stop signs, signage, intersections, and road rule knowledge
Performance	Slow cautious driving performance, demonstrating problem-solving, and anticipatory responses. Overtook vehicles and blocked road obstacle in appropriate manner. Too slow at times and demonstrated some difficulties with parking
Non-critical errors	*2× driving too slow, driving 45 km/h in 60 km/h zone. Parking: Unable to turn adequately to check if clear for reversing of car, however used mirrors satisfactory Disoriented when trying to find exit point from carpark*
Critical errors	Nil observed

The tests used here are a select few of a multitude available
MOCA Montreal Cognitive Assessment, *SDSA* Stroke Drivers Screening Assessment
[a]Regulatory standard
[b]Evidence-based screening tools

5   Case Example: Mr. Smith's Driving Assessment

A 75-year-old male sustained a right-hemispheric stroke lesion. Pre-stroke comorbidities included history of smoking, mild osteoarthritis of the spine, and hypertension. As per the hospital medical guidelines, Mr. Smith was advised not to drive for 1 month post event. In a follow-up visit with his neurologist, Mr. Smith was asked if he could resume driving; however, in that same visit, Mr. Smith's wife expressed concerns about this. The neurologist conducted a clinical assessment that included physical, visual, and cognitive tests. His visual acuity was tested as within the visual driving standards of 6/12 (20/40) in both eyes, and a confrontation visual field test did not suggest any peripheral difficulties. Mr. Smith scored 25/30 on the Montreal Cognitive Assessment (MoCA) indicating impairment (≤26 cutoff) (Nasreddine et al. 2005). The neurologist determined that Mr. Smith has ongoing mild left-sided hemiparesis and executive and visuospatial issues. He was uncertain about Mr. Smith's functional ability to drive, so referred him to a driving assessor for a fitness-to-drive determination.

Three weeks later, Mr. Smith underwent an off-road, clinical assessment and an on-road, practical assessment. The off-road clinical evaluation examines physical, visual, sensory, and cognitive abilities specific to driving and identifies any problem skill areas for the on-road test to focus on. Prior to both assessments, Mr. Smith's demographic data, driving particulars, relevant medical history was obtained, and he reviewed and signed the informed consent and release of information form. His driver's license was valid and standard, he drove a medium-sized automatic transmission car, avoided busy traffic times, and had been driving about 16,000 km annually prior to stroke event. He reported no history of traffic violations or motor vehicle crashes in the past 5 years. His falls history was documented as falls in older adults is associated with significantly increased risk of subsequent crash risk (Scott et al. 2017).

A battery of off-road tests was administered and some of these results are outlined in Table 2.

The on-road practical test took place on a separate day with the same occupational therapist driving assessor in a dual operated car. The test took 50 min to complete and included a standardized route with a residential area, strip mall with pedestrian crossings, traffic light intersections, stop sign intersections, roundabout, change of lanes, left and right-hand turns, and a forward single space car park between two parked cars. A competency and error checklist were used to record Mr. Smith's performance and covered: gap selection, follow distance, lane position, brake reaction, indicator/mirror use, speed observance, parking, intersections, road rule knowledge, driver interventions, and critical and non-critical errors.

5.1   Interpretation of Results

Physically, client is generally within functional standards for driving task. Range of motion issues was detected related to neck and torso turns which affect ability to safely perform over shoulder checks and looking behind vehicle for reversing.

Client meets visual standards in terms of visual acuity. Mildly impaired depth perception apparent.

Satisfactory cognitive results in relation to, Trail Making Test A, Rey Osterrieth Complex Figure, Road Sign Recognition, overall pass value of the SDSA, and Snellgrove Maze test. The results of Trail Making Test B, MoCA, Compass, and UFOV (divided and selective attention) demonstrated mild-to-moderate impairments in areas of visuospatial, memory, planning, attention, problem-solving, task switching, and mental flexibility.

Mr. Smith performed well on the on-road practical car test, demonstrating safe skills. He experienced difficulties with parking and was unable to turn and safely check rearview when reversing car, however, demonstrated satisfactory use of his mirrors. Could not remember the entry/exit point of carpark. Client has an older vehicle with no reverse sensor or camera technology and already has a disability parking card.

Recommendations:
1. Due to issues with range of movement in neck and torso, depth perception, planning, problem-solving, memory, and reduced attentional ability, the following is recommended: local area restriction, automatic transmission, blind spot mirrors, and reverse sensors or reverse camera technology installed. Mr. Smith was pro-

vided with contact details for purchase of equipment and a mechanic to install the recommended equipment.

2. Mr. Smith is to be provided with 3–4 rehabilitation training sessions to educate him on driving with specialized mirrors and reversing technology and practice parking.

3. Contingent on successful completion of rehabilitation training sessions, the following driving recommendations are provided to Mr. Smith: automatic transmission only, 10-km radius restriction from place of residence, and installation of blind spot mirrors and reverse technology.[1]

4. Reevaluation in 1 year or sooner if Mr. Smith's medical condition deteriorates or he experiences a secondary stroke.

Copies of the assessment report were sent to: Mr. Smith, Neurologist, and driving licensing agency (if appropriate).

6 Summary

The decision-making process of fitness-to-drive after stroke is multidisciplinary and complex. We recommend the use of evidence-based screening tools such as the Compass test, Road Sign Recognition Test, Trail Making Test B, and the Rey-Osterrieth Complex Figure to determine who should undergo a formal driving evaluation. A final decision on fitness-to-drive should be made after an on-road driving test, preferably complemented with a detailed battery of visual, motor, cognitive, and behavioral tests. If training is required, contextual training in a driving simulator may be more beneficial than non-contextual cognitive training.

References

Akinwuntan AE, Devos H (2017) Simulated driving performance of stroke survivors. In: Classen S (ed) Driving simulation for assessment, intervention, and training: a guide for occupational therapy and health care providers. AOTA Press, Bethesda, pp 251–261

Akinwuntan AE, De Weerdt W, Feys H et al (2005) Effect of simulator training on driving after stroke: a randomized controlled trial. Neurology 65:843–850

Akinwuntan AE, Feys H, De Weerdt W et al (2006) Prediction of driving after stroke: a prospective study. Neurorehabil Neural Repair 20:417–423

Akinwuntan AE, Devos H, Feys H et al (2007) Confirmation of the accuracy of a short battery to predict fitness-to-drive of stroke survivors without severe deficits. J Rehabil Med 39:698–702

Akinwuntan AE, Tank R, Vaughn I et al (2009) Normative values for driving simulation parameters: a pilot study. In: Proceedings of the fifth international driving symposium on human factors in driver assessment, training and vehicle design. Public Policy Centre, Iowa, pp 161–168

Akinwuntan AE, Gantt D, Gibson G et al (2013) United states version of the stroke driver screening assessment: a pilot study. Top Stroke Rehabil 20:87–92

---

[1] If the country's system provides for license conditions or restrictions, then X radius restriction and vehicle aids and equipment would be valid items to add to driver's license.

Aslaksen PM, Orbo M, Elvestad R et al (2013) Prediction of on-road driving ability after traumatic brain injury and stroke. Eur J Neurol 20:1227–1233

Austroads (2016) Assessing fitness to drive for commercial and private vehicle drivers: medical standards for licensing and clinical management guidelines. National Transport Commission, Sydney

Barco PP, Wallendorf MJ, Snellgrove CA et al (2014) Predicting road test performance in drivers with stroke. Am J Occup Ther 68:221–229

Blane A, Lee HC, Falkmer T et al (2017) Assessing cognitive ability and simulator-based driving performance in poststroke adults. Behav Neurol 2017(1378308):1–9. https://doi.org/10.1155/2017/1378308

Burns SP, Schwartz JK, Scott SL et al (2018) Interdisciplinary approaches to facilitate return to driving and return to work in mild stroke: a position paper. Arch Phys Med Rehabil 99:2378–2388

Canadian Medical Association (2017) CMA driver's guide: determining medical fitness to operate motor vehicles, 9th edn. Joule Inc., Ontario

Charlton JL, Koppel S, Odell M et al (2010) Influence of chronic illness on crash involvement of motor vehicle drivers. Report nr 300, 2nd edn. Monash University Accident Research Centre, Victoria

Crotty M, George S (2009) Retraining visual processing skills to improve driving ability after stroke. Arch Phys Med Rehabil 90:2096–3002

Davidse R (2006) Older drivers and adas—which systems improve road safety? SWOV Institute for Road Safety Research, Hague

Davidse RJ, Hagenzieker MP, van Wolffelaar P, Brouwer WH (2009) Effects of in-car support on mental workload and driving performance of older driver. Hum Factors 51:463–476

De Baets L, Ashford S, Devos H et al (2018) Complex case management. In: Stokes E, Stack E (eds) Physical management for neurological conditions, 3rd edn. Eslevier, London

Devos H, Akinwuntan A, Gelinas I, George S, Nieuwboer A, Verheyden G (2012). Shifting up a gear: considerations on assessment and rehabilitation of driving in people with neurological conditions. An extended editorial. Physiotherapy Research International 17:125–131

Devos H, Akinwuntan AE, Nieuwboer A et al (2011) Screening for fitness to drive after stroke: a systematic review and meta-analysis. Neurology 76:747–756

Devos H, Tant M, Akinwuntan AE (2014) On-road driving impairments and associated cognitive deficits after stroke. Cerebrovasc Dis 38:226–232

Dotzauer M, Caljouw SR, de Waard D, Brouwer WH (2013) Intersection assistance: a safe solution for older drivers? Accid Anal Prev 59:522–528

Driver and Vehicle Licensing Agency (2015) How many people hold driving licences in the UK, Swansea. https://www.gov.uk/government/organisations/driver-and-vehicle-licensing-agency. Accessed 3 May 2018

Driver and Vehicle Licensing Agency (2018) Assessing fitness to drive: a guide for medical professionals. Swansea, UK

Fastenau PS, Denburg NL, Hufford BJ (2010) Adult norms for the Rey-Osterrieth complex figure test and for supplemental recognition and matching trials from the extended complex figure test. Clin Neuropsychol 13:30–47

Federal Highway Administration (2011) Our nation's highways 2011, Washington, DC. https://www.fhwa.dot.gov/policyinformation/pubs/hf/pl11028/

George S, Crotty M (2010) Establishing criterion validity of the useful field of view assessment and stroke drivers' screening assessment: comparison to the result of on-road assessment. Am J Occup Ther 64:114–122

George S, Crotty M, Gelinas I et al (2014) Rehabilitation for improving automobile driving after stroke. Cochrane Database Syst Rev 2014(2):CD008357

Hird MA, Vetivelu A, Saposnik G et al (2014) Cognitive, on-road, and simulator-based driving assessment after stroke. J Stroke Cerebrovasc Dis 23:2654–2670

Hird MA, Vesely KA, Christie LE et al (2015) Is it safe to drive after acute mild stroke? A preliminary report. J Neurol Sci 354:46–50

Jang W, Man-Son-Hing M, Molnar FJ et al (2007) Family physicians' attitudes and practices regarding assessments of medical fitness to drive in older persons. J Gen Intern Med 22:531–543

Klavora P, Warren M (1998) Rehabilitation of visuomotor skills in poststroke patients using the dynavision apparatus. Percept Mot Skills 86:23–30

Kobayashi Y, Omokute Y, Mitsuyama A et al (2016) Predictors of track test performance in drivers with stroke. Turk Neurosurg 27:530–536

Lincoln NB, Fanthome Y (1994) Reliability of the stroke drivers screening assessment. Clin Rehabil 8:157–160

Lincoln NB, Radford KA, Nouri FM (2016) Stroke drivers screening assessment—SDSA manual (hebrew version). https://www.nottingham.ac.uk/medicine/documents/publishedassessments/sdsa-hebrew-translation.pdf. Accessed 7 Dec 2017

Lundberg C, Caneman G, Samuelsson SM et al (2003) The assessment of fitness to drive after a stroke: the nordic stroke driver screening assessment. Scand J Psychol 44:23–30

Lundqvist A, Gerdle B, Rönnberg J (2000) Neuropsychological aspects of driving after a stroke ± in the simulator and on the road. Appl Cogn Psychol 14:135–150

Marshall SC, Gilbert N (1999) Saskatchewan physicians' attitudes and knowledge regarding assessment of medical fitness to drive. CMAJ 160:1701–1704

Marshall SC, Molnar F, Man-son-hing M et al (2007) Predictors of driving ability following stroke: a systematic review. Top Stroke Rehabil 14:98–114

Mazer BL, Sofer S, Korner-bitensky N (2001) Use of the UFOV to evaluate and retrain visual attention skills in clients with stroke: a pilot study. Am J Occup Ther 55:552–557

Mazer BL, Sofer S, Korner-bitensky N (2003) Effectiveness of a visual attention retraining program on the driving performance of clients with stroke. Arch Phys Med Rehabil 84:541–550

Mazer B, Gélinas I, Duquette J et al (2015) A randomized clinical trial to determine effectiveness of driving simulator retraining on the driving performance of clients with neurological impairment. Br J Occup Ther 78:369–376

Michon J (1985) A critical view of driver behavior models: what do we know, what should we do? In: Evans L, Schwing RC (eds) Human behaviour and traffic safety. Springer, Boston, pp 485–524

Mielenz TJ, Durbin IL, Cisewski JA et al (2017) Select physical performance measures and driving outcomes in older adults. Inj Epidemiol 4:14

Murie-fernandez M, Iturralde S, Cenoz M (2014) Driving ability after a stroke: evaluation and recovery. Neurologia 29:161–167

Nasreddine ZS, Phillips NA, Bedirian V et al (2005) The Montreal Cognitive Assessment, MOCA: a brief screening tool for mild cognitive impairment. J Am Geriatr Soc 53:695–699

National Bureau of Statistics (2016) Number of registered drivers in china 2007–2016. https://www.statista.com/statistics/278430/number-of-drivers-in-china/. Accessed 7 Dec 2017

National Research Council US (2007) Preventing teen motor crashes: contributions from the behavioural and social sciences. National Academies Press, Washington

Newhouse R, Dearholt S, Poe S et al (2005) Evidence-based practice: a practical approach to implementation. J Nurs Adm 35:35–40

Nouri M, Lincoln NB (1993) Predicting driving performance after stroke. BMJ 307:482–483

OCEBM Levels of Evidence Working Group (2011). The Oxford 2011 levels of evidence. Oxford centre for evidence-based medicine. http://www.cebm.net/index.aspx?o=5653. Accessed 7 Feb 2018

Park MO (2015) A comparison of driving errors in patients with left or right hemispheric lesions after stroke. J Phys Ther Sci 27:3469–3471

Park M, Son J, Shin HK (2013) Development of the Korean stroke drivers screening assessment: a pilot study for adapting road sign recognition subtest. Jpn J Ergon 49:s463–s466

Platz T (2017) Practice guidelines in neurorehabilitation. Neurol Int Open 01(03):E148–E152. https://doi.org/10.1055/s-0043-103057

Ponsford AS, Viitanen M, Lundberg C et al (2008) Assessment of driving after stroke: a pluridisciplinary task. Accid Anal Prev 40:452–460

Ranchet M, Akinwuntan AE, Tant M et al (2016) Fitness-to-drive agreements after stroke: medical versus practical recommendations. Eur J Neurol 23:1408–1414

Sackett DL, Rosenberg WM, Gray JA et al (1996) Evidence based medicine: what it is and what it isn't. BMJ 312:71–72

Schünemann H, Brożek J, Guyatt G, Oxman A (2013) GRADE handbook for grading quality of evidence and strength of recommendations. The GRADE Working Group. Updated October 2013. www.guidelinedevelopment.org/handbook

Scott KA, Rogers E, Betz ME et al (2017) Associations between falls and driving outcomes in older adults: systematic review and meta-analysis. J Am Geriatr Soc 65:2596–2502

Selander H, Johansson K, Lundberg C et al (2010) The Nordic stroke driver screening assessment as predictor for the outcome of an on-road test. Scand J Occup Ther 17:10–17

Shaheen SA, Niemeier DA (2001) Integrating vehicle design and human factors: minimizing elderly driving constraints. Transp Res Part C 9:155–174

Soderstrom ST, Pettersson RP, Leppert J (2006) Prediction of driving ability after stroke and the effect of behind-the-wheel training. Scand J Psychol 47:419–429

Tombaugh TN (2004) Trail making test a and b: normative data stratified by age and education. Arch Clin Neuropsychol 19:203–214

Tucker DM, Bigler ED, Chelune GJ (1981) Reliability of the Halstead-Reitan battery in individuals displaying acutely psychotic behavior. J Behav Assess 3:311–319

Tupler IA, Welsh KA, Asare-Aboagye Y (1995) Reliability of the Rey-Osterrieth complex figure in use with memory-impaired patients. J Clin Exp Neuropsychol 17:566–579

Visual Awareness Research Group (2009) UFOV User's guide, version 6.1.4. www.visualawareness.com/Pages/UFOV_Manual_V6.1.4.pdf

Waller PF (1991) The older driver. Hum Factors 33:499–505

World Health Organisation (2016) Statistics of drivers worldwide 2006–2015. Statista. https://www.statista.com/topics/1197/car-drivers/. Accessed 7 Dec 2017

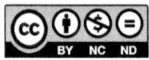

Healthcare Settings for Rehabilitation After Stroke

Sabahat A. Wasti, Nirmal Surya, Klaus Martin Stephan, and Mayowa Owolabi

1   Introduction

Stroke care has changed from being largely supportive to interventional with emphasis on reduction of both mortality and resultant disability (Schwamm et al. 2005; Powers et al. 2018). The development that started with integrated stroke units has evolved into hyperacute stroke care with emphasis on early diagnosis and revascularization, by either dissolving the clot or mechanically removing it (Marler et al. 2000; Rha and Saver 2007; Higashida et al. 2013; Powers et al. 2018). Alongside the early administration of recombinant tissue plasminogen activator and thrombectomy, one other intervention showing some promise in limiting the long-term disabling impact of stroke is early rehabilitation (Langhorne 2013; Momosaki et al. 2016; Coleman et al. 2017; Yagi et al. 2017). Furthermore, there is now an understanding that establishing a continuum of stroke rehabilitation provides for best possible outcome for stroke patients (NICE 2013). Therefore, it is important to define the service structure for rehabilitation, one that follows the patient through the course of stroke care continuum. This chapter deals with recommendations in this context.

S. A. Wasti (✉)
Neurorehabilitation, Cleveland Clinic, Abu Dhabi, UAE
e-mail: wastis@clevelandclinicabudhabi.ae

N. Surya
Surya Neuro Center, Mumbai, India

K. M. Stephan
SRH Gesundheitszentrum Waldbronn, Waldbronn, Germany
e-mail: KlausMartin.Stephan@gns.srh.de

M. Owolabi
Blossom Specialist Medical Center (First Center for Neurorehabilitation, East West and Central Africa), Ibadan, Nigeria

© The Author(s) 2021   261
T. Platz (ed.), *Clinical Pathways in Stroke Rehabilitation*,
https://doi.org/10.1007/978-3-030-58505-1_14

Stroke rehabilitation is a continuous process that starts at the time the patient first presents with impairments and may need to be provided throughout the rest of his or her living years (Teasell et al. 2018). In order to do so, it is imperative that rehabilitation encounters are appropriately defined in terms of timing, service structures and resource requirements. Furthermore, effective interventions at each level of care must also be identified. Based on current evidence, we recommend the following settings as components of the stroke rehabilitation continuum:

1. Early rehabilitation (hyperacute phase and acute phase).
2. Subacute rehabilitation.
3. Outpatient rehabilitation.
4. Home-based rehabilitation.
5. Community-based rehabilitation.
6. Long-term and sustained rehabilitation.

2   Methodological Considerations

We present the current best evidence and evidence-based recommendations for specific interventions addressing each target domain of rehabilitation in stroke patients. As outlined in chapter "Clinical Pathways in Stroke Rehabilitation: Background, Scope, and Methods", the focus is on best evidence and the corresponding recommendations, but not on explicit health system design prescriptions. Clinical pathways for health system designs depend largely on regional circumstances and have to be developed locally taking both the evidence-based recommendations and the local context and needs into consideration (Platz 2019).

Nevertheless, there is still a need for guidance on health system design for stroke rehabilitation. Whilst we acknowledge the need for regional adaptation of specific practice recommendations and hence have been reluctant to make very explicit recommendations on system design in other chapters, in this chapter, the global author group provides some more general guidance on how to build healthcare settings for stroke rehabilitation.

This chapter makes primarily recommendations on how (best) to organize health care for stroke rehabilitation on a continuum from stroke onset to the long-term situation of living with stroke sequelae. Since we know that such a continuum of care cannot be implemented in many regional settings, this chapter concludes with reflections on how to deal with the contextual limitations that exists in many low-income countries or rural settings. These limitations often include a severe shortage of trained staff and even most basic rehabilitative interventions often rely on the dedication of family members or other volunteers (see Sect. 3.7 for discussion).

In contrast to specific interventions, there is paucity of evidence addressing benefit, harm and cost-effectiveness of healthcare settings. Therefore, this chapter is largely based on clinical reasoning and experience from clinical practice in diverse settings ranging from low-income to high-income countries. Many recommendations made are expert opinions. When evidence is available, this is referenced and the level of evidence is then categorized according to the Oxford Centre for Evidence-Based Medicine—Levels of Evidence and rated with four categories according to "GRADE" ("Grades of Recommendation, Assessment, Development and Evaluation") (Owens et al. 2010):

- High quality: further research is unlikely to affect our confidence in the estimation of the (therapeutic) effect.
- Medium quality: further research is likely to affect our confidence in the estimation of the (therapeutic) effect and may alter the estimate.
- Low quality: further research will most likely influence our confidence in the estimation of the (therapeutic) effect and will probably change the estimate.
- Very low quality: any estimation of the (therapy) effect or prognosis is very uncertain.

Whenever possible, recommendations of existing guidelines and/or evidence-based reviews have been included.

3 Stroke Rehabilitation Continuum

3.1 Early Rehabilitation After Stoke

With reduction in stroke mortality (Seminog et al. 2019) and more patients surviving the acute phase, attention is now focused on reduction of morbidity and disability due to stroke. Revascularization with tPA or mechanical thrombectomy as well as protection of neural tissue by effective management of complications, such as haemorrhagic transformation of infarct or brain oedema, is directed at limiting the extent of brain damage and thereby the disabling effect of impairments. To support this effort, emphasis on recovery of function and prevention of secondary complications should be considered as the main goal of early rehabilitation (Winstein et al. 2016). When rehabilitation is provided in an intensive care setting immediately after stroke, it is best referred to as hyperacute, whilst ward-based or step-down unit level rehabilitation should be termed as acute rehabilitation. Early rehabilitation refers to both of these levels of care. It is advisable, however, to use the individual terms as these reflect the exact level of rehabilitation setting more distinctly. The provision for early rehabilitation is recommended in the American Heart Association Guidelines, with evidence for this recommendation graded at 1A (Winstein et al. 2016) corresponding to a strong recommendation (A) building on high-quality evidence.

In hyperacute setting, the stroke care team ought to include at least a physician with expertise in stroke rehabilitation, speech and language pathologist/therapist with expertise in swallow and early communication techniques, physical therapist, occupational therapist and stroke care–trained nurse specialists (Boulanger et al. 2018). In this setting, the main goal of rehabilitation should be to prevent early complications and assess safety and feasibility of early mobilization (Coleman et al. 2017). In this context the key domains of care are:

1. Complete assessment of patient with focus on the following:
   (a) Impact of stroke with particular focus on presenting impairments and their severity (impairment mapping).
   (b) Co-morbidities and their premorbid impact on function.
   (c) Pre-existing musculoskeletal conditions and/or deformities.
   (d) Pre-existing disability(ies).
   (e) Family setup and support.
   (f) Work and social status.
2. Protection of the airway and swallow assessment and management.
   (a) Early swallow assessment by speech and language therapist, who is adequately trained in dysphagia management or by another professional (nurse or doctor), is recommended (Palli et al. 2017). Although, as yet, evidence is not conclusive regarding efficacy of this practice in reducing the aspiration episodes (Smith et al. 2018), it is strongly recommended that screening should be carried out (Wolfe and Rudd 2011; Lakshminarayan et al. 2010) and in our judgement it should be adopted as part of acute stroke care.
   (b) The patient should not be fed orally or given medications unless cleared by swallow screening (Duncan et al. 2005).
   (c) The period within which this is to be conducted is difficult to specify as evidence in this respect does not support a standardized practice. However, currently, there is a consensus agreement that in patients who have signs of dysphagia, the assessment should be carried out within 24 h (Ellis and Adams 2016).
   (d) At present, there is no consensus on the instrument or instruments for the assessment, and we recommend that this should be agreed upon locally depending on resources, needs, availability, expertise and training (Donovan et al. 2013).
   (e) Enteral feeding should be initiated early in patients with dysphagia to avoid malnourishment. Whilst this should be considered as early as it is clinically established that patient is not able to swallow, the delay in introducing the enteral feeding should not exceed 3 days (Yamada 2015; Ojo and Brooke 2016).
   (f) Evidence indicate that early insertion of per-endoscopic gastrostomy tube should be avoided (George et al. 2017).
   (g) In patients requiring enteral feeding, nasogastric tube feeding is recommended for as long as 3 weeks, beyond which insertion of PEG may be considered (George et al. 2017). Please note that nasogastric tube feeding can be associated with regurgitation and aspiration if the patient lies down immediately after a meal. Therefore, the patient should remain seated for over 2 h (gastric emptying time) after each meal to avoid regurgitation and aspiration.

3. Very early or early mobilization (VEM/EM):
   (a) Currently, there is no evidence to support VEM (defined as out of bed activity within 24–48 h). Indeed, AVERT III showed negative impact on mortality at 3 months (Langhorne et al. 2018; Bernhardt et al. 2019).
      - In the light of lack of evidence for beneficial effect and evidence for negative impact at 3 months, we recommend that mobilization within 24 h after stroke cannot be recommended (Langhorne et al. 2018).
      - Mobilization within 48 h may be considered acceptable in patients who meet key safety parameters. However, there is still no convincing evidence for efficacy of this practice (Xu et al. 2017).
   (b) Early mobilization is recommended.
      - Currently there is no agreement on the definition of "EARLY". Mobilization within 72 h may be considered as such (Bernhardt et al. 2015).
      - On the basis of current evidence, mobilization after 24 h, unless otherwise contraindicated, is recommended. There are no studies to indicate that this practice is likely to harm patient and indeed, there is some evidence that it may be of some benefit (Li et al. 2018).
      - Dose, including intensity, frequency and duration should be commensurate to patient's clinical status. Dose should be incrementally increased in line with patient's tolerance and response (Yagi et al. 2017).
      - Specific motor rehabilitation focuses are head and trunk control, arm function, stance, gait and balance and should be addressed as individually indicated early after stroke.
      - Change, progress and outcome should be analytically recorded daily.
4. Communication and speech.
   (a) Early assessment of communication by a speech therapist is recommended.
   (b) Strategies for establishing communication early with stroke patients are recommended (National Institute for Health and Care Excellence (NICE) 2013).
   (c) The evidence for active speech and language therapy in early period after stroke, before 48 h, is not available (Nouwens et al. 2013).
   (d) There is some evidence that speech and language therapy when commenced from 2 days onwards has a beneficial effect on outcome (Mattioli et al. 2014). It is therefore, good practice to commence active speech and language therapy from 48 h onwards for dysphasic/aphasic patients.
5. Sensory and perceptual deficits.
   (a) Early detection of sensory and perceptual deficits is recommended.
   (b) There is evidence for introducing rehabilitation strategies for sensory deficit in early stroke rehabilitation (Pandian et al. 2014).
   (c) Given the current evidence, it is recommended that patients who are able to comprehend presence of deficits such as somatosensory deficits, visual field deficits, hemi-neglect or visual inattention should be made aware of these and rehabilitation strategies should be introduced early.

3.1.1   Prevention of Secondary Complications

An important role of rehabilitation team in early rehabilitation is prevention of complications. This has now been highlighted as key responsibility of rehabilitation teams in hyperacute and acute rehabilitation settings (Winstein et al. 2016).

The rehabilitation team must take steps to prevent, rapidly detect and treat

- Malnutrition and dehydration.
- Pressure sores.
- Aspiration-related chest infections.
- Over dependence on ancillary devices such as urinary catheter, tracheostomy tube and feeding tube.
- Contractures.
- Excessive muscle wasting.
- Shoulder pain and positional malalignment.
- Agitation and restlessness.
- Mood disorder/depression and social isolation.
- Urinary tract infection.

3.2   Subacute Stroke Rehabilitation

Subacute stroke rehabilitation is the next level of care for stroke patients. As shown for many of the target domains in this book and in national guidelines, in the subacute stage of stroke, interventions should be intensive, challenging and tailored towards the individual needs of the patients.

When a patient is deemed fit to be discharged or transferred from acute care, a decision has to be made by the treating team whether a safe discharge home is possible or the patient should be transferred to a specialized facility to continue structured multidisciplinary stroke rehabilitation. Subacute stroke rehabilitation units are either stand-alone services or may be part of larger acute care hospitals. There is some evidence in favour of this level of care of stroke patients (Rønning and Guldvog 1998). Several factors influence this decision: These include:

- Availability of required subacute stroke rehabilitation facilities (currently only developed healthcare systems consistently provide this level of care).
- Affordability of subacute rehabilitation.
  - State funded (most are eligible, but waiting lists and duration may be barriers).
  - Medical insurance (restrictive/selective).
  - Self-funding (expensive).
  - Charity funding (limited).
- Geographical location and accessibility to patient and his or her family.
- Medical capability of a facility, as this determines at what stage patient may be transferred. For example, if the patient has a tracheostomy tube and subacute rehabilitation facility that he or she can be transferred to does not have a clinical

set up to cater for tracheostomized patients then a safe transfer is not possible. This results in longer stay in acute care with limited access to subacute level of rehabilitation.

3.2.1 Transfer Criteria to Subacute Rehabilitation Facility

Whilst transfer criteria will differ from place to place and will depend on the services available at the subacute rehabilitation facility, some guiding criteria for transfer from acute to subacute level of rehabilitation may be applied:

1. All investigations required for determining the nature and cause of stroke have been completed.
2. All required interventions for secondary preventions have been optimized.
3. Medical stability has been achieved with satisfactory control of blood pressure and diabetes mellitus.
4. Patient continues to need close physician supervision.
5. Patient continues to need specialized nursing care.
6. Patient is cognitively able to engage meaningfully in therapies.
7. Patient is able to tolerate higher intensity of therapies.
8. Patient requires more than one therapy input daily.
9. Patient and family have been suitably counselled to accept lesser level of medical surveillance and higher intensity of rehabilitation.
10. Patient and family have agreed to the transfer and fully understand its need.

3.2.2 Subacute Rehabilitation Facility

The subacute rehabilitation facility for stroke patients should have integrated multidisciplinary set up for provision of this level of rehabilitation. The patient should be offered intensive therapies. We recommend that for optimal functioning a facility should at least meet the following standards:

- The physical space and environment should be optimal and conducive to adequately accommodate the number of patients a given facility is likely to serve.
- The multidisciplinary team should include the following categories of staff:
  - Physician(s) with expertise in neurorehabilitation.
  - Rehabilitation-trained nurses.
  - Neurological physical therapists.
  - Neurological occupational therapists.
  - Neurological speech and language therapist with expertise in dysphagia management and communication rehabilitation.
  - Dietician(s).
  - Social worker(s)/case manager(s).
- When available, the provision of neuropsychological and orthoptic services is recommended.

The facility should have links with or access to orthotic, neurological, urological, psychiatry, ophthalmology and general medical services.

- The facility should have all essential therapy equipment and aids.
- The facility should have dedicated therapy areas, e.g. for physiotherapy, occupational therapy and speech and language therapy.
- Social networking spaces and provision for community re-integration (shopping, leisure trips, etc.) are desirable.

The ideal staff to patient ratios have not been optimally evaluated and differ in various settings. We recommend that the following ratios be considered for planning such facilities:

- One physician (with expertise in neurorehabilitation) should not be expected to supervise the care of more than 20–25 inpatients.
- Nurse to patient ratio: No more than 5 patients to one nurse.
- Physiotherapist to patient ratio: No more than 10 patients to one physiotherapist.
- Occupational therapist to patient ratio: No more than 10 patients to one occupational therapist.
- Speech and language therapist to patient ratio: No more than 20 patients to one speech and language therapist.
- For each 40 patients one neuropsychologist is recommended.

3.2.3 The Transfer Process

The representative of the subacute rehabilitation facility should meet with patient and his or her family ahead of transfer and fully brief them about the nature of services offered and the level of care they should expect. The transfer process should also be clearly explained.

The transfer process should be well coordinated and adjusted to the patient's needs. The following standards should be adhered to:

- All required documentation including discharge summaries from each discipline involved in the care of the patient in the referring facility should be provided to the subacute rehabilitation facility.
- The discharge medications complete with doses and schedules should be clearly listed.
- Detailed nursing handover should be provided.
- All required equipment and devices (e.g. orthosis, splints, wheelchair) necessary for continued care of the patient should be provided.

3.2.4 Subacute Rehabilitation Programmes

After admission, the patient should have structured care provided to him or her. The facility should have standardized policies for all sessions and domains of care. These include:

- Mobility training including gait training and where necessary training for full or semi-independence from wheelchair.
- Management of cognitive impairment and cognitive rehabilitation.

- Management of perceptual deficits.
- Management of dysphagia with the aim of retraining for oral feeding where this is possible to do safely.
- Participation in activities of daily living.
- Neuropathic pain management.
- Spasticity management.
- Management of mood disorder.
- Adjustment and "beginning to live with disability" training.
- Readiness for discharge to home or modified living.

The policies should highlight minimum standard of care for each domain of care. There should be agreed timeline for initial assessments and care planning and goals set thereafter should be measurable and achievable in realistic time frame. The following are some guiding parameters in this context:

- Patient(s) should undergo full multidisciplinary team (MDT) assessment within 24–72 h of admission.
- The MDT should develop a goal-directed care plan with specified timelines.
- The patient and family should be fully briefed about the care plan and their suggestions and concerns taken into consideration and the care plan adjusted accordingly.
- The progress of the patient should be reviewed by the MDT at least every week and goals and care plan modified to adjust for change.
- Discharge planning should start early, preferably within 1 week of admission.
- Periodic patient and family meetings should be held to brief them about the progress.
- Discharge planning meeting must always be convened.

The aim of subacute rehabilitation is to achieve clinical stability and functional readiness for discharge to community, home or modified living facility. This entails gaining modified partial to full independence and predictability of care needs. The discharge should be appropriately planned and the patient should be transferred to either outpatient or home-based rehabilitation services.

The specific recommendations given above have been formulated on the basis of good practice and in line with those detailed in several existing guidelines (Winstein et al. 2016; Gittler and Davis 2018).

The overall evidence for the effectiveness of this level of rehabilitation is not robust for the whole group of stroke patients (García-Rudolph et al. 2019). Teasell and co-workers differentiated their analysis according to the severity of stroke (Teasell et al. 2018; evidence-based review of stroke rehabilitation):

- In **mildly affected patients**, the site of rehabilitation does not influence functional outcome (level of evidence 1A; high-quality evidence),
- For the subgroup of **patients with moderately severe stroke**, specialized rehabilitation in a subacute rehabilitation unit does improve functional out-

come compared to conventional care on a general ward (level of evidence 1A; high-quality evidence),

- **Patients with severe or moderately severe stroke** who receive treatment on a stroke rehabilitation unit have a lower risk of being dependent or dead/dependent compared with patients who receive little or no rehabilitation (level of evidence 1B; medium-quality evidence).

Not all patients will need treatment within a special subacute rehabilitation facility. Especially patients with mild or moderate functional deficits may prefer to attend specific rehabilitation modules on an outpatient basis or even at home using tele-therapeutic devices (see also Sect. 3.6).

3.3   Outpatient Stroke Rehabilitation Services

Patients may be discharged from acute care and subacute facilities with arrangement to receive ongoing rehabilitation as outpatients. Indeed, there is evidence that early supported discharge directly from acute care to community-based rehabilitation as well as integrated outpatient rehabilitation delivers good outcome for stroke survivors (Rice et al. 2016; Langhorne et al. 2017). Teasell et al. (2018) found level 1A evidence that stroke patients with mild-to-moderate disability, discharged early from an acute hospital unit, can be rehabilitated in the community by an interdisciplinary stroke rehabilitation team and attain similar or superior functional outcomes when compared to patients receiving inpatient rehabilitation (high-quality evidence).

The patient could be referred to an outpatient stroke rehabilitation service if:

- He/she is clinically stable and is able to tolerate transportation to and from outpatient rehabilitation facility.
- He/she has sufficient effort tolerance level and does not fatigue so much that precludes effective participation in therapy sessions.
- He/she is able to engage cognitively in therapy sessions, re-engage in subsequent sessions with demonstrable carry over.

The outpatient stroke rehabilitation facility should be designed to offer multidisciplinary team rehabilitation. Patients should have access to all required therapies and interventions. The available services should include:

- Access to physician(s) with expertise in neurorehabilitation for continued management of residual effects of stroke including spasticity and pain.
- Physiotherapy service with adequately designed treatment areas with availability of most required equipment.
- Occupational therapy service with capacity to attend to issues such as extended activities of daily living and vocational rehabilitation.
- Speech and language therapy services with capacity to work on issues related to dysphagia and communication.

- Neuropsychological therapy for the treatment of cognitive, behavioural and emotional post-stroke disorders is recommended when available.
- Optional or ancillary services include dietetics, orthotics and specialized nursing service particularly, continence management. These services may also be accessed through a referral arrangement.

If the patient is able to travel to and from the clinic and logistically it is possible to do so with the least level of disruption to family life, then outpatient rehabilitation is preferable to home-based rehabilitation. In less developed healthcare systems, cost and availability may limit access and this may be combined/supplemented with home-based rehabilitation.

3.4   Home-Based (Family-Based) Stroke Rehabilitation

Once patients with stroke have been discharged home, it is important to continue with rehabilitation. Home-based rehabilitation in the present context is defined as a form of rehabilitation, where the training is provided by members of the family. It may be beneficial as it realizes the actual need-based training true to the patient's living environment. Task shifting is an attractive solution for healthcare sustainability. The patient's family can be trained to provide task-based training, and members of the rehabilitation team can visit the patient at home as needed to provide required therapies. In low- and middle-income healthcare systems, this may be an effective way of providing ongoing rehabilitation. (Lindley et al. 2017), and the outcomes may be comparable to long-term rehabilitation in non-domiciliary facilities (Mayo 2016). However, home-based (family-based) rehabilitation is under stress where the joint families are disintegrating into nuclear families thereby shrinking the pool of family members who can attend to the rehabilitation of patient after stroke. Therefore, task shifting to family members may increase caregiving burden and stress. Nevertheless, family participation at home reduces the need for travelling for outpatient appointments in centres, especially when distant from patients' homes. Furthermore, the financial burden is lessened if therapists are not required to administer therapy at home and day-to-day life is not severely disrupted. This may contribute to reduction in patient's and caregiver's anxiety and improve quality of life of affected family. Conversely, though it can be argued that in patients with limited functional improvement, over long period of time, the situation may become burdensome and result in caregiver's fatigue (Sarı 2017).

Furthermore, the results of the ATTEND trial did not demonstrate any benefit of family-led domiciliary care (ATTEND Collaborative Group 2017). This is also consistent with the absence of benefit seen in a systematic review of trials of caregiver-mediated exercises to improve activities of daily living after stroke (Vloothuis et al. 2016). Overall, these findings do not support investment in new stroke rehabilitation services that shift tasks to family caregivers, unless new evidence emerges. (Level 2B evidence, moderate evidence against the establishment of new family-led therapeutic interventions without concomitant research.)

The absence of benefit of the family-rehabilitation intervention has important implications for stroke recovery research, behavioural change, and task shifting in general. A future avenue of research should be to investigate the effects of task shifting to healthcare assistants or team-based community care to offer care after discharge (ATTEND Collaborative Group 2017). Another option may be to combine family-led rehabilitation with outpatient care. This may help reduce the frequency of outpatient care required thus promoting affordability.

3.5   Community-Based Stroke Rehabilitation (CBR)

Over the last couple of decades, CBR has acquired a lot of interest. CBR programmes improve, facilitate, stimulate and/or provide services to people with disabilities (PWDs), such as stroke survivors, their families and caregivers within the locations of their families and communities through locally employed full or part time, paid or volunteer community rehabilitation workers, who are trained, followed up and managed within a certain organizational set up, that has rehabilitation philosophy as its core operational principle (Ru et al. 2017). Only few studies are available on CBR and its advantages and disadvantages have not been critically studied (Stephenson and Wiles 2000). However, it is possible to list some advantages on the basis of experience and current practice.

Advantages of CBR, compared to the institutional approach include:

- In time, and in theory, all the people living with disabilities in a community can be reached and their basic needs be met.
- "Tailor-made" rehabilitation programmes can be established, based on the individual's capacities and needs, and focused directly on integration into the family/community. "Disability" is not a stable situation. CBR can evolve and adapt to changing needs of patients.
- Family members can witness and participate in the progress of a relative living with disability, thus enhancing their faith in that person's abilities and potential and challenging their own prejudices.
- CBR services, apart from carrying out their core work in rehabilitation, can also contribute towards the prevention of secondary complications related to impairments and disabilities, through activities such as primary healthcare, vaccinations, nutrition and hygiene.
- CBR programmes can trace many people living with disabilities who would never have been found by institutions and, through referral, can make the work of other existing specialized services more effective.
- CBR can be more effective in tackling issues such as return to work and community access, including leisure activities and extended activities of daily living.
- CBR could be cost-effective (if well managed!).

Problems of CBR, compared to the institutional-based approach,

- The poor living conditions of most people with disabilities are also poor conditions for rehabilitation. The objectives of individual CBR programmes therefore have to be very realistic and must focus on essential needs.
- Community- and home-based services by community rehabilitation workers can sometimes be rather routine and boring, for the worker, client and family alike; this may be less challenging than training or education in a centre.
- Poor families' priorities may be at the level of survival rather than solving problems of a member with disability. Furthermore, the disability of one family member is not always problematic for other family members; therefore, it is sometimes very hard to enlist their active collaboration.
- The organization and management of CBR are complex and difficult due to organizational and political reasons and local priorities for funding.
- The educational level of the community rehabilitation workers (CRWs) may be low. Better-educated individuals are often difficult to engage in CBR work. Front-line CBR is a low-profile job, which does not offer notable social status to people with higher education.

These factors influence the type, level and quality of the services which can be provided at the community level through a CBR programme. Although, these factors have been determined through critical appraisal of the existing services, there are limited number of studies and it is difficult to provide firm structural basis for community rehabilitation.

In Europe (defined geographically), such structures are already implemented in some countries, e.g. in the UK and in France. As part of the NHS (e.g. in Milton Keynes), Stroke Clinical Specialists are available "to provide in-depth knowledge and expertise; consistent education, support and advice in accessing information and a full range of services from the NHS, social care and others. This service is available to people who have had a stroke/TIA, their relatives and carers, members of the general public, professionals and voluntary organisations" (NHS homepage Milton Keynes, accessed 28.12.2019).

In Germany, pilot studies are run to employ community rehabilitation workers (e.g. "Schlaganfall-Lotsen") by regional stroke associations (e.g. "Schlaganfall Allianz Sachsen-Anhalt") or by charities (e.g. "Stiftung Deutsche Schlaganfall-Hilfe"). Their main aims are to provide advice to patients and their relatives, to help to implement elements of effective secondary prevention and help to organize the continuum of stroke care and therapy after discharge from the primary hospital. Similar services are also available or in preparation in other European countries, in some American, Asian and African countries and well established in some areas of Canada and Australia.

The aim of these coordinators is always to guide and to augment the existing structures in the community, they cannot—and should not—substitute the existing medical and therapeutic resources.

In many countries, stroke support groups and stroke survivor organizations (e.g. the Stroke Alliance for Europe (SAFE), a non-profit–making organisation with members from 24 countries) support education and stroke research; they campaign to support the acute treatment and prevention of stroke and help to improve the quality of life of stroke survivors, their families and caretakers.

It is our recommendation that at this time, local realities and resources should determine the structure and extent of services that are possible to provide under this umbrella taking into account the specificities of government run, insurance governed and privately financed systems. In this way, rehabilitation centres can also be included into the structure as local and/or regional centres of excellence especially for more severely affected patients. Such an approach is likely to be useful in low-, middle- and high-income countries. If implemented its effect should be scientifically evaluated whenever possible.

3.6 Long-Term and Sustained Rehabilitation

A significant number of stroke patients survive with established disability and with age as well as ongoing comorbidities. The burden of disability often increases and results in significant loss of function and independence (Meyer et al. 2015). If left unattended, the burden of care may progressively escalate (Van De Port et al. 2006). This can result in loss of employment, social restriction, care providers fatigue as well as ever-increasing financial burden. To date, there is no consensus as to how to support or provide care for stroke survivors in the long term (Aziz et al. 2016). It is, however, important to establish a suitable network of surveillance in order to prevent decline in stroke survivor's functional status and level of participation over time.

It is recommended that there should be a long-term care support and sustained rehabilitation program for patients with stroke. We recommend that consideration be given to providing this via primary care centres in the community or delivered by a specialist nurse practitioner. In developing and less-developed healthcare systems, a model of care can be developed whereby trained community workers can maintain regular contact with patients and their families and advise them to request help when they deem this is necessary. Modern technology can also be utilized for this purpose and contact can be maintained with patients and their families via mobile phones or specially developed apps. Telemedicine is also being utilized for surveillance (Sarfo et al. 2018) and it is anticipated that this model of care is likely to become widely used for provision of long-term support and sustained rehabilitation for stroke survivors in future.

3.7 Adapting Clinical Pathways to Diverse Regional Healthcare System Contexts

More than 80% of the world's population live in over 100 developing countries. Delivery of neurologic care in developing countries varies depending on the needs and resources of the country and the availability of medical and paramedical personnel (WHO 2014). Medical insurance and government support are usually minimal or totally lacking. The financial burden is heavy and includes direct costs of inpatient care, outpatient care and therapy sessions, investigations, medications and transport (patients from rural areas often have to travel long distances to urban healthcare centres). The indirect cost includes the loss of earnings due to unemployment during illness and convalescence. In the large majority of these countries, there may be no access to financial support such as disability benefits (Disability and Development Report 2018; Singh 2013).

The availability of neurorehabilitation services is inconsistent and may range from highly sophisticated in developed countries to totally inadequate or lacking in developing and underdeveloped countries. Over 60% of the developing countries have no neurorehabilitation services. There is severe paucity of trained professionals. The task of managing patients with neurological impairments is often devolved to generic therapists and inadequately trained nursing and medical staff. The overall effect is that treatments are being provided by less than adequate professionals, possibly delivering outcomes for patients that fall short of their potential. Even in those developing countries, where some neurorehabilitation service is provided, the quality is rarely good enough due to a lack of a well-structured neurorehabilitation system which can provide comprehensive rehabilitation services. More often than not treatment is not provided (WFNR 2015).

As stated before, hospital-based interdisciplinary neurorehabilitation care should be provided as a first line service to facilitate rapid recovery after neurological injury. The home-based or community-based services are appropriate for settlement at home and community re-integration in the recovery phase. Community-based rehabilitation services are the most appropriate way forward in enhancing outcomes particularly in developing countries, with tailored and culturally sensitive education for the family, to help them participate in the rehabilitation of the patient (Pandian et al. 2015). There have been repeated concerns about the adequacy of the evidence-base regarding the efficacy, effectiveness and efficiency of CBR predominantly using local resource in the local community (Surya 2010, 2015). However, on balance, in developing countries, CBR may be one of the most effective ways of providing rehabilitation after the acute/subacute phase, especially when there is an intimate social system and family structure that helps to provide the necessary physical, emotional and spiritual support. Strong family bond helps to overcome the negative impact of the disability and large extended family system ensures that the physical, social and financial burden of disease is shared.

The role as therapy giver can be switched depending on the availability of family members. Even though, the ATTEND trial (2017) and the Cochrane review by Vloothuis et al. (2016) have not shown a clear-cut beneficial effect of (additional) therapy provided by family members, these family members are often the only people available to the patients. They provide valuable social, emotional and psychological support. In order to strengthen and improve their role in delivering rehabilitation, different models for training can be tried to ensure best possible outcomes. As many family members as possible can be trained by the therapist or through web-based teaching application. Use of mobile phone to record the exercises and progress and sharing with the patient/caregiver is useful as patients/caregivers can review them regularly at home to be implemented at home. Mobile phone records of exercises at home also make it possible for therapists to check whether family members are correctly following the programmes at home. The recorded exercise pattern on phone can be reviewed during outpatient visits and any modification or adjustment to the programme can be made. This application is most useful tool in family-based rehabilitation (Zhou et al. 2018).

Family-based and community-based rehabilitation settings are likely to become important models in future for delivery of rehabilitation after the acute/subacute phase of stroke not only in low- and middle-income countries but also in high-income countries. As telemedicine and technologies become more sophisticated, this form of rehabilitation will play a pivotal role in patient's recovery and improving outcomes.

4   Conclusions

Stroke care has advanced in the past two decades and more patients are surviving the acute stage. The mortality rates are reducing both in developed and developing countries, thereby resulting in increased disability burden (Feigin et al. 2019). In stroke care model, rehabilitation is now considered an integral component of all levels of stroke care (Fig. 1). Whereas, there may be a reduction in the individual level of disability in sophisticated healthcare systems due to timely interventions and reduction of the impact of disabling impairment because of appropriate level of rehabilitative care (Lees et al. 2016; Emberson et al. 2014; Campbell et al. 2015); in developing countries, prolonged survival is associated with heavier burden of disability. The continuum of stroke care, including the pillars of the stroke quadrangle

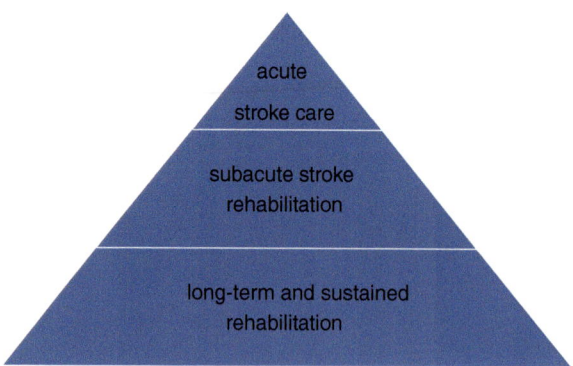

Fig. 1 Essential levels of stroke rehabilitation

(surveillance, prevention, acute care and rehabilitation), is lacking at many levels and contributes to poor outcome in the developing countries. It is imperative that despite the limitations of resources, appropriate efforts are made to improve services for stroke survivors and foundations are laid upon which an effective continuum of care can be developed. Some low-cost and simple measures can be put in place.

For developed countries, we recommend that the stroke care continuum should be reinforced with mechanisms in place for continual appraisal and improvement. A major challenge foreseen is the increasing demand for stroke rehabilitation that has to be met due to demographic changes with a higher proportion of elderly citizens who are at risk for cerebrovascular accidents.

For developing countries, we recommend that given the current evidence, early mobility, after 24 h, should be encouraged. Intensive care and acute care staff should be educated to pursue this objective. A simple measure of prescribing bed rest beyond 24 h only for those who require it and considering this as an exception may help to improve outcome. Deployment of physical therapists and other therapists in a multidisciplinary setting in hyperacute and acute care services must be considered vital. Training of all nursing staff in moving, handling and positioning of patients should be made mandatory. Furthermore, prevention of secondary complications must be diligently pursued (Scottish Intercollegiate Guidelines Network 2010). In fact, the healthcare cost savings through minimizing secondary complications should pay for any extra resource required to achieve this objective.

In the continuum of stroke care, subacute rehabilitation may be provided by specialized therapists on an outpatient or inpatient basis or in families in private homes, where most of the therapy will be provided by lay persons (Fig. 2). Although intensive and at the same time specific professional therapy after stroke is highly recommended in the subacute phase after stroke (see above), intermediate rehabilitation facilities may be difficult to provide in developing countries due to the cost of setting up and maintaining such facilities. However, where available, such facilities may also support community-based and family-based care by proving oversight and outpatient/inpatient multidisciplinary care as may be needed (see above).

We recommend the development of services in the community with investment in CBR and home-based rehabilitation, utilizing low-cost resources and—building on positive and negative conceptual experience—engaging family members as part of rehabilitation team not only in the subacute stage after stroke but also for long-term and sustained rehabilitation. To incorporate therapy into daily routine and practice is however an unsolved problem—both in developed and developing countries.

We have deliberately avoided explicit recommendations for technical rehabilitation interventions such as robotics, neuromodulation and other such expensive techniques and equipment which due to lack of availability and cost are difficult to generally recommend as necessary for rehabilitation. Furthermore, with regard to

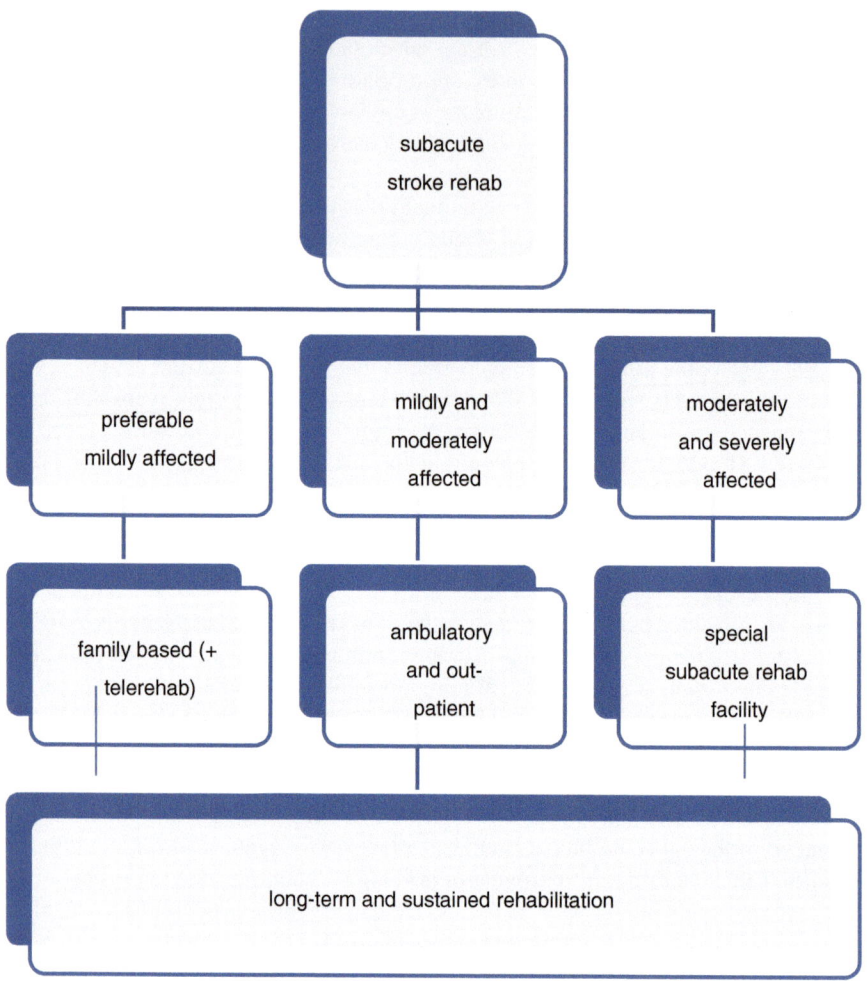

Fig. 2 Recommended stroke rehabilitation model for developing countries

recovery of function, the principles of functional brain recovery apply to both technology- and mankind-supported restorative treatment and training. Both approaches or their combination can be recommended based on their regional availability. Both feasibility and cost-effectiveness of purely therapist-led and technology-based rehabilitation vary according to regional socioeconomic circumstances and thus any hitherto decisions have to rest on their regional assessment.

Finally, it is our opinion that all healthcare systems, globally, must make stroke a priority and consider investing in continuum of care for stroke as doing so will result in lesser burden of care in the long-term and may indeed deliver net cost savings.

References

ATTEND Collaborative Group (2017) Family-led rehabilitation after stroke in India (ATTEND): a randomised controlled trial. Lancet 390(10094):588–599 . Epub 2017 Jun 27. https://doi.org/10.1016/S0140-6736(17)31447-2

Aziz NA, Pindus DM, Mullis R, Walter FM, Mant J (2016) Understanding stroke survivors' and informal carers' experiences of and need for primary care and community health services—a systematic review of the qualitative literature: protocol. BMJ Open 6(1):e009244. https://doi.org/10.1136/bmjopen-2015-009244

Bernhardt J et al (2015) Early mobilization after stroke: early adoption but limited evidence. Stroke 46(4):1141–1146. https://doi.org/10.1161/STROKEAHA.114.007434

Bernhardt J et al (2019) Very early versus delayed mobilization after stroke. Stroke 50:e178–e179. https://doi.org/10.1161/STROKEAHA.119.024502

Boulanger JM et al (2018) Canadian stroke best practice recommendations for acute stroke management: prehospital, emergency department, and acute inpatient stroke care, 6th edition, update 2018. Int J Stroke 13(9):949–984. https://doi.org/10.1177/1747493018786616

Campbell BCV, Donnan GA, Lees KR, Hacke W, Khatri P, Hill MD et al (2015) Endovascular stent thrombectomy: the new standard of care for large vessel ischaemic stroke. Lancet Neurol 14(8):846–854. https://doi.org/10.1016/S1474-4422(15)00140-4

Coleman ER et al (2017) Early rehabilitation after stroke: a narrative review. Curr Atheroscler Rep 19(12):59. https://doi.org/10.1007/s11883-017-0686-6

Disability and Development Report (2018) Realizing the sustainable development goals for persons with disabilities. https://doi.org/10.18356/6b539901-en

Donovan NJ et al (2013) Dysphagia screening: state of the art invitational conference proceeding from the state-of-the-art nursing symposium, international stroke conference 2012. Stroke 44(4):e24–e31. https://doi.org/10.1161/STR.0b013e3182877f57

Duncan PW et al (2005) Management of adult stroke rehabilitation care: a clinical practice guideline. Stroke 36(9):e100–e143

Ellis C, Adams RJ (2016) Improving stroke outcomes: a roadmap of care. Int J Neurorehabil 3:3. https://doi.org/10.4172/2376-0281.1000215

Emberson J, Lees KR, Lyden P, Blackwell L, Albers G, Bluhmki E et al (2014) Effect of treatment delay, age, and stroke severity on the effects of intravenous thrombolysis with alteplase for acute ischaemic stroke: a meta-analysis of individual patient data from randomised trials. Lancet 384(9958):1929–1935. https://doi.org/10.1016/S0140-6736(14)60584-5

Feigin VL, Nichols E, Alam T, Bannick MS, Beghi E, Blake N et al (2019) Global, regional, and national burden of neurological disorders, 1990–2016: a systematic analysis for the Global Burden of Disease Study 2016. Lancet Neurol 18(4):459–480. https://doi.org/10.1016/S1474-4422(18)30499-X

García-Rudolph A, Sánchez-Pinsach D, Salleras E, Tormos J (2019) Subacute stroke physical rehabilitation evidence in activities of daily living outcomes: a systematic review of meta-analyses of randomized controlled trials. Medicine 98:e14501. https://doi.org/10.1097/MD.0000000000014501

George BP et al (2017) Timing of percutaneous endoscopic gastrostomy for acute ischemic stroke. Stroke 48(2):420–427. https://doi.org/10.1161/strokeaha.116.015119

Gittler M, Davis AM (2018) Guidelines for adult stroke rehabilitation and recovery. JAMA 319:820. https://doi.org/10.1001/jama.2017.22036

Higashida R et al (2013) Interactions within stroke systems of care: a policy statement from the American Heart Association/American Stroke Association. Stroke 44(10):2961–2984. https://doi.org/10.1161/STR.0b013e3182a6d2b2

Lakshminarayan K et al (2010) Utility of dysphagia screening results in predicting poststroke pneumonia. Stroke 41(12):2849–2854. https://doi.org/10.1161/STROKEAHA.110.597039

Langhorne P (2013) Organised inpatient (stroke unit) care for stroke. Cochrane Database Syst Rev (4):CD000197. https://doi.org/10.1002/14651858.CD000197.pub3

Langhorne P, Baylan S, Trialists ESD (2017) Early supported discharge services for people with acute stroke. Cochrane Database Syst Rev 7(7):CD000443. https://doi.org/10.1002/14651858. CD000443.pub4

Langhorne P et al (2018) Very early versus delayed mobilisation after stroke. Cochrane Database Syst Rev (10):CD006187. https://doi.org/10.1002/14651858.CD006187.pub3

Lees KR, Emberson J, Blackwell L, Bluhmki E, Davis SM, Donnan GA et al (2016) Effects of alteplase for acute stroke on the distribution of functional outcomes: a pooled analysis of 9 trials. Stroke 47(9):2373–2379. https://doi.org/10.1161/STROKEAHA.116.013644

Li Z et al (2018) Effects of early mobilization after acute stroke: a meta-analysis of randomized control trials. J Stroke Cerebrovasc Dis 27(5):1326–1337. https://doi.org/10.1016/j.jstrokecerebrovasdis.2017.12.021

Lindley RI, Anderson CS, Billot L, Forster A, Hackett ML, Harvey LA et al (2017) Family-led rehabilitation after stroke in India (ATTEND): a randomised controlled trial. Lancet 390(10094):588–599. https://doi.org/10.1016/S0140-6736(17)31447-2

Marler JR et al (2000) Early stroke treatment associated with better outcome: the NINDS rt-PA Stroke Study. Neurology 55(11):1649–1655. https://doi.org/10.1212/WNL.55.11.1649

Mattioli F et al (2014) Early aphasia rehabilitation is associated with functional reactivation of the left inferior frontal gyrus a pilot study. Stroke 45(2):545–552

Mayo NE (2016) Stroke rehabilitation at home: lessons learned and ways forward. Stroke 47(6):1685–1691. https://doi.org/10.1161/STROKEAHA.116.011309

Meyer S, Verheyden G, Brinkmann N, Dejaeger E, De Weerdt W, Feys H et al (2015) Functional and motor outcome 5 years after stroke is equivalent to outcome at 2 months: follow-up of the collaborative evaluation of rehabilitation in stroke across Europe. Stroke 46(6):1613–1619. https://doi.org/10.1161/STROKEAHA.115.009421

Momosaki R et al (2016) Very early versus delayed rehabilitation for acute ischemic stroke patients with intravenous recombinant tissue plasminogen activator: a nationwide retrospective cohort study. Cerebrovasc Dis 42(1–2):41–48. https://doi.org/10.1159/000444720

National Institute for Health and Care Excellence (NICE) (2013) Stroke rehabilitation in adults. NICE clinical guidelines

NICE (2013) Stroke rehabilitation in adults. Guidance and guidelines, clinical guideline CG162

Nouwens F, Dippel DWJ et al (2013) Rotterdam Aphasia Therapy Study (RATS)-3: "The efficacy of intensive cognitive-linguistic therapy in the acute stage of aphasia"; design of a randomised controlled trial. Trials 14:24. https://doi.org/10.1186/1745-6215-14-24

Ojo O, Brooke J (2016) The use of enteral nutrition in the management of stroke. Nutrients 8(12):827. https://doi.org/10.3390/nu8120827

Owens DK et al (2010) AHRQ Series Paper 5: grading the strength of a body of evidence when comparing medical interventions-Agency for Healthcare Research and Quality and the Effective Health-Care Program. J Clin Epidemiol 63(5):513–523. https://doi.org/10.1016/j.jclinepi.2009.03.009

Palli C et al (2017) Early dysphagia screening by trained nurses reduces pneumonia rate in stroke patients: a clinical intervention study. Stroke 48(9):2583–2585. https://doi.org/10.1161/STROKEAHA.117.018157

Pandian JD, Arora R, Kaur P, Sharma D, Vishwambaran DK, Arima H (2014) Mirror therapy in unilateral neglect after stroke (MUST trial): a randomized controlled trial. Neurology 83(11):1012–1017. https://doi.org/10.1212/WNL.0000000000000773

Pandian JD, Felix C, Kaur P, Sharma D, Julia L, Toor G et al (2015) FAmily-led RehabiliTaTion aftEr stroke in INDia: the ATTEND pilot study. Int J Stroke 10(4):609–614. https://doi.org/10.1111/ijs.12475

Platz T (2019) Evidence-based guidelines and clinical pathways in stroke rehabilitation: an international perspective. Front Neurol 10:200. https://doi.org/10.3389/fneur.2019.00200

Powers WJ et al (2018) 2018 guidelines for the early management of patients with acute ischemic stroke: a guideline for healthcare professionals from the American Heart Association/American Stroke Association. Stroke 49(3):e46–e110. https://doi.org/10.1161/STR.0000000000000158

Rha JH, Saver JL (2007) The impact of recanalization on ischemic stroke outcome: a meta-analysis. Stroke 38(3):967–973. https://doi.org/10.1161/01.STR.0000258112.14918.24

Rice D, Janzen S, McIntyre A, Vermeer J, Britt E, Teasell R (2016) Comprehensive outpatient rehabilitation program: hospital-based stroke outpatient rehabilitation. J Stroke Cerebrovasc Dis 25(5):1158–1164. https://doi.org/10.1016/j.jstrokecerebrovasdis.2016.02.007

Rønning OM, Guldvog B (1998) Outcome of subacute stroke rehabilitation: a randomized controlled trial. Stroke 29(4):779–784. https://doi.org/10.1161/01.STR.29.4.779

Ru X, Dai H, Jiang B, Li N, Zhao X, Hong Z et al (2017) Community-based rehabilitation to improve stroke survivors' rehabilitation participation and functional recovery. Am J Phys Med Rehabil 96(7):e123–e129. https://doi.org/10.1097/PHM.0000000000000650

Sarfo FS, Ulasavets U, Opare-Sem OK, Ovbiagele B (2018) Tele-rehabilitation after stroke: an updated systematic review of the literature. J Stroke Cerebrovasc Dis 27(9):2306–2318. https://doi.org/10.1016/j.jstrokecerebrovasdis.2018.05.013

Sarı A (2017) Anxiety, Depression And Burnout Levels In Caregivers Of Stroke Patients In A Rehabilitation Hospital. Southern Clinics of Istanbul Eurasia. https://doi.org/10.14744/scie.2017.75046

Schwamm LH et al (2005) Recommendations for the establishment of stroke systems of care: recommendations from the American Stroke Association's Task Force on the Development of Stroke Systems. Circulation 111:1078–1091. https://doi.org/10.1161/01.CIR.0000154252.62394.1E

Scottish Intercollegiate Guidelines Network (2010) Management of patients with stroke: identification and management of dysphagia (SIGN guideline no 119). Scottish Intercollegiate Guidelines Network

Seminog OO et al (2019) Determinants of the decline in mortality from acute stroke in England: linked national database study of 795 869 adults. BMJ (Online) 365:l1778. https://doi.org/10.1136/bmj.l1778

Singh MB (2013) Neurologic disability: a hidden epidemic for India. Neurology 79(21):2146–2147

Smith EE et al (2018) Effect of dysphagia screening strategies on clinical outcomes after stroke: a systematic review for the 2018 guidelines for the early management of patients with acute ischemic stroke. Stroke 49(3):e123–e128. https://doi.org/10.1161/STR.0000000000000159

Stephenson S, Wiles R (2000) Advantages and disadvantages of the home setting for therapy: views of patients and therapists. Br J Occup Ther 63(2):59–64. https://doi.org/10.1177/030802260006300203

Surya N (2010) Neurorehabilitation in India. Neurorehabilitation News Spring; ASNR, p 3

Surya N (2015) Rehabilitation of multiple sclerosis patients in India. Ann Indian Acad Neurol 18(Suppl 1):S43–S47

Teasell R, Foley N, Hussein N, Speechley M (2018) The elements of stroke rehabilitation, evidence-based review of stroke rehabilitation

Van De Port IGL, Kwakkel G, Van Wijk I, Lindeman E (2006) Susceptibility to deterioration of mobility long-term after stroke: a prospective cohort study. Stroke 37(1):167–171. https://doi.org/10.1161/01.STR.0000195180.69904.f2

Vloothuis JDM, Mulder M, Veerbeek JM et al (2016) Caregiver-mediated exercises for improving outcomes after stroke. Cochrane Database Syst Rev 12:CD011058

WFNR (2015) Neurorehabilitation in developing countries time for action. http://wfnr.co.uk/education-and-research/position-statements/

WHO (2014) Neurological disorders associated with malnutrition. In: Neurological disorders: public health challenges. WHO, Geneva. https://doi.org/10.1037/e521482010-002

Winstein CJ, Stein J, Arena R, Bates B, Cherney LR, Cramer SC et al (2016) Guidelines for adult stroke rehabilitation and recovery: a guideline for healthcare professionals from the American Heart Association/American Stroke Association. Stroke 47(6):e98–e169. https://doi.org/10.1161/STR.0000000000000098

Wolfe CDA, Rudd AG (2011) Improvement of care in acute stroke units. Lancet 378:1679–1680. https://doi.org/10.1016/S0140-6736(11)61545-6

Xu T et al (2017) Efficacy and safety of very early mobilization in patients with acute stroke: a systematic review and meta-analysis. Sci Rep 7:6550. https://doi.org/10.1038/s41598-017-06871-z

Yagi M et al (2017) Impact of rehabilitation on outcomes in patients with ischemic stroke: a nationwide retrospective cohort study in Japan. Stroke 48(3):740–746. https://doi.org/10.1161/STROKEAHA.116.015147

Yamada SM (2015) Too early initiation of enteral nutrition is not nutritionally advantageous for comatose acute stroke patients. J Nippon Med Sch 82(4):186–192. https://doi.org/10.1272/jnms.82.186

Zhou X, Du M, Zhou L (2018) Use of mobile applications in post-stroke rehabilitation: a systematic review. Top Stroke Rehabil:1–11. https://doi.org/10.1080/10749357.2018.1482446

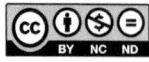